NAVELBINE ®
(vinorelbine)
UPDATE
and
NEW TRENDS

NAVELBINE ®
(vinorelbine)
UPDATE and NEW TRENDS

Scientific adviser

Philippe Solal-Celigny

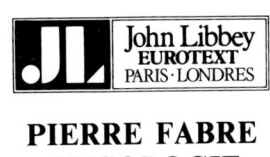

**PIERRE FABRE
ONCOLOGIE**

British Library Cataloguing in Publication Data
Solal-Celigny
Navelbine®
1. Man. Cancer. Drug therapy, Drugs
I. Title

616.994061

ISBN 0-86196-242-7

First published in 1991 by
John Libbey Eurotext Ltd
6, rue Blanche, 92120 Montrouge, France. (1) 47 35 85 52

John Libbey & Company Ltd
13 Smiths Yard, Summerley Street, London SW18 4HR, England. (1) 947 27 77

John Libbey CIC
Via Spallanzani 11, 00161, Rome, Italy

© John Libbey Eurotext. 1991. Il est interdit de reproduire intégralement ou partiellement le présent ouvrage — Loi du 11 mars 1957 — sans autorisation de l'éditeur ou du Centre français du Copyright, 6bis, rue Gabriel-Laumain, 75010 Paris.

Contents

List of participants IX

Preface. *M. Boiron* XV

Introduction. *M. Tubiana* XVII

PART I. Navelbine®, preclinical studies

1. **History of discovery of Navelbine®.** *P. Potier* 3

2. **Action of Navelbine® (NVB) on microtubules. Role of Tau and MAP$_2$ proteins.** *A. Fellous, V. Meininger, S. Binet, M. Chiche, T. Vacassin, C. Gagelin, H. Lataste, A. Krikorian, J.-P. Couzinier* 9

3. **Immunofluorescence study of the action of Navelbine®, vincristine and vinblastine on mitotic and axonal microtubules.** *S. Binet, E. Chaineau, A. Fellous, H. Lataste, A. Krikorian, J.-P. Couzinier, V. Meininger* 25

4. **Experimental antitumoral activity of Navelbine®.** *S. Cros, G. François, R. Guillon* 35

5. **Pharmacokinetics of Navelbine®.** *A. Krikorian* 43

PART II. Navelbine® and non small cell lung cancer

A. Non small cell lung cancer

6. **Introduction.** *J. Chrétien* 57

7. **Epidemiology and prognosis of non small cell lung cancer.** *B. Dautzenberg* ... 61

8. **Advantages of chemotherapy in non smal cell lung cancer.** *F. Soyez, J.-P. Kleisbauer* 69

9. **Combined radiotherapy and chemotherapy in non small cell lung cancer.** *R. Arriagada, B. Pellae-Cosset, E. Nasr, P. Berthaud, T. Le Chevalier* 79

10. Biological contributions to the study of lung cancer. *M.F. Poupon, F. Arvelo, M. Jacrot* 89

11. Design and analysis of phase II cancer clinical trials. Interest of the triangular test, a group sequential method. *E. Bellissant, J. Bénichou, Cl. Chastang* 101

B. Navelbine® : clinical results in non small cell lung cancer

12. Navelbine® and non small cell lung cancer. Some general remarks. *R.A. Joss* ... 129

13. Efficacy of Navelbine® and vinca alkaloids in the treatment of non small cell lung cancer (NSCLC). *A. Depierre, P. Jacoulet, G. Garnier*................. 133

14. Presentation of Navelbine® combinations in the treatment of non small cell lung cancer. *P. Carles, E. Quoix, J.C. Guérin, A. Tonnel, A. Bonnaud, G. Nouvet, D. Coetmeur* 137

15. Phase II study of Navelbine®-cisplatin in non small cell lung cancer. *B. Lebeau, J. Clavier, J.P. Kleisbauer, J.L. Rebishung, J.F. Muir, J.M. Brechot, A. Depierre*... 141

16. Phase I-II study of combination vinorelbine (Navelbine®)-cisplatin in advanced non small cell lung carcinoma. *P. Berthaud, T. Le Chevalier, M. Besenval, R. Arriagada, P. Ruffié* 147

17. Phase II study of combination of Navelbine® and mitomycin C in small cell lung cancer patients. *B. Milleron, C. Brambilla, F. Blanchon, F. Patte, E. Quoix, A. Taytard, H. Naman*.. 151

18. Alternatives to cisplatin : Phase II study of combined Navelbine® and etoposide. *E. Lemarié, A. Taytard, J.F. Muir, J.F. Cordier, G. Dabouis, L. Jeannin, A. Depierre*... 157

19. Alternatives to cisplatin : 5FU-Navelbine® combination. *J. Tredaniel, V. Dieras, C. Ferme, M. Marty, A. Hirsch* 163

20. Study of combined Navelbine®-cisplatin-VP16 in the treatment of non small cell lung cancer. *P. Jacoulet, A. Depierre, G. Garnier, J.C. Dalphin*............ 171

21. Combination Navelbine®-cisplatin-etoposide in bronchial adenocarcinomas. *J.L. Breau, J.F. Morere, C. Boaziz, L. Israel*.. 179

22. Navelbine® (vinorelbine) tolerance in non small cell lung cancer. *M. Besenval, F. Leray, F.M. Delgado, S. Merle, A. Krikorian, A. Herrera* 185

PART III. Navelbine® : perspectives

A. Advanced breast cancer

23. Phase II pilot study of Navelbine® in advanced breast cancer. *F.M. Delgado, L. Canobbio, F. Boccardo, F. Brema, V. Fosser* 199

24. Preliminary results of a phase II study of Navelbine® in the first line treatment of advanced breast cancer. *P. Fumoleau, T. Delozier, P. Kerbrat, F. Burki, A. Monnier, R. Keiling, Ph. Chollet, E. Garcia-Giralt, M. Namer, C. Brune, F.M. Delgado* 207

25. Phase II study of vinorelbine in first and second line treatment of advanced breast cancer. *J.M. Extra, S. Leandri, V. Dieras, C. Ferme, L. Mignot, F. Morvan, M. Espié, M. Marty* 213

26. Navelbine®-5-fluoro-uracil combination in first line treatment of advanced breast cancer. *V. Dieras, C. Varette, C. Louvet, M. Espié, P. Colin, M. Marty* ... 221

B. Advanced ovary cancer

27. Phase II study of Navelbine® as second or third line treatment in advanced ovarian carcinoma. *J.F. Héron, M.J. George, P. Kerbrat, J. Chauvergne, A. Goupil, D. Lebrun, J.P. Guastala, M. Namer, R. Bugat, Y. Ayme, C. Lhomme, C. Toussaint, S. Merle, M. Besenval, J.P. Burillon* 231

28. Study of the combination vinorelbine-hexamethyl-melamine (V-H) in advanced ovarian adenocarcinoma : preliminary results of a phase I-II study NHO-88, from the ARTAC multicentric ovarian carcinoma study group. *M.C. Pinel, G. Pinon, M.J. Goudier, B. Coiffier, M.H. Filippi, A. Goupil, B. Roullet, T. Facchini, L. Mignot, P. Tresca, F. Heritier, M. Delgado, D. Belpomme* 237

C. Lymphomas

29. Phase II study of vinorelbine (Navelbine®) in previously treated Hodgkin's disease and non - Hodgkin's lymphomas. *H. Eghbali* 253

30. Clinical study of Navelbine® activity in Hodgkin's disease. Phase II study. *S. Benchekroun, Z. Chouffai, M. Harif, A. Quessar, M. Laabid, A. Trachli, N. Benchemsi, M. Besenval, A. Herrera* 261

31. Navelbine® : Conclusions and new trends. *M. Marty* 265

List of participants

Arriagada R., Comité de pathologie thoracique, Institut Gustave Roussy, rue Camille Desmoulins, 94805 Villejuif, France.
Arvelo F., Biologie des métastases, CNRS, 7, rue Guy Mocquet, BP 8, 94802 Villejuif, France.
Ayme Y., Institut Paoli-Calmettes, 232, boulevard de Sainte-Marguerite, 13273 Marseille Cedex 9, France.
Bellissant E., Département de biostatistique et informatique médicale, Hôpital Saint-Louis, 1, avenue Claude Vellefaux, 75475 Paris Cedex 10, France.
Belpomme D., ARTAC, 38, rue de Silly, 92100 Boulogne, France.
Benchekroun S., Service d'hématologie et d'oncologie pédiatrique, CHU Ibn Rochd, Casablanca, Maroc.
Benchemsi N., Service d'hématologie et d'oncologie pédiatrique, CHU Ibn Rochd, Casablanca, Maroc.
Benichou J., Département de biostatistique et informatique médicale, Hôpital Saint-Louis, 1, avenue Claude Vellefaux, 75475 Paris Cedex 10, France.
Berthaud P., Comité de pathologie thoracique, Institut Gustave Roussy, rue Camille Desmoulins, 94805 Villejuif, France.
Besenval M., Laboratoires Pierre Fabre Oncologie, 192, rue Lecourbe, 75015 Paris, France.
Binet S., Laboratoire d'anatomie, faculté de médecine, 45, rue des Saints-Pères, 75270 Paris Cedex 6, France.
Blanchon, F., CHG, 6-8, rue Saint-Fiacre, 77104 Meaux Cedex, France.
Boaziz C., Service d'oncologie médicale, CHU Avicenne, 93000 Bobigny, France.
Boccardo F., Istituto nazionale per la ricerca sur cancro, viale Benedetto XV, n° 10, 16132 Genova, Italia.
Boiron M., Hôpital Saint-Louis, 1, avenue Claude Vellefaux, 75475 Paris Cedex 10, France.
Bonnaud F., CHRU, 2, avenue Alexis Carrel, 87000 Limoges, France.
Brambillat C., Hôpital des Sablons, BP 217, 38043 Grenoble, France.
Breau J.L., Service d'oncologie médicale, CHU Avicenne, 93000 Bobigny, France.
Brechot J.M., Hôtel-Dieu, 1, place du Parvis Notre Dame, 75181 Paris Cedex 4, France.
Brema F., Servizio di oncologia, ospedale San Paolo, corso Italia 30, Savona, Italia.
Brune C., Pierre Fabre Médicament/CRPF, 192, rue Lecourbe, 75015 Paris, France.
Bugat R., Centre Claudius Regaud, 20-24, rue du Pont-Saint-Pierre, 31052 Toulouse Cedex, France.
Burillon J.P., Pierre Fabre Médicament/CRPF, 192, rue Lecourbe, 75015 Paris, France.
Burki F., Institut Jean Godinot, 1, rue du Général Koening, BP 171, 51056 Reims Cedex, France.

List of participants

Canobbio L., Istituto nazionale per la ricerca sur cancro, viale Benedetto XV, n° 10, 16132 Genova, Italie.
Carles P., CHU Purpan, place du Dr Baylac, 31059 Toulouse Cedex, France.
Chaineau E., Laboratoire d'anatomie, faculté de médecine, 45, rue des Saints-Pères, 75270 Paris Cedex 6, France.
Chastang Cl., Département de biostatistique et informatique médicale, Hôpital Saint-Louis, 1, avenue Claude Vellefaux, 75475 Paris Cedex 10, France.
Chauvergne J., Fondation Bergonié, 180, rue de Saint-Genès, 33076 Bordeaux, France.
Chiche M., INSERM U96, Hôpital de Kremlin-Bicêtre, 94275 Bicêtre Cedex, France.
Chollet Ph., Centre Jean Perrin, 30, place Henri-Dunant, BP 392, 63011 Clermont-Ferrand Cedex, France.
Chouffai Z., Service d'hématologie et d'oncologie pédiatrique, CHU Ibn Rochd, Casablanca, Maroc.
Chrétien J., Service de pneumologie, Hôpital Cochin, 27, rue du Faubourg Saint-Jacques, 75014 Paris, France.
Clavier J., CHR, 5, avenue Foch, 29285 Brest Cedex, France.
Coetmeur D., CHR, 17, rue des Capucins, 22023 Saint-Brieuc, France.
Coiffier B., Hôpital Edouard Herriot, 5, place Arsonval, 69374 Lyon Cedex 08, France.
Colin-Trescat P., Service d'oncologie médicale, Hôpital Saint-Louis, 1, avenue Claude Vellefaux, 75475 Paris Cedex 10, France.
Cordier J.F., CHU, 28, avenue Doyen Lepine, 69394 Lyon Cedex, France.
Couzinier J.P., Centre de recherche Pierre Fabre, 17, avenue Jean Moulin, 81106 Castres, France.
Cros S., Laboratoire de pharmacologie et de toxicologie fondamentales du CNRS, 205, route de Narbonne, 31077 Toulouse Cedex, France.
Dabouis G., Hôpital Laënnec, BP 1005, 44035 Nantes Cedex, France.
Dalphin J.C., Service de pneumologie, CHR Besançon, 25000 Besançon, France.
Dautzenberg B., Service de pneumologie et de réanimation respiratoire, groupe hospitalier Pitié-Salpêtrière, 75651 Paris Cedex 13, France.
Delgado F.M., Pierre Fabre Médicament/CRPF, 192, rue Lecourbe, 75015 Paris, France.
Delozier T., Centre François Baclesse, route de Lion-sur-Mer, BP 5026, 14021 Caen Cedex, France.
Depierre A., Service de pneumologie, CHR Besançon, 25000 Besançon, France.
Dieras V., Service d'oncologie médicale, Hôpital Saint-Louis, 1, avenue Claude Vellefaux, 75475 Paris Cedex 10, France.
Eghbali H., Fondation Bergonié, 180, rue de Saint-Genès, 33076 Bordeaux, France.
Espié, M., Service d'oncologie médicale, Hôpital Saint-Louis, 1, avenue Claude Vellefaux, 75475 Paris Cedex 10, France.
Extra J.M., Service d'oncologie médicale, Hôpital Saint-Louis, 1, avenue Claude Vellefaux, 75475 Paris Cedex 10, France.
Facchini T., Centre hospitalier régional, 57038 Metz, France.
Fellous A., INSERM U96, Hôpital du Kremlin-Bicêtre, 94275 Bicêtre Cedex, France.
Ferme C., Centre médico-chirurgical de Bligny, 91640 Bris-sur-Forge.
Filippi M.H., Hôpital Bichat, 46, rue Henri Huchard, 75018 Paris, France.
Fosser V., Ospedale Vicenza San Bartolo, via Rodolfi, 36100 Vicenza, Italia.

List of participants

François G., Laboratoire de pharmacologie et de toxicologie fondamentales du CNRS, 205, route de Narbonne, 31077 Toulouse Cedex, France.
Fumoleau P., Centre René Gauducheau, quai Moncousu, 44035 Nantes Cedex, France.
Gagelin C., INSERM U96, Hôpital du Kremlin-Bicêtre, 94275 Bicêtre Cedex, France.
Garcia-Giralt E., Institut Curie, 26, rue d'Ulm, 75231 Paris Cedex 05, France.
Garnier G., Service de pneumologie, CHR Besançon, 25000 Besançon, France.
George M.J., Institut Gustave Roussy, rue Camille Desmoulins, 94805 Villejuif, France.
Goudier M.J., Centre hospitalier, 27, rue du Dr Lettry, 56100 Lorient, France.
Goupil A., Centre René Huguenin, 35, rue Dailly, 92211 Saint-Cloud, France.
Guastala J.P., Centre Léon Bérard, 28, rue Laënnec, 69373 Lyon Cedex, France.
Guérin J.C., Hôpital de la Croix Rousse, 93, Grand rue Croix Rousse, 69004 Lyon, France.
Guillon R., Laboratoire de pharmacologie et de toxicologie fondamentales du CNRS, 205, route de Narbonne, 31077 Toulouse Cedex, France.
Harif M., Service d'hématologie et d'oncologie pédiatrique, CHU Ibn Rochd, Casablanca, Maroc.
Herrera A., Laboratoires Pierre Fabre Oncologie, 192, rue Lecourbe, 75015 Paris, France.
Héron J.F., Centre François Baclesse, Route de Lion-sur-Mer, BP 5026, 14021 Caen Cedex, France.
Hirsch A., Service de pneumologie, Hôpital Saint-Louis, 1, avenue Claude Vellefaux, 75475 Paris Cedex 10, France.
Israël L., Service d'oncologie médicale, CHU Avicenne, 93000 Bobigny, France.
Jacoulet P., Service de pneumologie, CHR Besançon, 25000 Besançon, France.
Jacrot M., Laboratoire de cytogénétique, faculté de médecine de Grenoble, Domaine de la Merci, 38700 La Tronche, France.
Jeannin L., CHR La Trouhaude, rue Dr Calmette, 21000 Dijon, France.
Joss R.A., Division of oncology, Department of Medicine, Kantonspital, CH-6000 Luzern 16, Suisse.
Keiling R., Centre Paul Strauss, 3, rue de la Porte-de-l'Hôpital, 67085 Strasbourg Cedex, France.
Kerbrat P., Centre Eugène Marquis, Pontchaillou, 35011 Rennes Cedex, France.
Kleisbauer J.P., Hôpital Salvador, 249, boulevard Sainte-Marguerite, BP 51, 13274 Marseille Cedex 09, France.
Krikorian A., Pierre Fabre Médicament/CRPF, 192, rue Lecourbe, 75015 Paris, France.
Laabid M., Service d'hématologie et d'oncologie pédiatrique, CHU Ibn Rochd, Casablanca, Maroc.
Lataste H., Laboratoires Pierre Fabre Médicament/CRPF, 17, avenue Jean Moulin, 81106 Castres, France.
Leandri S., Service d'oncologie médicale, hôpital Saint-Louis, 1, avenue Claude Vellefaux, 75475 Paris Cedex 10, France.
Lebeau B., Hôpital Saint-Antoine, 184, faubourg Saint-Antoine, 75571 Paris Cedex, France.

List of participants

Lebrun D., Institut Jean Godinot, 1, rue du Général Koening, BP 171, 51056 Reims Cedex, France.
Le Chevalier T., Comité de pathologie thoracique, Institut Gustave Roussy, rue Camille Desmoulins, 94805 Villejuif, France.
Lemarie E., Service de pneumologie, CHU Bretonneau, 37044 Tours Cedex, France.
Leray F., Laboratoires Pierre Fabre Oncologie, 192, rue Lecourbe, 75015 Paris, France.
Lhomme C., Institut Gustave Roussy, rue Camille Desmoulins, 94805 Villejuif, France.
Louvet C., Service d'oncologie médicale, Hôpital Saint-Louis, 1, avenue Claude Vellefaux, 75475 Paris Cedex 10, France.
Marty M., Service d'oncologie médicale, Hôpital Saint-Louis, 1, avenue Claude Vellefaux, 75475 Paris Cedex 10, France.
Meininger V., Laboratoire d'anatomie, faculté de médecine, 45, rue des Saints-Pères, 75270 Paris Cedex, France.
Merle S., Pierre Fabre Médicament/CRPF, 192, rue Lecourbe, 75015 Paris, France.
Mignot L., Service d'oncologie médicale, CMC/Fondation médicale du Mont-Valérien, 40, rue Worth, 92151 Suresnes Cedex, France.
Milleron B., Hôpital Tenon, 4, rue de la Chine, 75970 Paris Cedex 20, France.
Monnier A., CHR Bouloche, rue du Dr Flamand, 25209 Montbéliard, France.
Morere J.F., Service d'oncologie médicale, CHU Avicenne, 93000 Bobigny, France.
Morvan F., Service d'oncologie médicale, centre René Dubos, avenue de l'Ile-de-France, 95301 Cergy-Pontoise, France.
Muir J.F., CHU, 76000 Rouen, France.
Naman H., Clinique Le Méridien, 93, avenue du Dr Picaud, 06150 Cannes, France.
Nasr E., Comité de pathologie thoracique, Institut Gustave Roussy, rue Camille Desmoulins, 94805 Villejuif, France.
Namer M., Centre Antoine Lacassagne, 36, voie Romaine, 06054 Nice Cedex, France.
Nouvet G., Hôpital Charles Nicolle, 1, rue Germont, 76031 Rouen, France.
Patte F., CHU, 350, avenue Jacques-Cœur, 86021 Poitiers Cedex, France.
Pellae-Cosset B., Comité de pathologie thoracique, Institut Gustave Roussy, rue Camille Desmoulins, 94805 Villejuif, France.
Pinel M.C., ARTAC, 38, rue de Silly, 92100 Boulogne, France.
Pinon G., Polyclinique de Courlancy, 30, rue de Courlancy, 51100 Reims, France.
Potier P., Institut des substances naturelles, CNRS, 91190 Gif-sur-Yvette, France.
Poupon M.F., Biologie des métastases, CNRS, 7, rue Guy Mocquet, BP 8, 94802 Villejuif, France.
Quessar A., Service d'hématologie et d'oncologie pédiatrique, CHU Ibn Rochd, Casablanca, Maroc.
Quoix E., CHU, 1, place de l'Hôpital, 67000 Strasbourg, France.
Rebishung J.L., Hôpital Saint-Joseph, 7, rue Pierre Larousse, 75674 Paris Cedex 14, France.
Roullet B., CHU Dupuytren, rue Alexis Carrel, 87000 Limoges, France.
Soyez F., Hôpital Salvador, 249, boulevard Sainte-Marguerite, BP 51, 13274 Marseille Cedex 09, France.
Taytard A., CHU, 146, rue Léo Saignet, 33076 Bordeaux Cedex, France.
Tonnel A., Hôpital Albert Calmette, boulevard Leclerc, 59037 Lille, France.

List of participants

Toussaint C., Institut Gustave Roussy, rue Camille Desmoulins, 94805 Villejuif, France.
Trachli A., Service d'hématologie et d'oncologie pédiatrique, CHU Ibn Rochd, Casablanca, Maroc.
Tredaniel J., Service de pneumologie, Hôpital Saint-Louis, 1, avenue Claude Vellefaux, 75475 Paris Cedex 10, France.
Tubiana M., Institut Gustave Roussy, rue Camille Desmoulins, 94805 Villejuif Cedex, France.
Vacassin T., INSERM U96, Hôpital de Kremlin-Bicêtre, 94275 Bicêtre Cedex, France.
Varette C., Service d'oncologie médicale, Hôpital Saint-Louis, 1, avenue Claude Vellefaux, 75475 Paris Cedex 10, France.

Preface

The first symposium on Navelbine® (vinorelbine) was held at the 13th Congress of ESMO in Lugano, Switzerland, in October 1988. One year later, after a more in-depth study of this new anticancer molecule, we are able to confirm the great hope that had been placed on it.

Since 1988, the originality of this semi-synthetic vinca alkaloid with respect to existing alkaloids, vincristine, vinblastine and vindesine, was evident : a) originality of the chemical structure since it is one of the first representatives of the 5' nor vinca-alkaloids, b) originality of its mechanism of action, which is selective for mitotic microtubules, axonal microtubules being virtually untouched, c) wide range of anti-tumor action in animals, d) low neurologic, hematologic and alopecic toxicities, and e) specific pharmacokinetic profile.

All these features were confirmed by studies reported during the Biarritz Symposium held on November 2-3, 1989. A study on the unique action of Navelbine® on the proteins associated with tubuline (weaker longitudinal bonds, less apparent spiralization, lower aggregation action and lower paracristal formation) was of particular interest.

Since 1988, we also thought that it was highly probable that Navelbine® had a spectrum of activity in human tumors, that was different from the existing vinca alkaloids. The significant results reported at the Biarritz Symposium make this evident. It is clear that Navelbine® is more than just a new vinca alkaloid derivative, it is a completely new anticancer drug. It is considered active in the following malignancies :

1) Non small cell lung cancer, with results showing activity in monotherapy and in various polychemotherapy combination studies.

2) Metastatic breast cancer (first line treatment or in pretreated metastatic disease), with significant results particularly with certain chemotherapy combinations, and especially in skin and nodal localizations. These results are so remarkable that Navelbine® has already been introduced in adjuvant and neoadjuvant chemotherapeutic schemas.

3) Hodgkin and non-Hodgkin lymphomas, where Navelbine® has already been introduced in combination chemotherapy for patients with relapse.

4) Ovarian cancer, with interesting results both in monotherapy and in combination chemotherapy.

Other studies also create interest, for example, the use of Navelbine® in other epidermoid cancers, adenocarcinomas and other hematologic malignancies.

Naturally, Navelbine®, like any other new anticancer drug, cannot avoid the test of proving its therapeutic efficacy against the wide variety of agents already in use for different cancer types. Performing this type of study poses a number of questions and problems to be examined specifically :

• deciding the mode of administration : bolus, continuous intravenous (IV), semi-continuous IV, oral administration, weekly vs every 3 weeks;

- the series of questions associated with combination chemotherapy :
  - Which therapeutic protocol ? For example, the combination of a spindle poison, an agent that is active on DNA or an agent that is active on topoisomerases.
  - Which methodology ?
  - Which should be the acceptable toxicity, and how can it be reduced by the administration of G-CSF ?
  - Which type of tumors ?
  - Which activity goals to be tested ?

These studies are under way and have already shown interesting preliminary results.

In conclusion, the discovery of Navelbine®, has reestablished the former interest in vinca alkaloids and mitotic spindle poisons. Its considerable antitumoral activity confirms the need for continuous research in this area and we hope that new developments will arise in the future. Pierre Potier, who is a well known chemist in this domain, has been the principal responsible, with his team from the Institute of Chemicals and Natural Substances of the CNRS, in the synthesis of Navelbine® and is worthy of both our admiration and respect.

M. Boiron
Hôpital Saint-Louis
Paris, France

Introduction

M. TUBIANA

Institut Gustave-Roussy, Hautes-Bruyères, rue Camille-Desmoulins, 94805 Villejuif Cedex, France

In France, life expectancy has risen from 44 years in 1900 to 76 years today. This is similar to USA figures, which report increases from 48 to 78 years for Caucasians, and 36 to 72 years for Blacks. Therefore, the fact that the rate of cancer deaths in industrialized countries is rising is no surprise since the probability of developing a cancer increases with age, especially for persons over 40. However in industrialized countries cancer incidence has remained constant for people of the same age, and the increase is entirely due to aging. The cancer death rate in France, which was 4 % in 1905, has reached a current rate of 24 %, due to the progressive ageing of the population. It is presumable that by the year 2000, 30 % of deaths in Western countries will be cancer-related, even if we take into account the greater number of patients being cured thanks to therapeutic developments.

This worldwide constancy of the cancer incidence for people of the same age hides significant variations for some cancer types. In the last 30 years the percentage of stomach cancer has dropped considerably (most probably owing to a diet richer in fruits and vegetables and poorer in cured or smoked meat and fish), as has the incidence of uterine cancer (due to improved gynecologic care and hygiene). Since the beginning of the century, the age-specific rate of lung cancer for non-smokers has been relatively uniform, which shows that atmospheric pollution is not a major factor. However the proportion of tobacco-related cancer quintupled since the end of the Second World War which explains constancy of cancer age corrected rate on an international scale. During this time the cost of National Health Care budgets rose significantly : in the US, for example, from 5.9 % of the gross national product (GNP) in 1965 to 11.1 % in 1987, which is the highest figure in the world. In France, the percentage of the GNP spent on Health Care is somewhat lower (10.4 %), but apart from the US, it is one of the highest worldwide, and the highest in the European Economic Community. It is practically twice that of Great Britain and slightly higher than in Germany.

In the face of economic problems, the heavy burden these expenditures place on budgets has led governments to use any means necessary to slow down and perhaps even stabilize the increasing cost of National Health Care. Some doctors and economists believe that the inevitable accretion of such expenditures, which is due to the lenghthening of life expectancy and more sophisticated diagnostic and therapeutic technology, might be compensated by curtailing superfluous expenditure.

The latter, according to certain experts, can be accredited with a major percentage of the overall cost. Cancer causes about 25 % of deaths but accounts for only 5 to 10 % of expenditure. Treatment cost for cancer patients is on the average far less expensive than that of patients suffering from other chronic diseases, chronic renal insufficiency or AIDS for example. The average cost of treatment for cancer, however, depends largely on the localization. Lung cancer treatment is among the most expensive, especially considering the small reported success due to poor therapeutic results.

This is one of the main reasons for placing current emphasis on prevention for this type of cancer, in essence, the fight against tobacco. For many other cancer types the current tendancy is also to focus on prevention. Nevertheless we should also aim at developing effective treatments in the near future; thus we must pursue efforts on therapeutic research. Unfortunately, results for most solid tumors have currently reached a plateau. The sophistication of radiotherapeutic and surgical treatment in specialized centers has reached the level where there is little hope of any spectacular developments. We still have a lot of ground to cover to ensure the highest level of care in all treatment centers, but this is mainly a problem of education, the consolidation of techniques and of quality control.

In monotherapy, chemotherapy is the origin of cure in 4 to 5 % of cancer cases. Used in association with radiotherapy or surgery it plays an important role in approximately 15 % of cures and helps reduce treatment mutilations. This relatively low rate can be explained, for example, by the limited efficacy of cytotoxics for epidermoid carcinoma. Even those which initially seem to be chemosensitive are rarely chemocurable because of the fairly rapid emergence of chemoresistant cell lines. Thus even for clinically chemosensitive tumors, combination radio/chemotherapy remain useful [4]. Under the present circumstances there is a strong need for three kinds of research :

1) Those aiming to understand better the *mechanisms of chemoresistance.* These are numerous; some are related to enhancement of detoxification systems. Others are induced by mutations making the cell chemoresistant. In the latter, the probability of the appearance of resistant lines is linked to the genetic instability of malignant cells, and is therefore greater in certains types of cancer such as non small cell lung cancer, where instability is particularly high.

Many recently published studies focusing on spontaneous or acquired chemoresistance have been comprehensively reviewed, and therefore I shall not elaborate on them [1, 2, 3].

2) The addition of *biologicals agents* to chemotherapy. Some (e.g. growth factors of hematopoietic tissues, such as CSF) are capable of helping to achieve more rapid repair of normal tissues damaged by cytotoxic drugs, which allows higher doses to be given or a shortening at the intervals between two successive cycles. Others, such as immunomodulators, stimulate human anti-cancer defense mechanisms. Ever since S. Rosenberg proved the clinical efficacy of adoptive immunotherapy., immunomodulators have progressively become more important. Apart from IL-2, interest in other standard immunomodulators (levamisole, polyA-polyU, etc.) has been renewed since controlled clinical trials suggest that they may play a useful role against subclinical malignant cancer foci.

3) The development of new *cytotoxic agents,* either more active or less toxic than those used presently while having similar efficacy, or without cross resistance. The

Introduction

absence of cross resistance has two fundamental advantages : to increase the response rate and the probability of cure during the initial treatment, and to prolong the cytotoxic efficacy. All new types of cytotoxics, especially when they are active on solid tumors, should be of fundamental interest.

In this manner we can acknowledge the progress that Navelbine® appears to embody. Information presented in the course of the symposium suggest both greater efficacy and better tolerance for this drug. Still remaining to be done are *in vitro* and *in vivo* studies on cross resistance with other derivatives of vinca alkaloids. Certain results, however, lead us to believe that Navelbine® may even be effective in patients who have previously been treated by chemotherapy which is very encouraging.

In conclusion, I would like to emphasize one final point. The discovery and development of this cytotoxic agent is the result of an exemplary collaboration between research laboratories and the pharmaceutical industry. Having been for a number of decades a strong advocate for this type of cooperation, both at the Institut Gustave-Roussy and the EORTC, it is my sincere pleasure to congratulate both Professor Potier and Pierre-Fabre Laboratories for the success of their joint project. Without any doubt, future discussions will illustrate the benefits that mutual collaborative efforts, uniting the scientific rigor of university researchers and the dynamism of the industry, are able to produce.

References

1. Tubiana M. The role of radiotherapy in the treatment of chemosensitive tumors. *Int J Radiation Oncology* 1989; 16 : 763-774.
2. Calvo F, de Gremoux P. Gène de la résistance multidrogue. *Bull Cancer* 1989; 76 : 973-977.
3. Jacquemin-Sablon A. Résistance multifactorielle à certains agents antitumoraux. *Bull Cancer* 1989; 76 : 967-971.
4. Tubiana M. Chimiorésistance des tumeurs. Facteurs liés à la cinétique tumorale et à l'apparition de cellules résistantes. *Bull Cancer* 1989; 76 : 959-965.

PART I

Navelbine®, preclinical studies

1

History of the discovery of Navelbine®

P. POTIER

Institut de Chimie des Substances Naturelles, avenue de la Terrasse, BP 1, 91198 Gif-sur-Yvette Cedex, France

Introduction

The insulin research conducted at the Western University of Ontario, London, Canada, between 1920 and 1935 by Banting, Best, Noble, etc., has received tremendous recognition and acclaim. The extension of this work to encompass antidiabetic and hypoglycemic substances of natural and particularly plant origin resulted in the investigation of a wide variety of plants used empirically in these therapeutic fields.

One such plant is the Madagascan periwinkle, *Catharanthus roseus* (G. Don), a member of the *Apocynaceae* family, also known erroneously as *Vinca rosea*. *Vinca* and *Catharanthus* are characterised by morphologic (and genetic) features which, though similar, are sufficiently different to justify botanic classification into two genera.

The Canadian investigators discovered hitherto unsuspected properties in extracts from the stems, leaves, and roots of the Madagascan periwinkle. While they were unable to demonstrate any antidiabetic properties, they observed that the laboratory animals to which the extracts were administered died of infections related to severe leukopenia. This effect was soon attributed to the action of certain alkaloids present in the plant extracts.

The discovery of such leukopenic properties in certain compounds used as toxic gases during the First World War (nitrogen mustards such as yperite, lewisite, etc.) led to the synthesis of a series of new antitumor drugs, the alkylating agents. Similarly, the Canadian team decided to test the leukopenic alkaloids isolated from *Catharanthus roseus* in the treatment of cancers and leukemias.

At the same time, American researchers at the Eli Lilly Laboratories, Indianapolis, USA, discovered antitumor properties in certain alkaloids isolated from the leaves of the Madagascan periwinkle while systematically screening plant extracts for antitumor properties.

The American and Canadian teams opted to pool their resources in order to develop these novel substances, which were eventually added to the chemotherapeutic arsenal (including other natural products such as colchicine and podophyllotoxin and their derivatives) available in the fight against tumors and leukemias. Their findings have been reported previously in several detailed reviews [1, 2, 3]. Essentially, their combined efforts soon resulted in the isolation of a variety of active alkaloids : vinblastine 1, vincristine 2, leurosine 6 and leurosidine 7.

Unfortunately, the yields of these products obtained by contemporary extraction methods were disappointingly low, ranging from a few hundred milligrams to several grams of active substance per ton of dry leaves.

These results prompted several chemists, including those at the Eli Lilly Laboratories, to develop a production method (synthetic or semisynthetic) for these substances, especially the two alkaloids soon to be in great demand on the pharmaceutical market : vinblastine 1 and vincristine 2, sold under the names of Velbe® and Oncovin® respectively and estimated at a market value of $US 70 million. A number of other compounds such as vindesine have also been prepared from the same natural sources.

Discovery of vinorelbine (INN) or Navelbine®

Attempts to synthetize the complex alkaloids in the vinblastine group proved unsuccessful until 1974. The first synthesis was finally achieved at the CNRS, Institute for Chemistry of Natural Products, Gif-sur-Yvette, France [4-7]. It was based on a chemical reaction developed at those laboratories, the modified Polonovski reaction. This reaction was applied to the N_b-oxide of catharanthine 3 in the presence of vindoline 4, and generated high yields of anhydrovinblastine 5.

Anhydrovinblastine 5 is a natural intermediate in plant biogenetic pathways producing most of the complex alkaloids of the vinblastine group. The mere action of ambient oxygen converts anhydrovinblastine 5 to leurosine 6, for example [8, 9]. We were also able to convert anhydrovinblastine to leurosidine 7 [10] and vinblastine 1 [11]. During this research, we demonstrated that the fragmentation reaction, discovered at our laboratories for the indole series, was able to produce two new types of compounds : $C_{5'}$-$C_{6'}$ seco-derivatives A, and nor-5' derivatives B [12, 13] and, finally, vinorelbine (INN) or Navelbine® (NVB) (nor-5' anhydrovinblastine 8).

Evidence of the biological activity of vinorelbine (INN) or Navelbine®

We have been investigating new antitumor agents obtained from natural sources since 1968. Among them are the "spindle poisons", the archetype spindle poison being the

Discovery of Navelbine®

	R_1	R_2	R_3	R_4
1	CH_3	OH	C_2H_5	H
2	CHO	OH	C_2H_5	H
5	CH_3	C_2H_5		Δ
6	CH_3	C_2H_5		$-O-$
7	CH_3	C_2H_5	OH	H

$4 = V$

A

B

8 R· = H

well-known substance colchicine. Long recognized as an inhibitor of cell division, the mechanism of action of colchicine has been shown to involve binding of the alkaloid to a ubiquitous protein present in all eukaryote cells, tubulin [13]. Other natural substances such as those in the vinblastine *1* group also bind to tubulin, inducing polymerization to form microtubules and microfilaments and inhibiting spindle formation. These observations formed the basis for the simple preliminary screening assay for spindle poisons developed by Shelanski and adapted by ourselves [14, 15].

The activity of Navelbine® was subsequently elucidated in the following manner. A tiny fraction (7 %) obtained from the anhydrovinblastine 5 fragmentation reaction and subjected to the modified Polonovski reaction proved active in the tubulin test [15]. Consequently, we decided to improve the yield of that product obtained by using different reagents and this step enabled us to direct the reaction towards the formation of Navelbine® [16].

The biological properties of Navelbine® justified further research involving collaboration with the Institute of Cancerology and Immunogenetics, Villejuif, France (G. Mathé, R. Maral, E. Chenu), resulting in confirmation of the *in vivo* antitumor activity of Navelbine®. These studies were extended to include a collaborative effort with the CNRS Fundamental Pharmacology and Toxicology Laboratories, Toulouse, France (Directors : Cl. Paoletti, J. Cros) [3].

Systematic investigation of Navelbine® activity subsequently gave rise to preclinical and then clinical studies of the new antitumor substance, vinorelbine (Navelbine®), which is now used in antitumor chemotherapy following invaluable collaboration with the Pierre Fabre Laboratory (P. Fabre, F. Fauran, J.P. Couzinier *et al.*). Although the interaction with tubulin is evident and lies at the heart of its activity, the mechanism of action of vinorelbine has not yet been fully elucidated. We still require more precise information on the nature of this interaction since tubulin is linked with "microtubule-associated proteins" (MAP$_s$), the nature of which vary according to the cellular origin of the "tubulins".

Conclusion

By solving the chemical difficulties implied in the synthetic preparation of complex vinblastine alkaloids and by studying their reactivity, we were able to discover a new structural type, the "nor-vinblastine" derivatives, which exhibit interesting biological properties. These derivatives have not yet been detected under natural conditions, an observation that can be explained by the fact that they generally act as spindle poisons; the vinblastine derivatives in particular are toxic substances which interact with the tubulin present in cells. These plants do not perish. The "spindle poisons" they biosynthesize are formed within the vacuolar system which thus prevents their interaction with the cytoskeletal element (that is, tubulin) present in the cytoplasm. But that is another story...

References

1. Noble RL. Symposium *Lloydia* 1964; 27 : 280.
2. De Conti RC, Creasey WA, *In* : Taylor WI and Farnsworth NR. The Catharanthus alkaloids, New York, Marcel Dekker, 1975.

3. Cros S, Potier P. *In* : Barton D, Ollis WD, Advances in medicinal phytochemistry. London, John Libbey, 1986.
4. Langlois N, Guéritte F, Langlois Y, Potier P. Application of a modification of the Polonovski reaction to the synthesis of vinblastine-type alkaloids. *J Am Chem Soc* 1976; 98 (22) : 7017-24.
5. Potier P. Modified Polonovski reaction. *Rev Latinoam Quim* 1978; 9 (2) : 47-54.
6. Potier P. *In* : Bartmann W, Winterfeldt E, *Stereoselective synthesis of Natural Products*, Amsterdam, Oxford, *Excerpta Medica*, 1978; 457 : 17.
7. Potier P. Synthesis of the antitumor dimeric indole alkaloids from Catharanthus species (vinblastine group). *J Nat Prod* 1980; 43 (1) : 72-86.
8. Langlois N, Potier P. Antitumor alkaloids of the vinblastine-type : is leurosine an artefact ? *J Chem Soc Chem Commun* 1978; 3 : 102-103.
9. Langlois Y, Langlois N, Mangeney P, Potier P. Hemisynthesis of leurosine, an antitumor alkaloid, isolated from Catharanthus roseus G Don (Apocynaceae). *Tetrahedron Lett* 1976; 44 : 3945-3948.
10. Langlois Y, Potier P. Hemisynthèse de la leurosidine, alcaloïde antitumoral isolé de *Catharanthus roseus* G Don (Apocynacées). *Tetrahedron Lett* 1976; 14 : 1099-1102.
11. Mangeney P, Andriamialisoa RZ, Langlois N *et al.* Preparation of vinblastine, vincristine and leurosidine, antitumor alkaloids from Catharanthus species (Apocynaceae). *J Am Chem Soc* 1979; 101 (8) : 2243-2245.
12. Mangeney P, Andriamialisoa RZ, Langlois N *et al.* A new class of antitumor compounds : 5'-nor and 5', 6'-seco derivatives of vinblastine-type alkaloids. *J Org Chem* 1979; 44 (22) : 3765-3768.
13. Mangeney P, Andriamialisoa RZ, Lallemand JY, *et al.* 5'-Noranhydrovinblastine. Prototype of a new class of vinblastine derivatives. *Tetrahedron* 1979, 35, (18) : 2175-2179.
14. Snyder JA, McIntosh RJ. Biochemistry and physiology of microtubules. *Ann rev Biochem* 1976; 45 : 699.
15. Potier P, Guenard D, Zavala F. Current results in the field of vinblastine antitumor alkaloids. Biochemical studies. *CR Seances Soc Biol. Ses Fil* 1979; 173 (2) : 414-424.
16. Gueritte F, Pouilhes A, Mangeney P *et al.* Antitumor compounds in vinblastine group : nor-5'-anhydrovinblastine derivatives. *Eur J Med Chem Chim Ther* 1983; 18 (5) : 419-424.

2

Action of Navelbine® (NVB) on microtubules. Role of Tau and MAP$_2$ proteins

A. FELLOUS[1], V. MEININGER[2], S. BINET[2], M. CHICHE[1], T. VACASSIN[1], C. GAGELIN[1], H. LATASTE[3], A. KRIKORIAN[3], J.-P. COUZINIER[3]

[1] *INSERM U96, Hôpital de Kremlin-Bicêtre, 94275 Bicêtre Cedex, France.*
[2] *Laboratoire d'Anatomie, Faculté de médecine, 45, rue des Saints-Pères, 75270 Paris Cedex 06, France.*
[3] *Laboratoires Pierre Fabre Médicament CRPF, 17, avenue Jean-Moulin, 81106 Castres Cedex, France.*

Summary

Navelbine® (NVB, 5'nor-anhydro-vinblastine) is distinguished from other vinca alkaloids, such as vinblastine (VBL) or its derivative, vincristine (VCR), by its spectrum of antitumor activity and its very low neurotoxicity. This *in vitro* study compares the mechanisms of action of NVB, VBL and VCR. Sub-stoichiometric concentrations of NVB inhibited tubulin assembly to form microtubules, but inhibition was less effective than that of VBL or VCR. Stoichiometric concentrations of NVB, VBL and VCR all caused aggregation of tubulin when it was bound to Tau proteins, to produce paracrystalline structures. But the aggregating effects of the three drugs differed quantitatively and qualitatively. Aggregation was slower and less complete with NVB than with VCR or VBL. When certain isoforms of Tau were bound to tubulin they reduced the aggregating capacity of NVB. These forms are present in tissues containing a high proportion of mitotic cells and may be associated with the microtubules involved in mitosis.

These differences, together with electron microscope data, indicate that the anticancer drug NVB can have very different effect on microtubules, depending on the type of microtubules involved. A model of NVB action is proposed which explains the differential role of Tau isoforms in NVB-induced tubulin aggregation and the greater sensitivities of certain types of tumors to NVB.

Introduction

The semi-synthetic vinblastine (VBL) derivative, Navelbine® (5' nor-anhydrovinblastine) (NVB), was first produced by Potier et al., in 1979 [1]. It is a double-indole alkaloid, like the other vinca derivatives, vincristine (VCR), vinblastine (VBL) and vindesine. The antitumor effects of VCR, VBL and vindesine, via destruction of the mitotic spindle, have been well documented [2, 3]. They also have an overall antimicrotubule action which varies according to the type of microtubule, and hence, an action on the wide range of biological functions which are dependent on the cytoskeleton [2, 3]. Vinca alkaloids such as VCR or VBL can disrupt microtubular organization by depolymerizing microtubules or inhibiting tubulin assembly to form microtubules, or by causing tubulin to aggregate into very regular birefrigent paracrystalline structures [4-6]. Vinca alkaloids can cause tubulin crystallization in vitro [7-9] and in isolated cells [4-6]. Tubulin aggregation produces abnormal, irreversible structures, which may give rise to numerous secondary effects during cancer chemotherapy. It is, therefore, most important to know how microtubule aggregation or disruption occurs.

We have previously shown that the VBL-induced crystallization of tubulin is catalyzed by Tau proteins and inhibited by MAP_2 proteins [7-9]. Tau and MAP_2 proteins are two families of proteins associated with tubulin, named MAP_s, in certain types of microtubules. They can both exist as a mixture of numerous isoforms, which varies with the stage of cell differentiation [10]. Thus the effects of Tau and MAP_2 proteins may vary according to the isoforms in the cell at a particular time. The various isoforms of Tau and MAP_2 appear to have no differential effect on VBL or VCR-induced tubulin crystallization [9]. But NVB may act differently since its pharmacological properties differ from those of VCR and VBL. NVB frequently has a greater antitumoral effect than VCR and VBL in certain cancers of the lung, ovary and breast [11-13]. Also, patients treated with NVB suffer from few, or minor neuropathies, in contrast to patients treated with VBL or VCR [14]. This study was therefore carried out to compare the effects of NVB, VBL and VCR on microtubule aggregation or disassembly. A very close link was found between the heterogeneity of certain microtubular components and the effects of NVB.

Materials and methods

Products

VBL and VCR were purchased from Sigma (St Louis, USA); NVB ditartrate was provided by Pierre Fabre Médicament, Toulouse, France.

Methods

Microtubules were prepared from rat brains by a modification [15] of the *in vitro* temperature-dependent assembly-disassembly procedure of Shelanski *et al.* [16]. Tubulin was purified by a modification [15] of the method of Weingarten *et al.* [17]. MAP_2 were extracted from microtubules of drug-induced aggregates by thermal denaturation, and MAP_2 and Tau were isolated by gel filtration [15].

Stock solutions of microtubule proteins, NVB, VCR and VBL were prepared in the following buffer: 100 mmol/L 2 N-morpholino-ethanesulfonic acid, pH 6.4, 1 mmol/L ethylene glycol bis (b-amino-ethyl ether) N-N', N-N' tetracetic acid, 0.1 mmol/L ethylene-diamine-tetraacetic acid, 0.5 mmol/L $MgCl_2$, 1mmol/L guanosine-5'- triphosphate, 1 mmol/L b-mercaptoethanol, 1 mmol/L PMSF.

The MAP_2 extracted from vinca alkaloid-induced paracrystals were analyzed by SDS (10 %) PAGE (10 %) [18].

Microtubule and paracrystal formation was assayed by light scattering in a Uvicon (Kontron, France) spectrophotometer equipped with a thermostated (37°C) automatic six-sample charger. Turbidity (optical density at 350 nm) was determined every 30 seconds.

Samples for electron microscopy were placed on Formvar-coated copper grids, stained with 1 % unanyl acetate, and examined in a Philips CM 12 electron microscope [8].

Results

Inhibition of tubulin assembly by NVB, VCR and VBL

All three alkaloids inhibited tubulin assembly induced by Tau proteins (*Figure 1*) or MAP_2 proteins (*Figure 2*) isolated from the brains of adult rats (*Figures 1, A-B et 2, A-B*) or 9-day-old rats (*Figures 1, C-D and 2, C-D*). Low concentrations of NVB (0.2 µM) did not inhibit tubulin assembly induced by Tau protein from adult rat brain (*Figure 1A*), while this concentration of VBL or VCR caused 20 % inhibition. A higher concentration (0.5µM) of NVB was inhibitory, but still less effective than VBL or VCR (*Figure 1B*). The inhibitory effects of all three alkaloids were greater when tubulin assembly was induced with Tau proteins from 9-day-old rats, but NVB remained less effective than VBL or VCR (*Figure 1 C-D*).

The inhibitory effects of the alkaloids on tubulin assembly induced by adult or young rat MAP_2 proteins (*Figure 2*) were very similar to those on Tau-induced microtubule assembly. NVB inhibited microtubule formation with 9-day MAP_2 more strongly (*Figure 2 C-D*) than microtubule formation with adult MAP_2 (*Figure 2 A-B*), but the effects of NVB were always smaller than those of VBL and VCR.

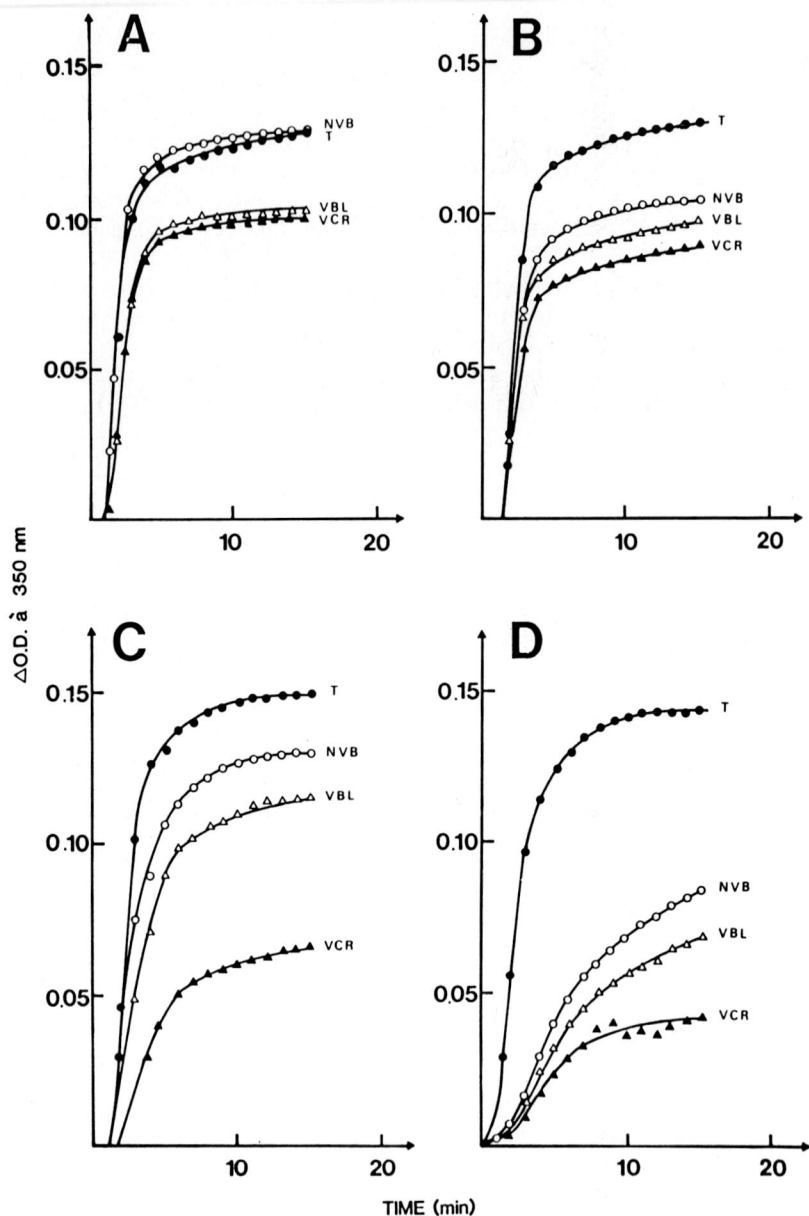

Figure 1. Inhibition of Tau-induced tubulin assembly by VCR, VBL and NVB. The drugs (0.2 µM in A and C, and 0.5 µM in B and D), were added at time 0 to mixtures of purified tubulin and Tau extracted from the brains of adult (A and B) and 9-day-old (C and D) rats.

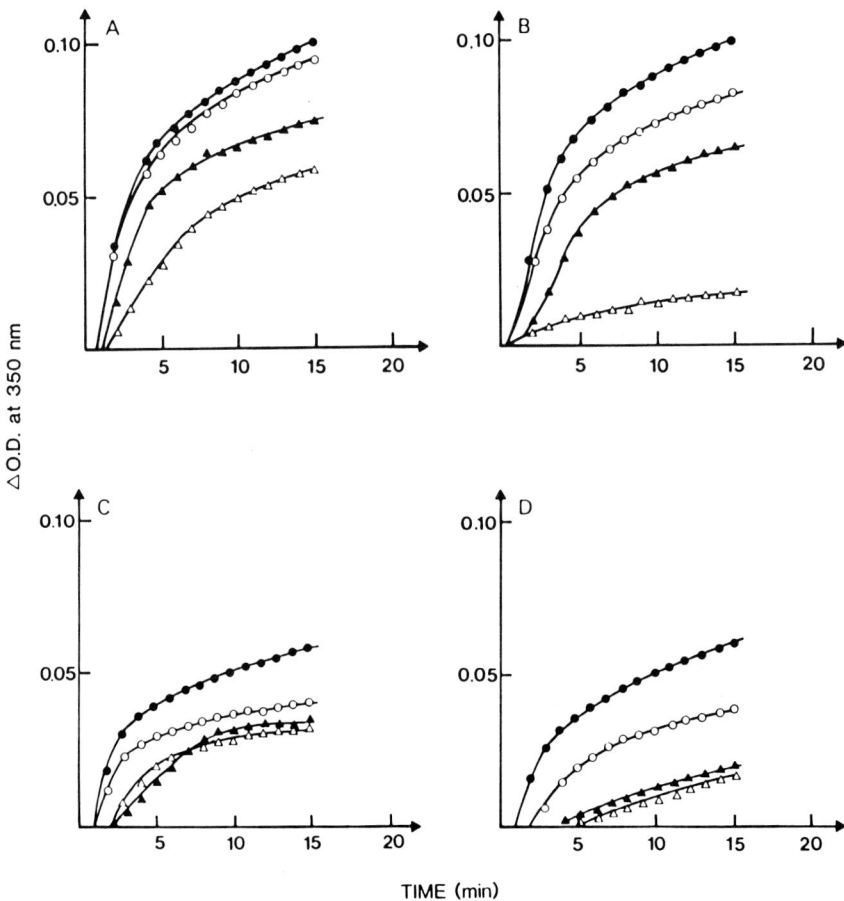

Figure 2. Inhibition of MAP$_2$-induced tubulin assembly by VCR, VBL and NVB. The drugs (0.2 µM in A and C, and 0.5 µM in B and D), were added at time 0 to mixtures of purified tubulin and MAP$_2$ extracted from the brains of adult (A and B) and 9-day-old (C and D) rats.

Aggregation of tubulin induced by NVB, VBL and VCR

Addition of a high concentration (60µM) of VCR to microtubules formed by incubating purified tubulin with purified Tau proteins produced a large increase in turbidity (*Figure 3A*). The increase in A_{350} was proportional to the amount of tubulin aggregated to form birefringent paracrystals (*Figure 3A, insert*). No increase in A_{350} occurred when tubulin was incubated with MAP$_2$ proteins instead of Tau. MAP$_2$ proteins do not catalyze the formation of dense tubulin aggregates in presence of VCR. This difference between the activities of Tau and MAP$_2$ was also seen in the

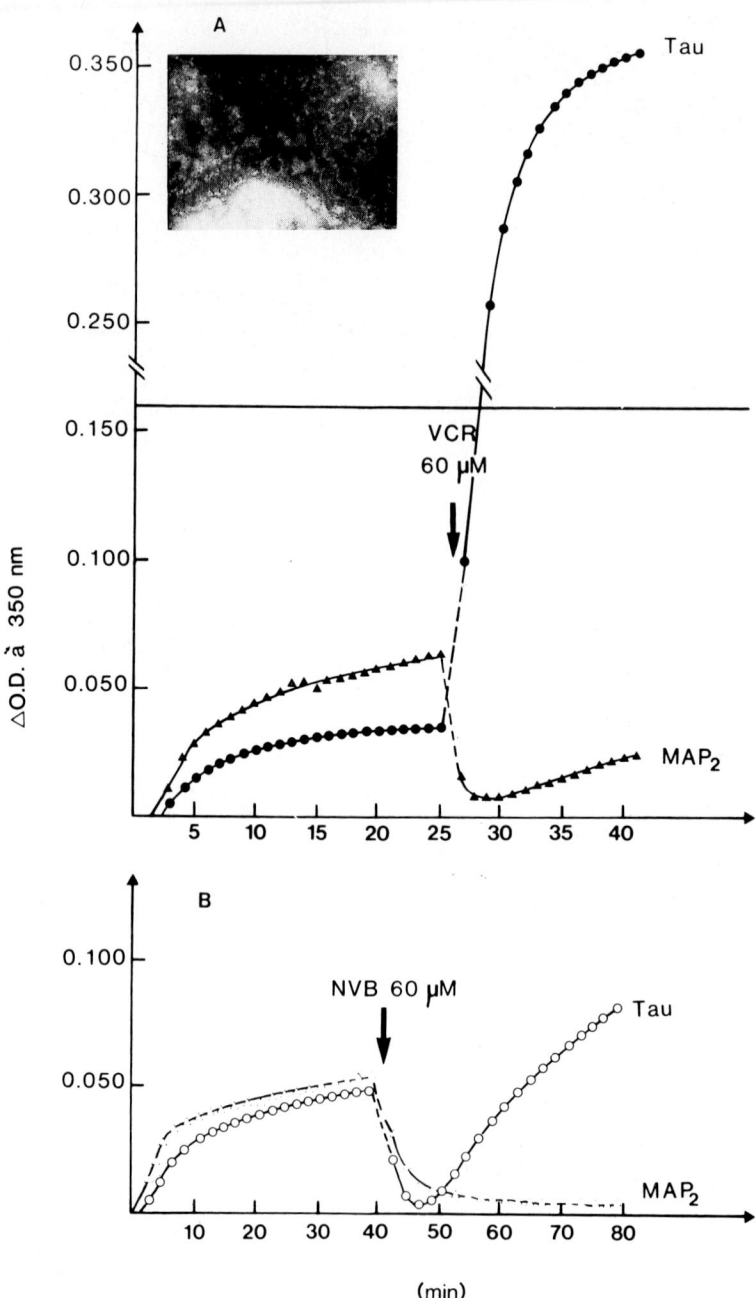

Figure 3. Effects of MAP$_2$ and Tau proteins on tubulin aggregation induced by VCR and NVB. Mixtures of purified tubulin and Tau or MAP$_2$ extracted from adult rat brains were pre-incubated at 37°C for 25 min (3A) or 40 min (3B). The drugs VCR (A) or NVB (B) were then added (concentration 60 µM) and incubation continued for a further 15 to 40 min. Samples of the reaction mixtures were then removed and prepared for electron microscopy. The insert shows an electron micrograph of Tau-induced microtubules treated with 60 µM VCR (× 50,000).

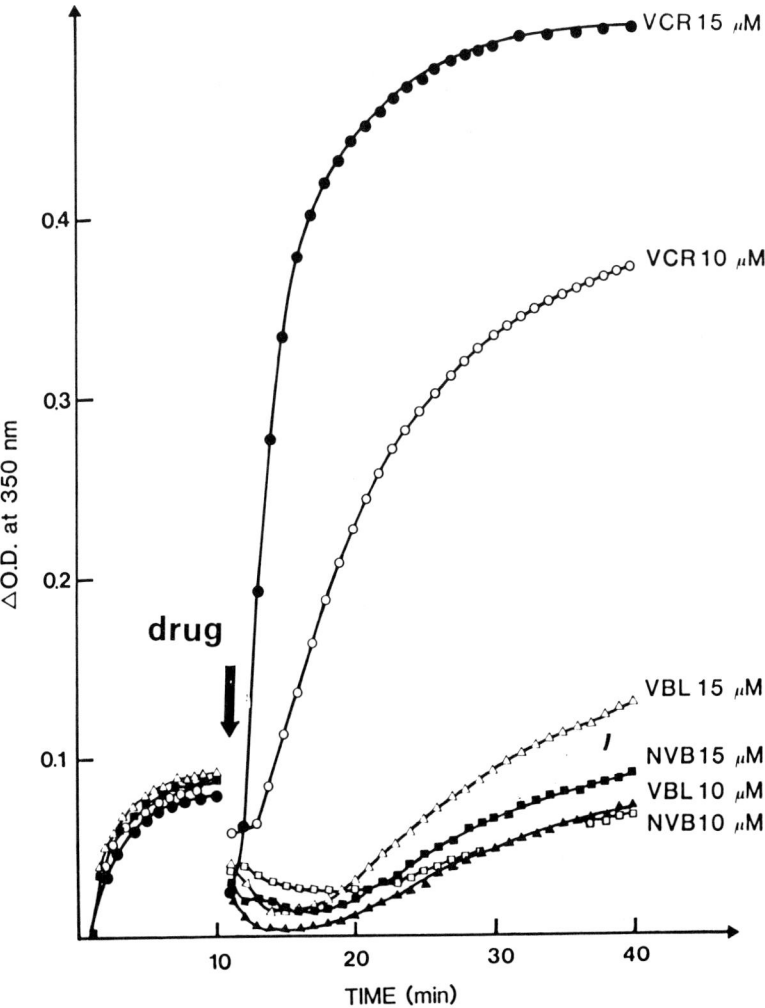

Figure 4. Effect of two concentrations of VCR, VBL and NVB on tubulin aggregation induced by « adult » Tau. The drugs were added to mixtures of purified tubulin and Tau extracted from the brains of adult rats.

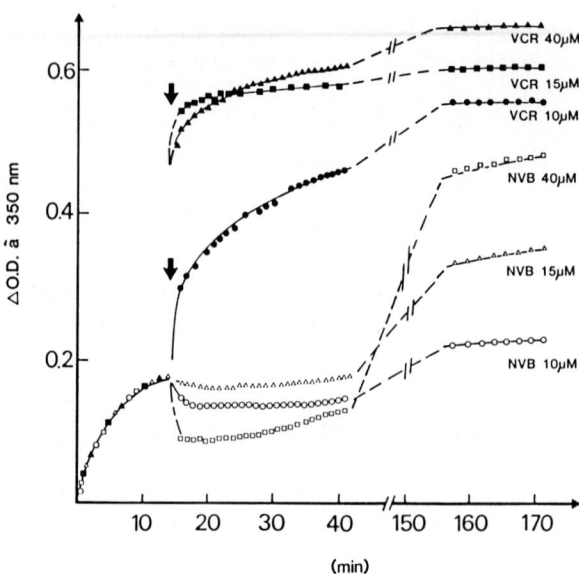

Figure 5. Effect of three concentrations of VCR and NVB on tubulin aggregation induced by « young » Tau. VCR and NVB (10, 15 or 40 μM) were added to reaction mixtures containing purified tubulin from adult rat brains and Tau extracted from the brains of 9-day-old rats.

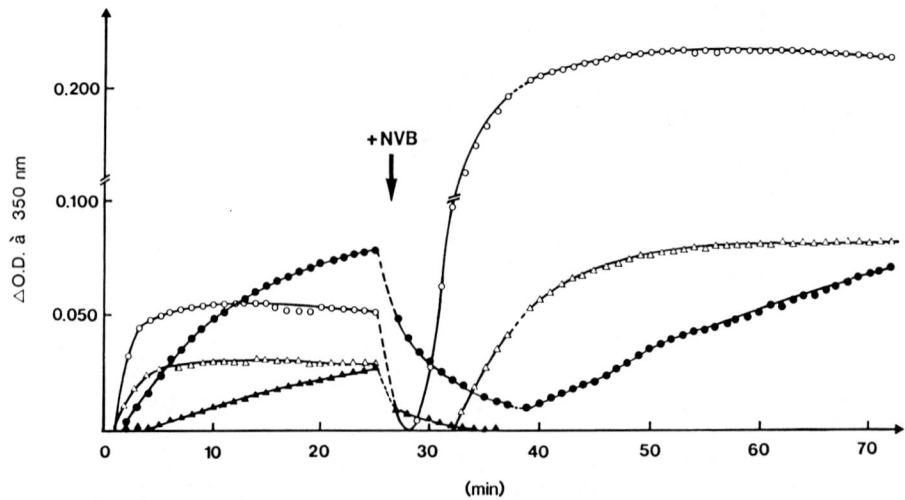

Figure 6. Effects of « adult » and « young » Tau on NVB-induced tubulin aggregation. Tubulin was pre-incubated with either « adult » or « young » Tau for 25 min at 37°C before adding NVB (20 μM).
△ — △ tubulin + adult Tau (75 μg)
○ — ○ tubulin + adult Tau (100 μg)
▲ — ▲ tubulin + young Tau (75 μg)
● — ● tubulin + young Tau (100 μg)

presence of NVB (*Figure 3B*). However, the aggregating capacity of NVB was less effective than that of VCR. *Figure 4* shows that the aggregating effect of NVB remained less important than that of VCR and VBL at low (10 and 15 µM) concentrations. The proteins from adult rat brains were used to obtain the results shown in *Figures 3 and 4*.

Similar experiments with Tau proteins from 9-day-old rat brains also induced tubulin aggregation (*Figure 5*), but aggregation was very much slower than that induced by adult Tau. Optical density also increased much slowlier in systems containing tubulin, "young" (75 or 100 µg/ml) Tau and 20 µM NVB than in equivalent systems containing "adult" Tau (*Figure 6*). This figure also shows that more "young" Tau proteins are needed to catalyze tubulin aggregation than are "adult" Tau.

Electron micrographs of VCR and NVB-induced tubulin aggregates

Very dense aggregates were formed when VCR (10 µM or 40 µM) was added to microtubules formed from purified tubulin and "young" Tau proteins and negatively

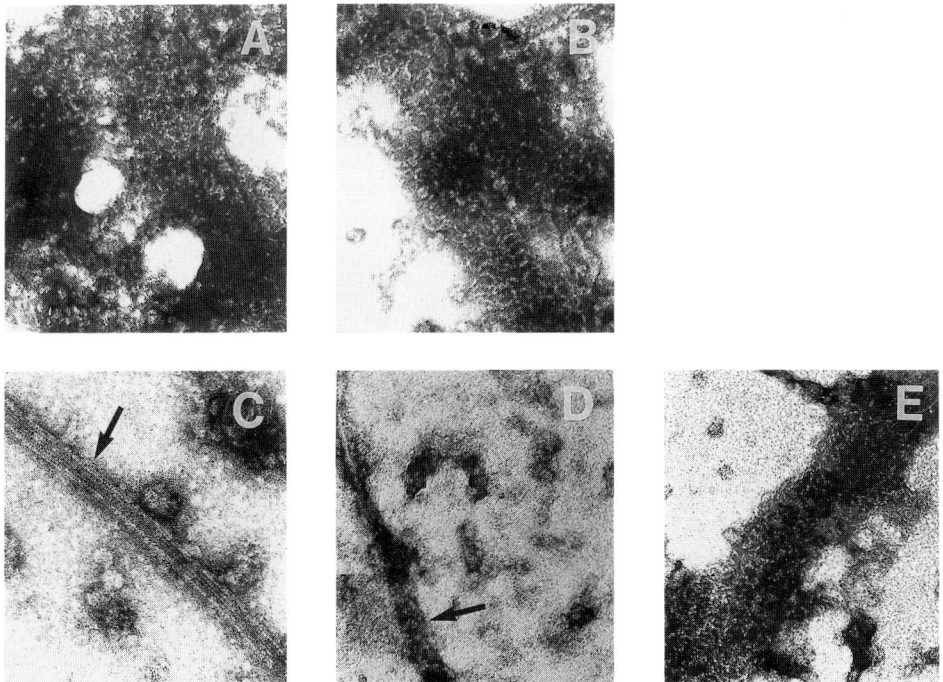

Figure 7. Electron micrographs of microtubule preparations treated with VCR or NVB. Purified tubulin and « young » Tau were pre-incubated for 15 min at 37°C. 10 µM (A) or 40 µM (B) VCR, or 10 µM (C), 15 µM (D) or 40 µM NVB (E) were then added and incubation continued for 60 min. One drop of each mixture was then taken for electron microscopy.

stained (*Figure 7 A-B*). These aggregates were made up of very dense paracrystalline structures, which are themselves formed by the association of tightly spiralled tubulin protofilaments. VCR treatment resulted in aggregation of almost all the tubulin, while the effects of NVB were concentration-dependent. Only some of the tubulin was aggregated at NVB concentrations of 10 and 15 µM. These aggregates were small and lay close to unmodified microtubules (10 µM NVB, *Figure 7C*) or in contact with microtubules which had begun to be altered (15 µM NVB, *Figure 7D*). A high concentration (40 µM) of NVB induced massive tubulin aggregation (*Figure 7E*).

Effects of Tau isoforms on the NVB-induced formation of tubulin paracrystalline structures

Differences were found between the interaction of "young" Tau with tubulin in presence of VCR or NVB. The profiles of "young" Tau proteins copolymerizing with tubulin aggregates induced by 10, 15 or 40 µM VCR were essentially the same (*Figure 8, lanes a,c and e*). But aggregates induced with 10 or 15 µM NVB contained low concentrations of certain low molecular weight Tau proteins (*Figure 8, lanes b, d*). These "fast" Tau proteins remained either free or associated with tubulin subunits or small aggregates. The "fast" Tau proteins were associated with more concentrated aggregates of tubulin at high concentrations of NVB (40 µM) (*Figure 8, lane f*). On the other hand, "adult" Tau proteins appeared to have the same capacity to copolymerize with the tubulin aggregates induced by 10, 15 or 40 µM VCR or 10, 15 or 40 µM NVB. The electrophoretic patterns of "adult" Tau proteins associated with tubulin induced by VCR or NVB were essentially the same (*Figure 8, lanes h-m*).

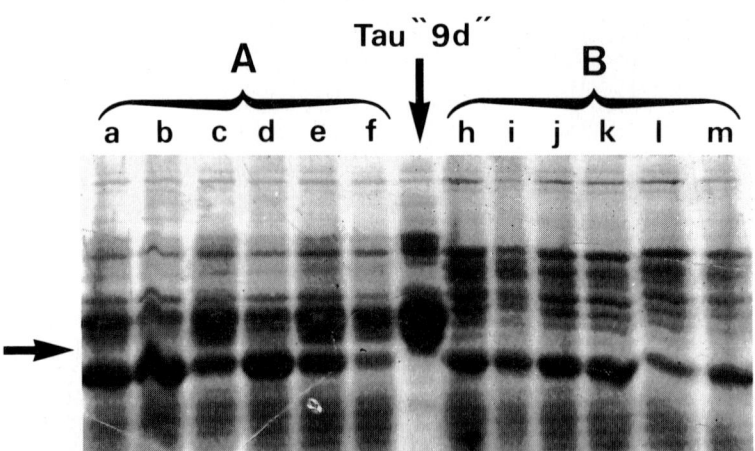

Figure 8. Electrophoretic mobilities of Tau isoforms extracted from VCR- or NVB- induced paracrystals. Paracrystals were separated from soluble microtubule components and very small aggregates by centrifugation at 15,000 rpm for 30 min. « Young » (A) or « Adult » (B) Tau isoforms were extracted from paracrystals induced with 10 µM (a,h), 15 µM (c,j) or 40 µM (e,l) VCR, or 10 µM (b,i), 15 µM (d,k) or 40 µM (f,m) NVB by thermal denaturation and analysed by SDS-PAGE.

Effect of NVB on tubulin aggregation in high Mg^{++} concentrations

Tubulin aggregation by NVB depends directly on the nature of the polymerization promoter. The promoter Mg^{++} is an excellent catalyst of NVB-induced tubulin aggregation. There was a large increase in A_{350} when 20 µM was added to tubulin purified in the presence of Mg^{++} ions (*Figure 9*). The rise in A_{350}, correlated with the formation of tubulin aggregates, increases *pari passu* with the concentration of Mg^{++} ions. For concentrations of Mg^{++} as low as 4.5 mM, the amplitude of tubulin aggregation is large with respect to that obtained in presence of Tau proteins. These aggregates are not simply tubulin precipitates. The aggregates formed by NVB and Mg^{++} could be dissociated by the anti-microtubule drug, maytansine (*Figure 9*), as can the paracrystalline tubulin structures formed with Tau and VBL [15].

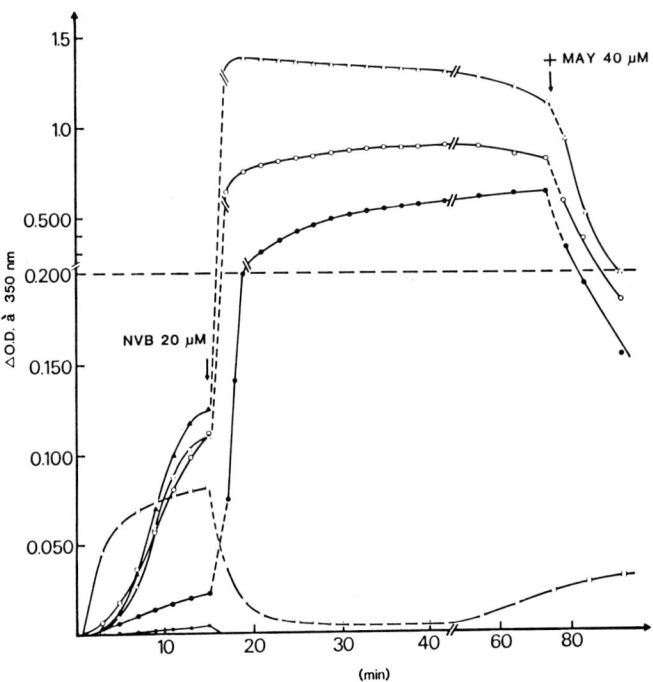

Figure 9. Effect of Mg^{++} on NVB-induced tubulin aggregation. Purified tubulin was preincubated with either Mg^{++} or « young » Tau for 15 min. NVB (20 µM) was then added and incubation continued for a further 60 min. Finally, maytansine (40 µM) was added to the samples containing Mg^{++} and NVB.

●—● 4.5 mM Mg^{++}
○—○ 8.5 mM Mg^{++}
△—△ 12.5 mM
▲—▲ 16.5 mM Mg^{++}
□—□ 100 µg/ml « young » Tau

Discussion

This study of the inhibition of tubulin polymerization by NVB, VCR and VBL shows that NVB is a less effective inhibitor than the other two alkaloids, regardless of the polymerization promoter used. The lower inhibitory capacity occurred at all NVB concentrations tested (only the results at 0.2 and 0.5 µM are shown). This suggests that NVB has a lower affinity for tubulin than the other two alkaloids tested. The tubulin site implicated in inhibition is known to be a high-affinity site [20], but there is very little difference in the affinity of this site for VCR and VBL [21]. Our preliminary studies have also shown that there is a marginally significant difference in the site's affinity for VBL and NVB. Thus the difference in the inhibiting activity of NVB and the other vinca alkaloids is better explained by postulating that the isomers of Tau or MAP$_2$ can modulate or alter the high affinity site differently for each alkaloid. If this is true, then certain classes of microtubules would have a selective sensitivity to vinca alkaloids, so that certain Tau or MAP$_2$ proteins would either confer resistance to low doses of NVB or amplify the effects of these low doses.

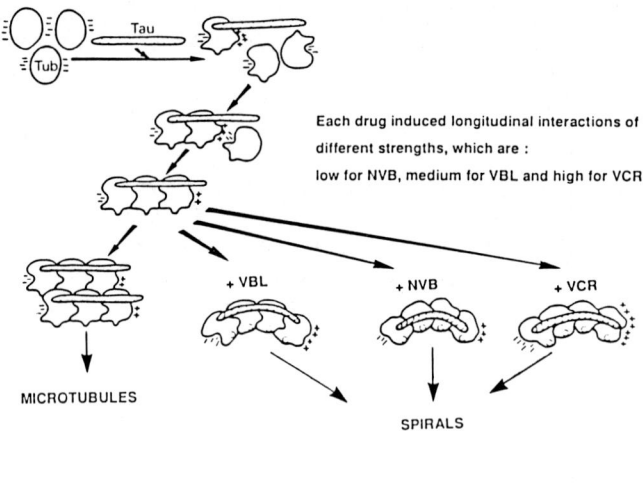

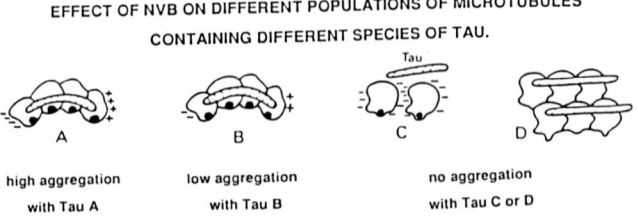

Figure 10. Model of VCR, VLB and NVB action on different classes of microtubules.

The modulation of the effects of vinca alkaloids by Tau or MAP_2 proteins appears most clearly in the process of tubulin crystallization, which involves the low affinity drug-binding site [20]. MAP_2 proteins cannot promote the formation of paracrystalline structures from tubulin and the three alkaloids. Several explanations have been proposed, such as a change in conformation of the tubulin molecule induced by binding MAP_2, resulting in either an altered, non-functional, low affinity site, or a tubulin-MAP_2-alkaloid complex which is unsuitable for aggregation.

The role of the Tau proteins in aggregation seems to be more complex, as shown in the model outlined in *Figure 10*. Each given species of Tau protein will provide a different degree of tubulin aggregation, depending on the alkaloid involved. Thus VCR is the most powerful aggregator and NVB the least. This may be because NVB has the lowest affinity for the low affinity site on tubulin, or because of the formation of tubulin-Tau-NVB, tubulin-Tau-VBL and tubulin-Tau-VCR complexes having different aggregation capacities. The heterogeneity of Tau proteins could modulate the aggregation activity of the vinca alkaloid. Such a role has not been demonstrated for VBL or VCR. With VCR, for example, all the species of Tau proteins seem to have the same capacity to catalyze tubulin aggregation. Almost all the tubulin in contact with the drug aggregates to form paracrystals containing all the isoforms of Tau proteins added to the reaction mixture, even at low concentrations of VCR (10 or 15 µM). This indicates that the different classes of microtubules formed with different species of Tau proteins may be modified in the same way by VCR. Thus, axonal microtubules containing certain Tau isoforms [22] and mitotic spindle microtubules also containing Tau isoforms [23], but which are probably different, may be aggregated by the same or very similar concentrations of VCR. However, the influence of Tau heterogeneity is much greater with NVB. There are both quantitative and qualitative differences, in the effects of NVB on microtubules formed with different types of Tau proteins. Tau proteins from young rats have a much poorer aggregating effect than Tau proteins from adult rats. This does not necessarily mean that all the isoforms of Tau proteins isolated at early stages of development are less efficient, on a mole-for-mole basis, at inducing tubulin crystallization. At low (10-15 µM) concentrations of NVB certain isoforms from "young" Tau proteins cause tubulin crystallization while others cannot. These non-aggregating Tau proteins, which are not present in the adult Tau population, may be involved in cell division.

The differing actions of Tau isoforms may be due to charge differences. The most powerful aggregating Tau proteins would be those whose binding to tubulin caused a conformational change unmasking the greatest number of positive charges. This idea seems to be supported by the experiments showing that binding of Mg^{++} ions to tubulin causes aggregation of tubulin so that aggregation increases with the Mg^{++} concentration. The position on tubulin of the positive charges, induced either by the Tau proteins or by Mg^{++} binding, would be polarized, as in *Figure 10,* allowing formation of a long tubulin protofilament which could then form a spiral in the presence of NVB. Thus the properties of the alkaloid and the tubulin aggregation promoter would modulate the speed and extent of the tubulin aggregation.

This process of aggregation, which results in very dense paracrystalline structures both *in vitro* and in cultured or isolated cells, may appear very different in the cells of an organism treated with vinca alkaloids. Paracrystalline structures are not observed in these organisms, but similar structures, such as small hard-to-dissociate aggregates of tubulin might be formed after alkaloid treatment. These can destroy microtubule function over what may be a very long time. NVB would be able to alter certain microtubules by both alkaloid-specific routes leading to either depolymerization or aggregation. Up to certain drug concentrations at least, this property would affect only a few classes of microtubules, some of which might be involved in mitosis. As Tau heterogeneity acts as a modulator, then NVB should affect differentiated and mitotic cells differently. This heterogeneity of Tau proteins could also lead to differential NVB effects on different types of mitotic cells. The results of these interactions would explain why NVB is a better anti-cancer agent for certain types of cancers.

Acknowledgement

We thank P. Gounon for taking electron micrographs, A. Lefèvre and M. Bahloul for assistance in manuscript preparation.

References

1. Potier P, Guenard D, Zavala F. Résultats récents dans le domaine des alcaloïdes antitumoraux du groupe de la vinblastine. Etudes biochimiques. *CR Soc Biol* 1979; 47 : 414-424.
2. Olmsted JB, Borisy GG. Microtubules. *Ann Rev Biochem* 1973; 42 : 507-540.
3. Margulis L. Colchicine-sensitive microtubules. *Int Rev Cytol* 1973; 34 : 333-361.
4. Bryan J. Vinblastine and microtubules. I. Induction and isolation of crystals from sea urchin oocytes. *Exp Cell Res* 1971; 66 : 129-136.
5. Bryan J. Vinblastine and microtubules. II. Characterization of two protein subunits from the isolated crystals. *J. Mol Biol* 1972a; 66 : 157-168.
6. Bryan J. Definition of three classes of binding sites in isolated microtubule crystals. *Biochemistry* 1972b; 11 : 2611-2616.
7. Luduena RF, Fellous A, Francon J, Nunez J, McManus L. Effect of Tau on the vinblastine induced aggregation of tubulin. *J Cell Biol* 1981; 89 : 680-683.
8. Luduena RF, Fellous A, McManus L, Jordan MA, Nunez J. Contrasting effects of Tau and microtubule-associated protein 2 in the vinblastine-induced aggregation of tubulin. *J Biol Chem* 1984; 259 : 12890-12898.
9. Fellous A. Ohayon R, Mazie JC, Rosa F, Luduena R, Prasad V. Tau microheterogeneity : an immunological approach with monoclonal antibodies. *Ann Acad Sci* 1986; 466 : 240-256.
10. Francon J, Lennon AM, Fellous A, Mareck A, Pierre M, Nunez J. Heterogeneity of microtubule-associated proteins and brain development. *Europ J Biochem* 1982; 129 : 465-471.
11. Depierre A, Lemarie E, Dabouis G, Garnier G, Jacoulet P, Dalphin JC. Efficacy of navelbine (NVB) in non small cell lung cancer (NSLCLC) *Semin Oncol* 1989; 16 : 26-29.

12. George MJ, Heron JF, Kerbrat P, et al. Navelbine® in advanced ovarian epithelial cancer : a study of the french oncology centers. *Semin Oncol* 1989; 16 : 30-32.
13. Canobbio L, Boccardo F, Pastorino G, et al. Phase-II study of Navelbine® in advanced breast cancer. *Semin Oncol* 1989; 16 : 33-36.
14. Besenval M, Delgado M, Demarez JP, Krikorian A. Safety and tolerance of Navelbine® in phase I-II clinical studies. *Semin Oncol* 1989; 16 : 37-40.
15. Shelanski ML, Gaskin F, Cantor CR. Microtubule assembly in the absence of added nucleotides. *Proc Natl Acad Sci USA* 1973; 70 : 765-768.
16. Fellous A, Francon J, Lennon AM et al. Microtubule assembly *in vitro*. Purification of assembly promoting factors. *Eur J Biochem* 1977; 78 : 167-174.
17. Weingarten MD, Lockwood AH, Hwo Sy et al. A protein factor essential for microtubule assembly. *Proc Natl Acad Sci USA* 1975; 72 : 1858-1852.
18. Laemmli UK. Cleavage of structural proteins during the assembly of the head of bacteriophage T4. *Nature* 1970; 227 : 680-685.
19. Fellous A, Luduena RF, Prasad V et al. The effects of Tau and MAP_2 on the interaction of maytansine with tubulin-poisonous effects of maytansine on vinblastine-induced aggregation of tubulin. *Cancer Res* 1985; 45 : 5004-5010.
20. Bhattacharayya B, Wolff J. Tubulin aggregation and disaggregation : mediation by two distinct vinblastine-binding sites. *Proc Natl Acad Sci USA* 1976; 73 : 2375-2378.
21. Owellen RJ, Owens AM, Donigian DW. The binding of vincristine, vinblastine and colchicine to tubulin. *Biochem Biophys Res Commun* 1972; 47 : 685-691.
22. Tytell M, Brady ST, Lassek RJ. Axonal transport of a subclass of Tau proteins : evidence for the differential differenciation of microtubules in neurons. *Proc Natl Acad Sci USA* 1984; 81 : 1570-1574.
23. Connolly JA, Kalnis VI, Cleveland DW, Kirschner MW. Immunofluorescent staining of cytoplasmic and spindle microtubules in mouse fibroblasts with antibody to Tau protein. *Proc Natl Acad Sci USA* 1979; 14 : 2437-2440.

3

Immunofluorescence study of the action of Navelbine®, vincristine and vinblastine on mitotic and axonal microtubules

S. BINET[1], E. CHAINEAU[1], A. FELLOUS[2], H. LATASTE[3],
A. KRIKORIAN[3], J.-P. COUZINIER[3], V. MEININGER[1]

[1] *Laboratoire d'Anatomie, UER Biomédicales des Saints-Pères et Broussais-Hôtel-Dieu, 45, rue des Saints-Pères, 75270 Paris Cedex 06, France*
[2] *INSERM U96, Hôpital du Kremlin-Bicêtre, 94275 Bicêtre Cedex, France*
[3] *Pierre-Fabre Médicament CRPF, 17, avenue Jean-Moulin, 81106 Castres Cedex, France*

Summary

Among the various non-naturally occurring vinca alkaloid compounds, nor-anhydro-vinblastine (Navelbine®, NVB) has been shown in preliminary clinical studies to have a broader anti-tumor activity and less neurotoxicity than vinblastine (VBL) and vincristine (VCR). The action of these three vinca alkaloids on axonal and mitotic microtubules has been experimentally studied in a specific model, the tectal plate anlage of mouse embryos at the earliest stages of neuronal differentiation. Postimplantation embryos were cultured *in toto* in a medium containing increasing concentrations of drugs. Microtubules were stained using immunofluorescence with a tubulin-specific polyclonal antibody in semi-thin sections after embedding in high molecular weight polyethylene glycol. All three drugs induced a depolymerization of both interpolar and mitotic microtubules and a cell blockage at metaphase at the same concentration, of 2 µM. Increasing the concentrations led to a progressive depolymerization of kinetochore microtubules; however, NVB was the only drug that was able to induce a complete depolymerization of these microtubules. The activity of the three compounds on axonal microtubules was identical; they induce a depolymerization of a labile pool of microtubules. This action was observed at higher concentrations with NVB than with the two other vinca alkaloids. These results demonstrate that in this model NVB is as active on mitotic microtubules and less active on axonal microtubules than VCR and VBL. The difference between the three compounds observed with regard to the range of concentrations active on the two types of microtubules suggests that their mechanism of action may be mediated by microtubule ligands other than tubulin, probably the microtubule-associated proteins.

Introduction

The *Catharanthus* alkaloids, vincristine sulfate (VCR) and vinblastine sulfate (VBL), are widely used cancer chemotherapeutic agents. Although their chemotherapeutic effects are different, *in vivo* and *in vitro* studies demonstrated that their mechanism of action appears identical and is mediated, at least in part, through their action on microtubules. They induce a disruption of mitotic microtubules, causing the dissolution of cell mitotic spindles and the arrest of the cells at their metaphase [1, 2], these cells being called "c-mitosis".

Therapeutic uses of these drugs could appear to be limited by their toxicity. Most symptoms of "toxicity" observed with vinca alkaloids result from the inhibition of mitotic growth in the bone marrow, the intestine and the hair follicle bulb. However, the most limiting toxicity is neurotoxicity, as these drugs commonly produce a mixed sensorimotor neuropathy [3]. The pathogenesis of the neuropathy is poorly defined, but it seems likely that they are related to microtubule modifications and to alteration of the axonal transport, a microtubule-dependent process [4].

These limitations led to the development, either by identification of synthesis, of drugs having at least the same antitumor spectrum and less neurotoxicity. In preliminary studies, a recently discovered hemisynthetic alkaloid agent, nor 5'-anhydrovinblastine or Navelbine® (NVB), has been demonstrated to have both properties and to be a potentially good candidate in cancer chemotherapy.

The aim of the present study was to compare the action of NVB with that of VBL and VCR on microtubules using a specific model, the tectal plate anlage of the postimplanted mouse embryo cultivated in a rotatory display as described by New [5]. As previously demonstrated [6, 7], this region of the embryonic nervous system is basically composed of two cell types at the earliest stages of neuronal differentiation : a progenitor cell, which is epithelial in nature — the bipolar neuroepithelial cell (BNC)- and the postmigratory young neurons with their growing axons. The well-known fact that the BNC undergoes complete cell cycles [6], including mitosis, explains the observation that various types of microtubules coexist in the neuroepithelium : mitotic, in the mitotic phases of the cell cycle, interphasic, and axonal, in the growing axons.

In the present study, we used this model to analyze the effects of the three drugs on mitotic and axonal microtubules stained by immunofluorescence after embedding in polyethylene glycol (PEG).

Materials and methods

Materials

Mouse embryos were collected at stage E11, eleven days after a vaginal plug was noted (stage E0) in random-bred mice of CD1 strain (Ch. River, France). Mice were mated between 8.00 and 10.30 a.m. Dams were killed by cervical dislocation. Uterine horns were carefully removed and rinsed in Hank's solution at room temperature.

Methods

Culture

Embryos were dissected free of maternal tissue and the Reichert's membrane, leaving the ectoplacental cone and the yolk sac intact [8]. The dissection was performed in Hank's balanced salt solution with fine forceps under aseptic conditions. A small aperture was carefully opened in the yolk sac to ensure good penetration of the drug at the point of contact with the embryo. For each concentration tested, 5 embryos were cultivated in a medium containing the tested agent and 5 embryos were cultivated in a drug free medium as control. Embryos in culture displayed all characteristics of embryos at stage E11. Embryos damaged during dissection and embryos displaying abnormalities before culture were discarded.

The culture medium consisted of heat-inactivated filtered (0.22 μm, Flow Pore D26) rat serum free of antibiotics. Vincristine sulfate, vinblastine sulfate and 5'-noranhydrovinblastine ditartrate (NVB) were freshly dissolved in sterile distilled water and added at increasing concentrations to 2 ml of medium.

Each test vial (25 ml) containing one embryo and 2 ml of medium was gassed with a mixture of 95 % O_2 and 5 % CO_2, placed on a rotator and rotated at 40 rpm in an incubator at 37°C for 90 min, this time corresponding to a complete cell cycle at this stage [9]. At the end of the culture period, embryos were removed and examined for viability, appraised by the presence of yolk sac circulation and a heartbeat. Non-viable embryos were discarded.

Immunocytochemistry

Embryos were gently perfused either through the umbilical vein of through the cardiac anlage using a fixative solution containing 0.5 % glutaraldehyde (EM grade, Agar Aids) and 4 % paraformaldehyde in a 0.1 M phosphate buffer (pH 7.4; 1250 mOsm), at room temperature. Clearing of the cerebral vessels ensured the quality of the perfusion.

Well perfused embryos were immersed *in toto* for 90 min in the fixative solution after which the tectal plates were dissected out and immersed in a fresh fixative solution at room temperature for another 90 min.

Embedding was carried out after the blocks has been thoroughly rinsed in the 0.1 M phosphate buffer for 30 min. PEG embedding medium was used for immunocytochemistry and embedment was performed according to Meininger and Binet [7].

Semi-thin sections with a nominal thickness of 0.5 μm and 1 μm were obtained on an Ultrotome V (LKB)R using glass knives and mounted on Chrome-Alum-gelatine coated slides using 20 % PEG 200 in distilled water (v/v). Sections were rinsed with distilled water and exposed to freshly prepared sodium borohydride (0.5-1.0 mg/ml in distilled water) for 20 min with gentle agitation. Slides were rinsed in 0.1 % BSA buffer (20 mM Tris, 0.5 M NaCl, pH 8.3 containing 0.1 % BSA, type V, Sigma). Sections were treated for 30 min with NGS (Normal Goat Serum, Nordic) and exposed for 2h in a moist chamber to an affinity-purified primary rabbit antitubulin antibody, specific for microtubules [10] (kindly provided by M. de Brabander, Janssen Pharmaceutica), diluted at 1 μg/ml in the 0.1% Tris-BSA buffer containing 1 % NGS. Slides were washed in the 0.1 % Tris-BSA buffer and exposed to a FITC-labeled goat antiserum to rabbit IgG (GAR/FITC, Nordic) diluted 1:40 in 0.1 % Tris-BSA for 1 h at room temperature in a moist chamber. Slides were then rinsed, mounted in Gelvatol (Monsanto), examined and photographed through a Nikon microscope under epifluorescence illumination using an objective aperture of 1.4 and light source of 515 nm wavelength as suggested by Weber and Osborn [11].

Results

The appearance of the tectal plate anlage at stage E11 has already been described [6, 7]. It looks like a thin veil of tissue, 100 to 150 μm thick, covering the dorsal part of the ventricle, exhibiting three zones from the basal, or ventricular surface, to the apical, or pial surface. A clear-cut identification of mitotic and neuronal cells was allowed on the basis of their appearance, their location in one of these zones and their orientation. The ventricular zone, the largest one, contains the mitotic cells in contact with the ventricular surface. These cells are round-shaped and contain mitotic microtubules stained by the antitubulin antibody. The intermediate zone is located near the apical surface and is characterized by tangentially oriented young neurons and axonal profiles. In these profiles, axonal microtubules appear as dense bundles brightly stained by the antitubulin antibody.

Embryos were exposed at increasing concentration of the three drugs, these concentrations ranging from 0.01 μM to 50 μM. Embryolethal effects probably related to cardiac cells toxicity were observed after exposure to concentrations above 20 μM with VCR 30 μM with VBL and 50 μM with NVB.

Mitotic cells *(Figure 1)*.

All three drugs were active at the same concentration, 0.1 μM. At this concentration, all mitotic figures are observed but there is an increase in the number of mitotic cells.

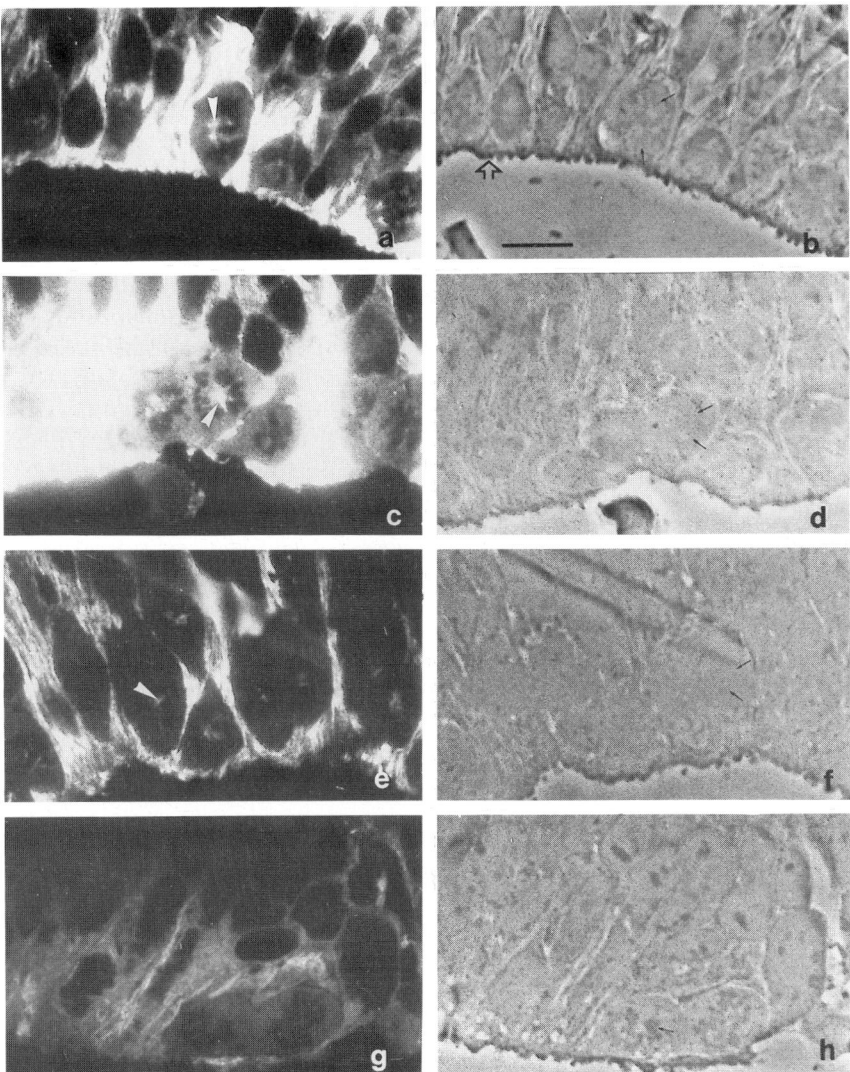

Figure 1. Ventricular zone of the tectal plate of embryos at stage E11; PEG embedding, 0.5 μm semi-thin sections (nominal thickness). In a, c, e and g, immunostaining using a polyclonal specific antitubulin antibody; in b, d, f and h, corresponding phase-contrast photographs. In **a** and **b**, VBL 5 μM treated embryos. The ventricular zone is enriched in round-shaped cells with characteristic appearance of « c-mitosis ». In a, the white arrow head points to a centrally located centriolar apparatus. In b, the small arrows point to peripherally located chromosomes. The open and large arrow head designates the ventricular surface. In **c** and **d**, VCR 5 μM treated embryos. The appearance is identical to VBL treated embryos with characteristic « c-mitosis ». In **e** and **f**, NVB 5 μM treated embryos. The « c-mitosis » are identical to the other vinca alkaloids treated embryos. In **g** and **h**, NVB 30 μM treated embryos. No kinetochore microtubules, nor centrioles are stained. Cells are arrested in pro-metaphase state. Bar = 10 μM (for all photographs).

At 2 µM, all three drugs induced a cell blockade at metaphase, with the appearance of the characteristic morphology called "c-mitosis". These pseudo-metaphase arrested cells were characterized by chromosomes located at the periphery of the cells and one or more densely fluorescent central spots corresponding to centrioles. Fluorescent microtubules linking these centrioles to the chromosomes and corresponding to kinetochore microtubules were present, whereas the long microtubules linking the centrioles (the interpolar microtubules) were not seen, suggesting that they were depolymerized.

Increasing the concentrations led to 1) a progressive increase in the number of mitotic cells and the presence of numerous round mitotic cells arrested at metaphase; and 2) a depolymerization of the kinetochore microtubules. Depolymerization of these microtubules was observed at 2 µM in the case of VCR and at 5 µM in the case of VBL and NVB. However, VBL and VCR induced only incomplete depolymerization with persistence of fluorescent spots at the contact of chromosomes. At high concentrations of NVB (25 µM), scattered chromosomes and fluorescent central centrioles were not observed, suggesting that cells were attested at the end of pro-metaphase and that all kinetochore microtubules were depolymerized.

Axonal microtubules (*Figure 2*)

All three drugs induced alterations of these microtubules, but the effective concentration was different. VCR was active at 5 µM, VBL at 30 µM and NVB at 40 µM.

The number of immunofluorescent microtubules was dramatically reduced in drug-treated embryos and contrasted with the persistence even at high concentrations of small and brightly fluorescent spots located in the axonal profiles.

Discussion

Our results demonstrate that VCR, VBL and NVB are active on both axonal and mitotic microtubules, but that the effect on axonal microtubules is concentration-dependent. Compared with VCR and VBL NVB is effective on mitotic microtubules at the same concentration, but its activity on axonal microtubules occurs at higher concentrations.

Since the pioneer work of Weber [12], Brinkley *et al.* [13] and Sato *et al.* [14], it has been clearly demonstrated that immunofluorescence is a powerful tool in analysing the spatial organization of microtubules, at least in cell culture. Using culture of post implantation mouse embryos [6] and immunofluorescence with a tubulin-specific polyclonal antibody on semi-thin sections after PEG embedding [15] of the tectal plate at the earliest stages of neuronal differentiation, we recently demonstrated that this technique permits different types of microtubules (mitotic, at all stages of mitosis, and axonal) to be analyzed *in situ*.

The three vinca alkaloids analyzed in this study appear to act identically on mitotic microtubules. The two-step loss of mitotic microtubules suggest that the mechanism

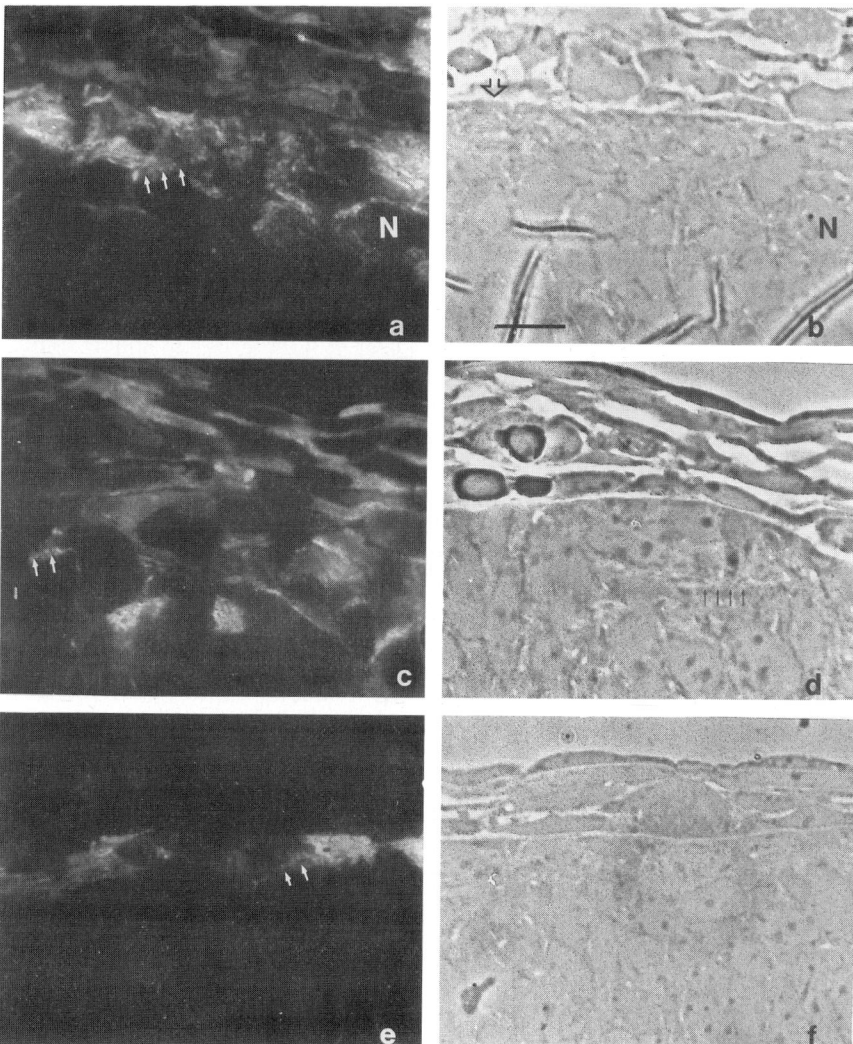

Figure 2. Apical zone of the tectal plate of embryos at stage E11; PEG embedding, 0.5 μm semi-thin sections (nominal thickness). In a, c and e, immunostaining using a polyclonal specific antibulin antibody; in b, d and f, corresponding phase-contrast photographs. In **a** and **b**, VBL 30 μM treated embryo. Small spots are observed in a (white arrow heads) corresponding to small fragments of microtubules. N is a tangential young neuron. The open and large arrow head in b indicates the apical surface. In **c** and **d**, VCR 10 μM treated embryo. The number and appearance of microtubules are identical to the VBL 30 μM treated embryo. In d, small arrows point to a characteristic axonal profile. In **e** and **f**, NVB 40 μM treated embryo. The region contains less axonal profiles but the number and appearances of the axonal microtubules are identical to the two other vinca alkaloid-treated embryos. The only one difference is the concentration at which these images are observed. Bar = 10 μM (for all photographs).

of action is mediated by a depolymerization at low concentrations of interpolar microtubules and a higher concentrations of kinetochore microtubules. The depolymerization of interpolar microtubules seems to induce the blockade of cells at metaphase and the appearance of pseudo-metaphase characterized by centrally located centrioles linked by intact kinetochore microtubules to scattered chromosomes located at the periphery of the cells. These images have been already described in colchicine and vinca alkaloid-treated material, largely in cell culture [2]. The consistency of our own results both with the images observed and with the concentrations used in cell cultures prove the model used in the present study to be valuable in the analysis of the activity of these drugs. The existence of two or more centrioles in "c-mitosis" confirm the well-known fact that vinca alkaloids have no effect on the reduplication of centrioles [2]. In our material, NVB was the only agent which at high concentrations blocked the cells at pro-metaphase and induced a complete depolymerization of kinetochore microtubules.

All drugs tested acted on axonal microtubules, inducing a depolymerization of these microtubules as demonstrated by the decrease in number of the fluorescent bundles of microtubules in the axonal profiles. All three drugs were characterized by the persistence of small fluorescent spots in the axonal profiles of the intermediate zones even at high drug concentrations. Similar observations have been reported in vincristine-treated rat sciatic nerves [3], namely a shift toward shorter lengths and reduced numbers of microtubules per square of axonal areas. As suggested by Sahenk et al. [3], and by our own observations [6], these spots appear identical to the fragments of microtubules observed after cold treatment. These observations suggest that microtubules, at least in axons, consist of both stable and labile portions. Under conditions that depolymerize microtubules, such as cold, vinca alkaloids, the labile portion is selectively affected, leaving the stable portions unaffected. These portions account for our observations of the persistence of small fluorescent spots in the axonal profiles of the treated embryos.

The characteristic concentration-dependent activity of vinca alkaloids on axonal and mitotic microtubules raises the question of the mechanism of action of these drugs on these two types of microtubules. Most authors [16-18] agree that, at least in vitro and in the case of vinblastine, the action of the drug is associated with and may be due to the binding of vinblastine to a high affinity site on tubulin. However, the difference of the range of concentrations active on mitotic and axonal microtubules observed between the three vinca alkaloids suggest that the mechanism of action of the three drugs may not be unique. Besides a possible difference in the affinity of the drugs for tubulin, it is possible to suggest another hypothesis. As previously observed by Wilson et al. [16], the activity of vinblastine differs dramatically in crude supernatant fractions of bovine brain homogenates from that in purified microtubule brain preparations. This result suggests that this difference may be related to the presence of important regulatory ligands such as microtubule-associated proteins in crude preparations which may play a key role in the action of vinca alkaloids. These proteins are present in living material, such as our material. It may be postulated that the different composition in microtubule-associated proteins of mitotic and axonal microtubules may account for the differences in activity of the various vinca alkaloids observed in the present study.

Aknowledgements

We thank Blandine Soudière for technical assistance with immunocytochemistry and Michel Soudière for photographic services.

References

1. Deconti RC, Creaey WA. Clinical aspects of the dimeric *Catharanthus* alkaloids. In : Taylor WI, Farnsworth NR (eds). *The Catharanthus alkaloids, botany, chemistry, pharmacology and clinical use.* New York, M. Dekker, 1975 : 237-27.
2. Dustin P. *Microtubules.* Berlin, New York, Springer-Verlag, 1978.
3. Sahenk Z, Brady ST, Mendell JR. Studies on the pathogenesis of vincristine-induced neuropathy. *Muscle Nerve* 1987; 10 : 80-84.
4. Brimijoin S. Microtubules and the capacity of the system for rapid axonal transport. *Federation Proc* 1982; 41 : 2312-2316.
5. New DAT. Whole-embryo culture and the study of mammalian embryos during organogenesis. *Biol Rev* 1978; 53 : 81-122.
6. Meininger V, Binet S. Characteristics of microtubules at the different stages of neuronal differentiation and maturation. *Int Rev Cytol* 1989; 114 : 21-79.
7. Meininger V, Binet S. Spatial organization of microtubules in various types of cells in the embryonic tectal plate of mouse using immunofluorescence after PEG embedding. *Biol Cell* 1988; 64 : 301-308.
8. New DAT, Coppola P. Development of a placental blood circulation in rat embryos *in vitro*. *J Embryol Exp Morphol* 1977; 37 : 227-235.
9. Jacobson M. *Developmental neurobiology.* New York, Plenum, 1978.
10. De Brabander M, Geuens G, de Mey J, Joniau M. Light microscopic and ultrastructural distribution of immunoreactive tubulin in mitotic mammalian cells. *Biol Cell* 1979; 34 : 213-226.
11. Weber K, Osborn M. Intracellular display of microtubular structures revealed by indirect immunofluorescence microscopy. In : Roberts K, Hyams JS (eds). *Microtubules.* London, Academic Press, 1979 : 279-313.
12. Weber K. Visualisation of tubulin-containing structures by immunofluorescence microscopy : cytoplasmic microtubules, mitotic figures and vinblastine-induced paracrystals. In : Goldman R, Pollart T, Rosenbaum J (eds). *Cell motility.* New York, Cold Spring Harbor lab, 1976, vol A : 403-417.
13. Brinkley BR, Fuller GM, Highfield DP. Tubulin antibodies as probes for microtubules in dividing and nondividing mammalian cells. In : Goldman R, Pollard T, Rosenbaum J (eds). *Cell motility.* New York, Cold Spring Harbor Lab, 1976, vol A : 436-456.
14. Sato H, Ohnuki Y, Fujiwara K. Immunofluorescent antitubulin staining of spindle microtubules and critique for the technique. In : Goldman R, Pollard T, Rosenbaum J (eds). *Cell motility.* New York, Cold Spring Harbor Lab, 1976, vol A : 419-435.
15. Wolosewick JJ, de Mey J, Meininger V. Ultrastructural localization of tubulin and actin in polyethylene glycol embedded rat seminiferous epithelium by immunogold staining. *Biol Cell* 1983; 49 : 219-226.

16. Wilson L, Jordan MA, Morse A, Margolis RL. Interaction of Vinblastine with steady-state microtubules *in vitro*. *J Mol Biol* 1982; 159 : 125-149.
17. Jordan MA, Margolis RL, Himes RH, Wilson L. Identification of a distinct class of vinblastine binding sites on microtubules. *J Mol Biol* 1986; 187 : 61-73.
18. Na GC, Timasheff SN. Interaction of Vinblastine with calf brain tubulin : multiple equilibria. *Biochemistry* 1986; 25 : 6214-6222.

4

Experimental antitumoral activity of Navelbine®

S. CROS, G. FRANÇOIS, R. GUILLON

Laboratoire de Pharmacologie et de Toxicologie Fondamentales du CNRS, 205, route de Narbonne, 31077 Toulouse Cedex, France

Navelbine® (NVB) (Vinorelbine®), or 5'-nor-anhydrovinblastine, is a new semi-synthetic antitumoral molecule of the vinca alkaloid family [1]. Its molecular target is tubuline, where it acts to inhibit the formation of microtubules [2, 3]. Its very low neurotoxicity, compared to its naturally occurring analogues, vincristine (VCR) and vinblastine (VBL), can be explained by its stronger affinity for mitotic microtubules than for axonal microtubules [4].

In a preliminary study, we have shown evidence that NVB has antitumoral activity against a wide spectrum of experimental murine tumors [5, 6, 7]. NVB was particularly active in L1210 leukemia, P388 leukemia, and B16 melanoma both intraperitoneally (ip) and subcutaneously (sc), even though the latter is generally refractory to chemotherapy [8].

Its activity has also been established in different human lung and stomach cancer nude mouse xenografts by Morimoto [6]. In these preclinical studies NVB demonstrated an equal or greater efficacy than other vinca alkaloids.

The object of the work we are presenting here is to expand the knowledge concerning the optimal conditions of the utilization of NVB. We describe the results obtained in P388 leukemia in mice after treatment by NVB, both intravenously (iv) and orally (po). Finally, from the standpoint of clinical phase III polychemotherapeutic studies, we looked for combinations with other agents likely to potentiate antitumoral effects in P388 and L1210 leukemias.

Material and methods

Drugs

Navelbine® is distributed by Pierre Fabre Médicament. It was used in monotherapy or in combination with mitomycin C (MTC-Choay), cisplatin (CDDP-synthesized by ourselves) and etoposide (VP16-Sandoz).

Murine tumors

P388 and L1210 leukemias were provided by the laboratory of G. Atassi (Institut Jules Bordet, Brussels) and the protocols of the National Cancer Institute were used in the evaluation tests of the drugs [9].

Tumors are maintained by weekly passages in the original DBA/2 line, and the experiments are done on female hybrid CDF1 mice (Balb/C females X DBA/2 males) of $20 \pm 2g$.

Tumor cells are implanted ip or iv on day 0 : 10^6 cells (P388 ip), 10^5 cells (either P388 iv or L1210 ip). Mice are randomized and separated in groups of 10 for each treatment series, the number of controls being equivalent to $2\sqrt{N}$ where N is the total number of animals treated.

The NVB is administered ip or iv 1 day after the inoculation of leukemic cells. For drug combination studies, the mice receive 1, 2 or 3 injections of the study agents ip, NVB always being given first. When the molecule is administered orally (po), different schedules are employed.

The agents are dissolved in water (NVB, MTC) or physiologic saline (CDDP, VP16). Solution concentration is adjusted for an injection of 0.1 ml/10 g of mouse weight.

The ratio T/C (median survival in days for the treated group compared with the control group) and the number of survivors on day 60 are the basis for the evaluation of treatment efficacy. Depending on the criteria defined by the NCI, the T/C % should be ≥ 125 in order for the antitumoral activity to be considered significant.

For drug combinations, we have used the increase in average lifespan over controls (ILS = T/C-100). Significant antitumoral activity is detected when the ILS is equal or greater than 25 %.

Results and discussion

Activity of Navelbine® in P388 leukemia

The stability of the P388 model is well established [10]. We have focused our study on the influence of different factors, such as the implant site of tumor cells, the mode of administration, on the antitumoral activity of the molecule.

Antitumoral activity of Navelbine®

Navelbine® was administered iv in a comparative study with VBL and VCR. Regardless of the mode of graft of tumor cells (ip or iv), the results are similar (*Figure 1*). By iv NVB is remarkably active. VCR and VBL never reached the same level of activity (T/C) as NVB, which moreover cured up to 50% of the mice.

The fact that NVB is not only active, but also curative in the ip-iv model proves that the molecule is effectively absorbed from the peritoneal cavity, which usually predicts with high probability the existence of clinical activity.

This "biodisposibility" of Navelbine® is discovered when it is given orally. Its activity is demonstrated in P388 leukemia by ip or iv grafts (*Table I*). It remains active in different treatment schedules D2, D2, 5, 8, D1, 7, 13 (P388 ip) or D1 (P388 iv). These results are in favor of the absorption of NVB from the digestive tract of mice.

Activity of Navelbine® in association with other cytostatics

The validity of murine leukemias has already been established. In addition to more effective schedules of administration of an antitumoral molecule, therapeutic combinations allow predictions for phase III studies of polychemotherapy.

We have researched the activity of Navelbine® in binary combinations with 10 cytostatics in P388 leukemia.

The combination of NVB-CDDP and NVB-VP16, at identical doses to those of each agent given in monotherapy, appears to be particularly promising [5]. However,

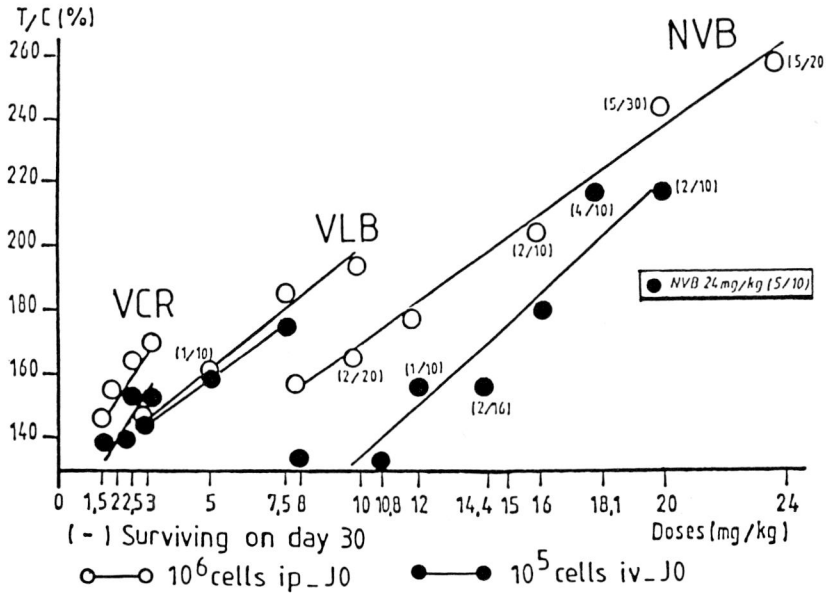

Figure 1. Effect of Navelbine®, vincristine and vinblastine (iv route on day 1) against P388 leukemia.

Table I. Antitumoral activity of Navelbine® by po route against P388 Leukemia.

Implantation site (nber of cells)	Treatment (day)	Total dose (mg/kg)	Body weight change in g (J1-J5)	T/C (%)
ip 10^6	1	36.1	−4.9	187
		28.9	−3.9	175
		21.7	−1.6	164
		14.4	−0.2	142
		7.22	+0.8	115
iv 10^5	1, 7, 13	65.1	−2.2	168
		54.3	−0.7	179
		43.2	−0.3	153
		32.4	0	140
		21.6	−0.4	111

before being able to claim a synergistic effect, it is necessary to compare the results for the agents given in monotherapy with those given in combination, at an optimal dose, *i.e.*, that with the highest activity. We have therefore started this study with the use of the binary combination of NVB-MTC in P388 leukemia. From the results obtained at a variety of dose levels, we were able to gauge the optimal dose for each experimental series (*Figure 2*). We note that by the 30th day all of the mice had died,

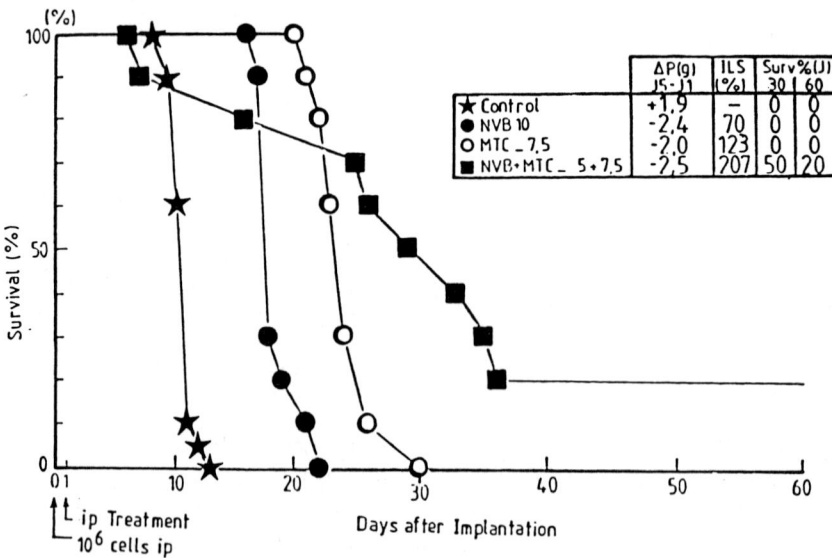

Figure 2. Combination of Navelbine® with mitomycine C against P388 leukemia. Comparison of results is based on optimal doses in each experimental series.

Table II. Combination of Navelbine® with cisplatin and etoposide against P388 leukemia.

Drug (mg/kg)			0	CDDP			VP16		CDDP+VP16		
				3	6	10	18	60	3+18	6+60	10+60
N A V E L B I N E®	0	Tox. J5 (%) ΔP(g) J1–5 ILS (surv) %	– – –	0 –0.2 65(0)	0 –1.9 74(0)	0 –4.6 123(10)	10 0 139(20)	10 –6.0 139(30)	0 –1.4 >161(60)	40 Toxic	60
	5	Tox. J5 (%) ΔP(g) J1–5 ILS (surv) %	0 –0.5 74(10)	0 –1.7 143(40)	– – –	0 –6.7 >161(60)	0 –2.2 135(20)	50 Toxic	0 –1.8 >161(100)	–	–
	10	Tox. J5 (%) ΔP(g) J1–5 ILS (surv) %	0 –3.5 100(10)	20 –3.3 178(40)	– – –	– – –	20 –4.6 >161(50)	– – –	20 –5.1 >161(70)	–	–
	15	Tox. J5 (%) ΔP(g) J1–5 ILS (surv) %	10 –5.6 87(0)	10 –5.5 139(40)	– – –	– – –	30 –5.5 217(40)	– – –	– – –	–	–

10^6 tumor cells are injected ip on day 0.
Treatment is administered ip on day 1, Navelbine® being given first.
Evaluation : 60 days.

except those treated by combination therapy where, without increasing toxicity (variations in mouse weight D1-D5), 50 % of the mice survived. At 60 days there were still 20 % survivors. These results, with an increase in life span value superior to the sum of the individual effects of each agent, permits the conclusion that NVB antitumoral activity is potentiated by combination with MTC.

The same experimental protocol applied in L1210 leukemia, less sensitive to NVB and to vinca alkaloids in general than P388 leukemia, demonstrated identical results : 20 % of survivors at 60 days without changes in toxicity.

With different combinations the percentage of cures can be increased. This is the case with the tri-combination NVB-CDDP-VP16 applied in P388 leukemia (*Table II*). At the optimal dose (*Figure 3*) the first mouse died on day 31 and on day 60, 80 % of the mice were still alive. There was also no sign of toxicity : no premature deaths, and a weight loss of 1.8 g between D1 and D5, usually higher in other experimental series.

This study was extended to L1210 leukemia (*Table III*). From a comparison of the optimal doses (*Figure 4*) it becomes evident that while NVB in monotherapy only prolongs survival by 39 %, the binary combination NVB-CDDP increased 60 day survival to 70 % and the triple combination NVB-CDDP-VP16 cured all the mice.

Thus, there is a potentiation of the effects using the NVB-CDDP-VP16 combination without an increase in toxicity, which can be explained by the fact that these three molecules do not act on the same molecular targets.

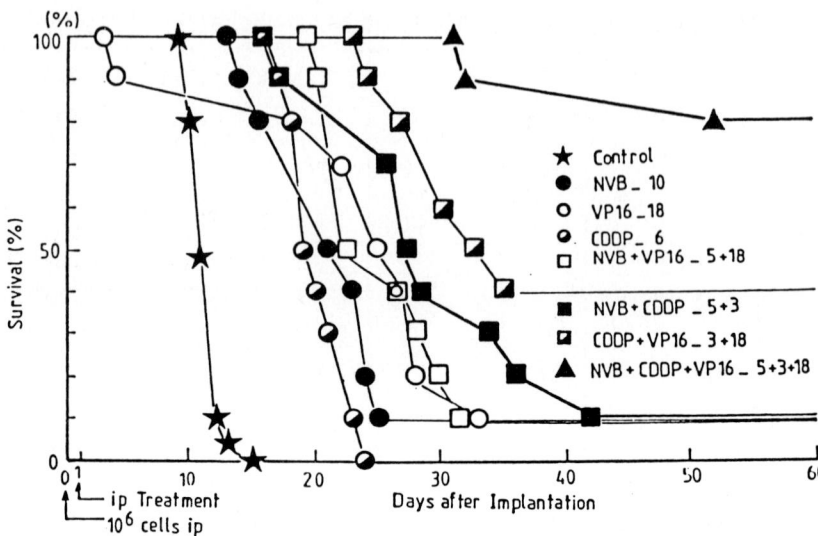

Figure 3. Combination of Navelbine® with cisplatin and etoposide against P388 leukemia. Comparison of results is based on optimal doses in each experimental series.

Tableau III. Combination of Navelbine® with cisplatine and etoposide against L1210 leukemia.

Drug (mg/kg)			0	CDDP		VP16		CDDP+VP16	
				3	10	18	60	3+18	10+60
N A V E L B I N E®	0	Tox. J5 (%) ΔP(g) J1−5 ILS (surv) %	— — —	0 +0.9 77(10)	0 −3.7 133(20)	0 −1.1 101(0)	0 2.5 243(40)	0 −0.8 184(30)	0 −6.4 >609(50)
	5	Tox. J5 (%) ΔP(g) J1−5 ILS (surv) %	0 −0.4 26(0)	0 −1.9 102(10)	0 −4.8 609(7)	0 −1.2 80(10)	10 −4.0 130(10)	0 −2.2 >609(70)	—
	10	Tox. J5 (%) ΔP(g) J1−5 ILS (surv) %	0 −3.1 39(0)	0 −4.3 109(10)	—	10 −4.2 71(0)	—	0 −4.2 >609(100)	—
	15	Tox. J5 (%) ΔP(g) J1−5 ILS (surv) %	10 −4.6 43(0)	0 −4.8 77(0)	—	20 −5.5 65(0)	—	—	—

10^5 tumor cells are injected ip on day 0.
Treatment is administered ip on day 1, Navelbine® being given first.
Evaluation : 60 days.

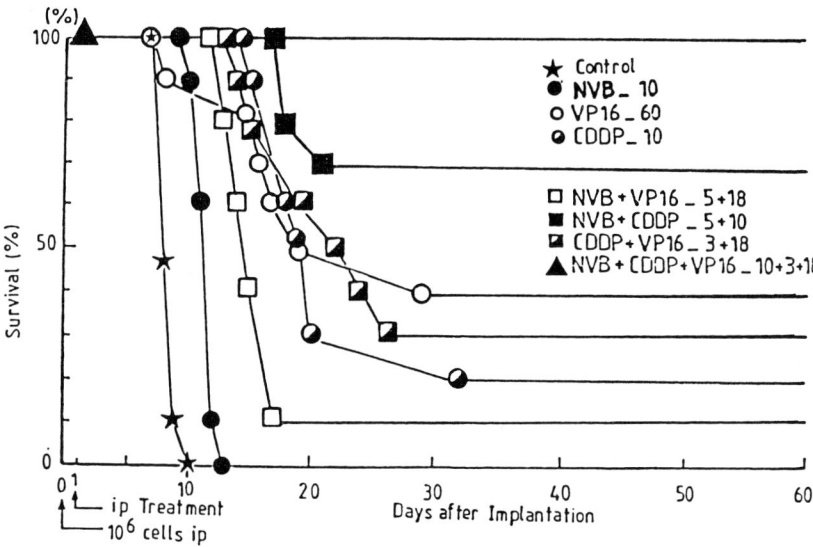

Figure 4. Combination of Navelbine® with cisplatin and etoposide against L 1210 leukemia. Comparison of results is based on optimal doses in each experimental series.

Conclusion

The first results of antitumoral pharmacology were able to demonstrate that NVB had an equal or greater activity than the other vinca alkaloids [5]. Further studies of this type highlighted the remarkable activity of Navelbine® given intravenously, regardless of the implantation site of tumor cells. The level of activity, high T/C and the significant number of surviving mice for a wide range of doses, confirms the evident superiority of NVB over VBL, VCR and the majority of other antitumoral molecules in current use.

The best mode of administration for Navelbine® at the present time is intravenous, which is used in human therapy.

The activity of Navelbine® by oral administration, at doses similar to those of other routes of administration (ip or iv), indicates good absorption of Navelbine® in mice. Pharmacokinetic studies have confirmed these results. They have also established that the biodisposibility of Navelbine® was higher in humans than in rodents, justifying the clinical development of this mode of administration for the molecule (A. Krikorian, personal communication).

The antitumoral effects of Navelbine® can be potentiated by different agents used in anticancer chemotherapy. The triple combination NVB-CDDP-VP16 cured up to 80% (P388) and 100% (L1210) of mice. These results, in accordance with the preliminary clinical studies of Navelbine® in polychemotherapy, underline the anticipated interest of these experimental models for studies of cytostatic combinations in man.

In conclusion, Navelbine® appears to be a new antitumoral molecule whose preclinical results suggest that it will be an effective treatment weapon against cancer.

Références

1. Langlois N, Gueritte F, Langlois Y, Potier P. Applications of a modification of the Polonovski reaction to the synthesis of vinblastine-type alkaloids. *J Amer Chem Soc* 1976; 98 : 7017-7024.
2. Potier P, Guénard D, Zavala F. Résultats récents dans le domaine des alcaloïdes antitumoraux du groupe de la vinblastine. Etudes biochimiques. *C R Soc Biol* 1979; 173 : 414-424.
3. Cros S, Takoudju M, Schaepelynck-Lataste H, *et al*. Comparative *in vitro* and *in vivo* study of Navelbine® ditartrate (nor-5'-anhydrovinblastine) with the two antitumor compounds vinblastine and vincristine. *In* : Ishigami J, ed. *Recent Advances in Chemotherapy, Anticancer Section 1*. Tokyo : University Press, 1985 : 477-478.
4. Binet S, Fellous A, Lataste H, *et al. In situ* analysis of the action of Navelbine® on various types of microtubules using immunofluorescence. *Semin Oncol* 1989; 16, n° 2, suppl 4 : 5-8.
5. Cros S, Wright M, Roussakis C *et al*. Etude expérimentale de l'activité antitumorale et anti-microtubulaire de la Navelbine® (5'-nor-anhydrovinblastine). *Deuxièmes journées de Pharmacocinétique Clinique Oncologique*, 1988, Lille, 20-21 octobre.
6. Cros S, Wright M, Morimoto M, *et al*. Experimental antitumor activity of Navelbine®. *Semin Oncol* 1989; 16, n° 2, suppl 4 : 15-20.
7. Cros S, François G, Garès M, Wright M. La Navelbine®, un nouvel agent antitumoral : activités précliniques. *Bull Cancer (Paris)* 1989; 76 : 549-550.
8. Venditti JM. Relevance of transplantable animal-tumor systems to the selection of new agents for clinical trial. *In* : Williams and Wilkins eds : *Pharmacological Basis of Cancer Chemotherapy*. Baltimore : *Collect Pap Annu Symp Fundam Cancer Res*, 1975 : 245-270.
9. Geran RI, Greenberg NH, MacDonald MM, *et al*. Protocols for screening chemical agents and natural products against animal tumors and other biological systems. Third edition. *Cancer Chemother Rep* 1972; part 3, 3 : 7-57.
10. Marsh JC, Shoemaker RH, Suffness M. Stability of the *in vivo* P388 leukemia model in evaluation of antitumor activity of natural products. *Cancer Treat Rep* 1985; 69 : 683-685.

5

Pharmacokinetics of Navelbine®

A. KRIKORIAN

Pierre Fabre Médicament CRPF, 17, avenue Jean-Moulin, 81106 Castres Cedex, France

Introduction

We first began investigating the pharmacokinetics of vinorelbine (Navelbine® or NVB) with great interest. Since this complex molecule is sensitive to both thermal and chemical breakdown, especially oxidation, and is highly lipophilic, we predicted that it would show highly complex behavior patterns in the body.

We also decided to investigate the pharmacokinetics of Navelbine® in an attempt to explain the considerable differences observed between species in terms of their sensitivity to the toxic effects of Navelbine® and the specific features of the molecule which distinguish it from other vinca alkaloids, previously confirmed in animal pharmacology and preliminary clinical studies.

Methods

We used 3 different approaches to study the pharmacokinetics distribution and metabolism of NVB :

1) Determination of total radioactivity by liquid scintigraphy or oxidation following an injection of tritium labelled NVB on the catharanthine moiety (*Figure 1*). The metabolic marker remained stable in this position, as verified by the detection of very small quantities of tritiated water in the body fluids.

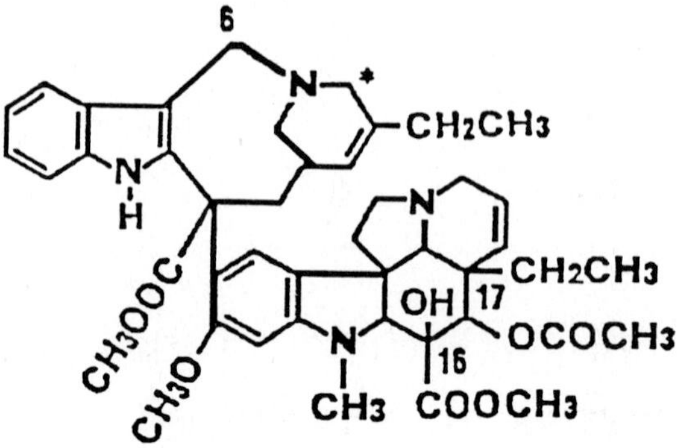

Figure 1. Labeling of the molecule. 3H-labeled NVB (synthesized by CEA laboratory). Specific activity 7.4 and 5.0 Ci/mmol.

2) The radioimmunoassay technique developed by Rahmani et al. [1] is both very sensitive (lower limit of detection : 10 fmols/ml) and exhibits minimal cross-reactivity with other analogs.

3) Specific determination of the unchanged product was recently made possible by the development of new high performance liquid chromatography techniques (Jehl et al. [2], Nicot et al. [3]). These methods are currently being assessed and the results will soon be available.

Pharmacokinetics of Navelbine®

Human pharmacokinetics

Radioactivity study

Following an iv injection of ^{3}H-NVB (30 mg/m^2) to 2 patients [4], plasma concentrations determined using radioactivity and radioimmunoassay techniques showed a dramatic fall (> 90 %) from their initial level during the first hour (*Figure 2*). The pharmacokinetic profile is best described by a tricompartmental model including a prolonged elimination phase. Excellent correlation was seen between total radioactivity and RIA levels, suggesting that most of the drug circulates in its unchanged form during the first 4 hours. After 4 hours, the plasma kinetics showed markedly different profiles with the 2 methods used : while the levels obtained by RIA continued to fall, radioactivity levels remained high for a considerable time, indicating the extensive formation of circulating metabolites not recognized by the epitope of the antibody used in the radioimmunoassay method. While 80 % of Navelbine® was initially bound to plasma proteins, this figure had fallen to 50 % after 96 hours.

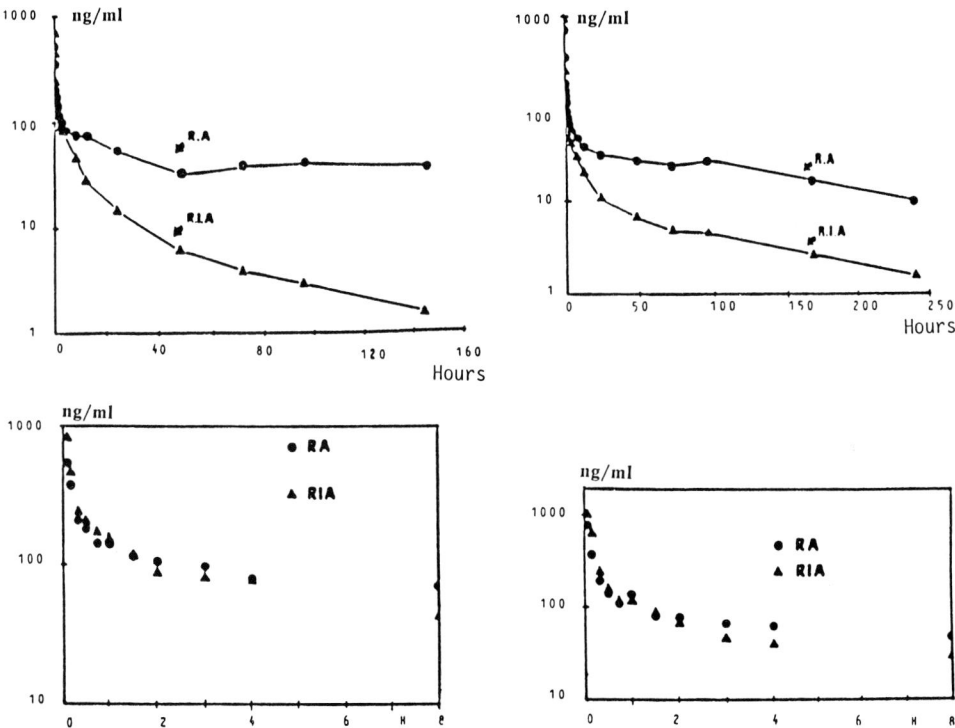

Figure 2. Plasma kinetics of ^{3}H-NVB in cancer patients. Reprinted with permission.

Radioimmunoassay determination [5]

Eleven patients received Navelbine® at doses of 15 mg/m^2, 30 mg/m^2 and 30 mg/m^2 (bolus) in this study designed to determine the pharmacokinetic parameters of this drug (*Table I*). Navelbine® demonstrated a high plasma clearance (0.71 l/h/kg), a large distribution volume and a prolonged half-life during the apparent elimination phase. Like other vinca alkaloids, Navelbine® showed a high degree of inter- and intra-subject variability in its pharmacokinetic profile.

Comparison with other vinca alkaloids

The clinical experience already acquired with antimitotic vinca alkaloids shows that, notwithstanding their marked chemical similarity, VCR, VDS and VLB exhibit considerable differences with respect to maximum tolerated dose and nature of dose-limiting toxicity (neutropenia with VDS and VLB *vs* neurotoxicity with VCR). Pharmacokinetic comparison of these 3 drugs using RIA methodology [6] demonstrated a strong correlation between plasma clearance and toxicity, on which the

Table I. Comparison of pharmacokinetics of VCR, VDS, VBL and NVB in cancer patients.

	VCR*	VDS*	VBL*	NVB†
Weekly dose (mg/m²)	1.4	3.5	8	30
Plasmatic clearance (1/h/kg)	0.106	0.252-0.53	0.740	0.72-0.92
Elimination $t_{1/2}$ (h)	85	23.2	24.8	39.5

* Data from Nelson et al. [6].
† Data from Rahmani et al. [10].

therapeutic dose is based. The author postulates that the increased neurotoxicity of VCR can be explained in terms of the longer half-life of this drug.

It would appear that the correlations established in the series presented in *Table II* are no longer applicable to Navelbine®. The maximum tolerated dose of Navelbine® is 4 times that of vinblastine for equal plasma clearance and its terminal half-life falls between those of VDS and VCR. The consequent implication that Navelbine® may prove more neurotoxic than VDS seems to contradict clinical experience.

These multiple comparisons show that structural modification of the catharanthine moiety of Navelbine® significantly affects its properties and therefore invalidates the excellent correlations established between the pharmacokinetics and clinical effects of VCR, VDS and VLB.

Interspecies comparison

The significant interspecies variability observed in sensitivity to the toxic effects of NVB is undoubtedly related to different pharmacokinetic profiles (*Table II*). The rat, for instance, which can tolerate a dose of 10 mg/kg iv eliminates NVB much faster

Table II. Interspecies differences in pharmacokinetics of NVB.

Species	Dosage by RIA					
	Dose (mg/kg)	C_{max} (ng/mL)	T_{max} (min)	AUC (ng/mL/h)	Clearance (L/h/kg)	$t_{1/2}$ of Main Phase
Rat*	1.5	128	5 min (0-24 h)	447	2.2	10 h
Monkey †	0.35	6500	3 min (0-120 h)	1971	0.53	35 h
Human ǂ	0.85	1168	5 min	2250	0.41	79 h
	0.4-0.8	1100	5 min	ND	0.7	40 h (extremes 22-68 h)

Values for the C_{max} were observed at the first analysis, i.e., 3 min or 5 min.
* Data from Rahmani et al. [1].
† Data from Bromet et al. [8].
ǂ Data from Bore et al. [4].

than the monkey, for which a dose of 4 mg/kg will prove lethal. Comparison of various pharmacokinetic parameters reported to the same dose of 1 mg/kg shows that clearance is 4 times greater in the rat than the corresponding value obtained in the monkey, while half-life is only 1/3 that seen in the monkey.

It has also been shown that the doses tolerated in the monkey and in man are very similar (approximately 0.5-1 mg/kg). This finding is consistent with very similar results obtained in pharmacokinetic studies. The rhesus monkey is consequently an excellent model in which to conduct toxicology studies of Navelbine®, as previously shown with other vinca alkaloids [7].

Tissue distribution

Autoradiographic study in the mouse [8]

A very impressive autoradiographic technique using scintigraphy and image analysis has been used to obtain a quantitative evaluation of the tissue distribution of NVB. As implied by the large distribution volume, NVB is intensely taken up by the tissues (*Figure 3*), with highest concentrations in the liver, followed by the lungs, spleen,

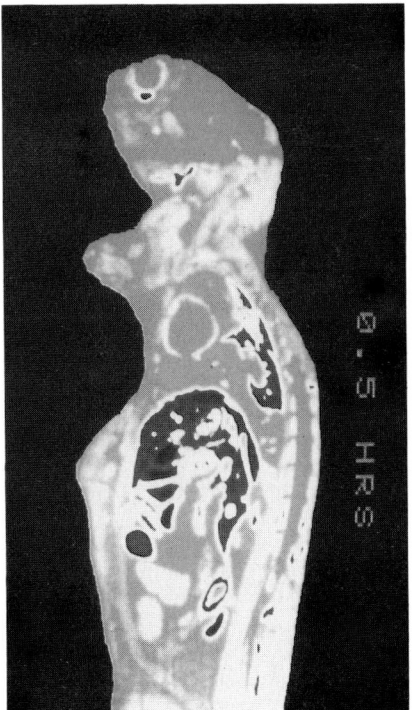

Figure 3. Autoradiographic study in the mouse : tissue uptake of the molecule.

lymphatic organs and femur. The radioactivity easily penetrates tumor tissue (P388 S/C). Brain tissue shows very little penetration. A 6-day follow up study revealed persistently high concentrations in the lung.

Quantitative and comparative study in the rat (Figure 4)

As predicted on the basis of the highly lipophilic nature of NVB, a comparative study conducted by Cano et al. showed tissue concentrations of NVB to be markedly higher than those of VDS and VCR. The largest differences were found in the lung (3.4 and 14.8 times higher than with VDS and VCR respectively), while only minor differences were seen in adipose and GI tissues. These results stimulated the initial research into NVB activity in lung cancer.

Quantitative study in the monkey [9] *(Table III)*

Following an injection of ^{3}H-NVB at a dose of 1.5 mg/kg iv, the animals were sacrified after 24 hours, 3 days and 5 days. The conclusions drawn on the basis of quantitative analysis of the radioactivity present in the major organs and tissues showed good agreement with those obtained in the rat and mouse studies described above :
— high tissue radioactivity concentrations, with a high tissue : blood ratio of 20: 80, even after 5 days;
— significant and prolonged pulmonary fixation;
— absence of specific cardiac retention; radioactivity uptake by the heart comparable to that of striated muscle;
— low concentrations in adipose, brain and bone marrow tissue;
— conversely, biliary concentrations were extremely high, reflecting the high proportion of elimination *via* this route.

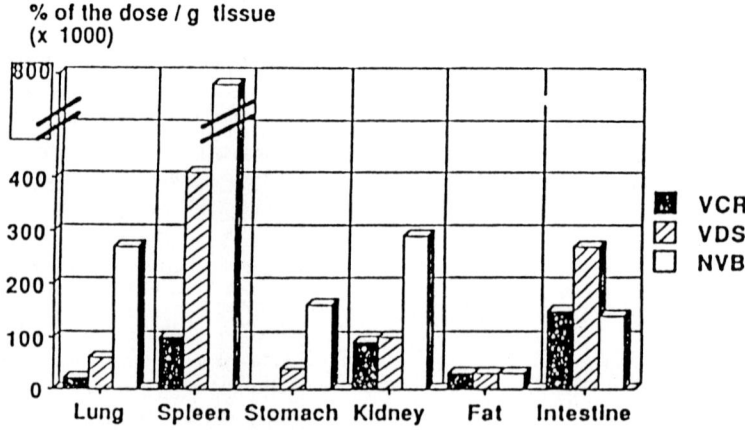

Figure 4. Tissue distribution of VCR, VDS and NVB in rats (24 hours). Reprinted with permission.

Tableau III. Tissue distribution ^{3}H-NVB in *Macaca mulata*.

	As % Dose g/tissue × 1000		
	24 h	72 h	120 h
Spleen	142	36	39
Liver	77	16	25
Kidney	65	10	22
Lung	52	66	16
Thymus	40	19	46
Heart	35	7	9
Muscle	21	9	6
Fat	18	1	1
Brain/cerebellum	7	4	5
Bone marrow	3	ND	2
Bile	1989	3400	446
Total blood	7	4	0.5

NVB IV, 1.5 mg/kg, one animal at each time. Reprinted with permission.

Metabolism

When human hepatocytes [10] were incubated *in vitro* with ^{3}H-NVB at therapeutic concentrations, rapid and intense intracellular uptake of radioactivity was observed. 55 % of the radioactivity was taken up within 1 minute and the concentration gradient between the intra- and extracellular compartments ranged from 134 to 370 (*Figure 5*).

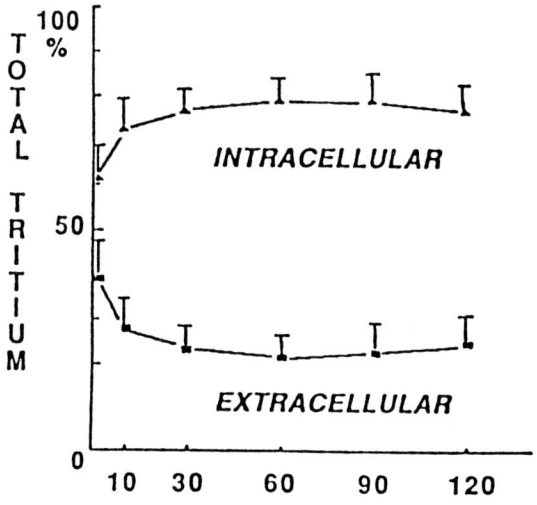

Figure 5. Human isolated hepatocytes (^{3}H-NVB, 5.10^{-7} mol/l). Reprinted with permission.

Considerable metabolization was observed in the extracellular compartment, with unchanged NVB accounting for a mere 18 % of total activity and the remaining 78 % in the form of 2 or 3 metabolites, as yet unidentified. In the intracellular compartment, however, 90 % of the total activity was represented by unchanged NVB, suggesting that only the active molecule was present (*Figure 6*).

This model also indicates avid binding of the molecule and cells; when the 30-minute incubation was followed by a 75-minute washing period, the majority (93.5 %) of radioactivity was still present in the hepatocytes.

HPLC analysis of the extracellular compartment and comparison with standard retention times suggests that the NVB may be metabolized to give the N-oxide and desacetyl-Navelbine®. Traces of desacetyl-Navelbine® were recently detected in human urines.

Excretion

The elimination profile of Navelbine® in different animal species is generally comparable to that in man, showing low urinary excretion (< 20 %) and extremely high fecal elimination related to the massive biliary elimination seen in the distribution studies (*Figure 7*). Urinary excretion, though only a minor elimination route, is rapid and is almost complete in 3-5 days. Fecal excretion, on the other hand, is extremely slow (3-4 weeks in monkey and man).

The interspecies quantitative differences in excretion profiles show good correlation with the pharmacokinetic data : elimination is relatively fast in the rat and mouse

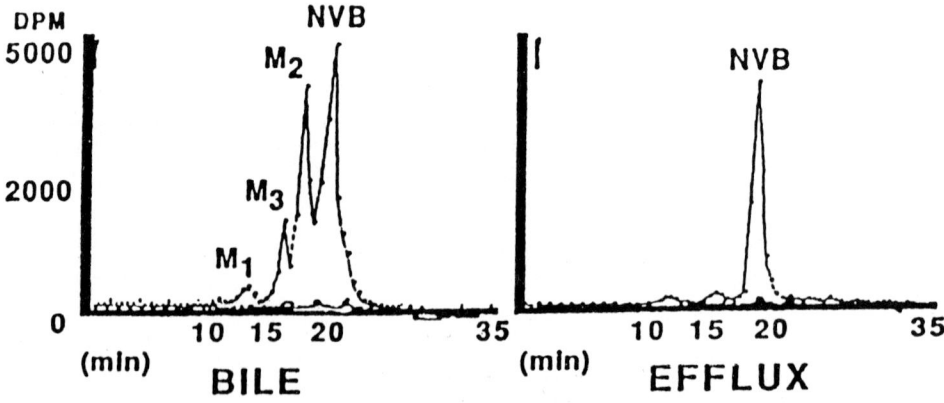

Figure 6. HPLC analysis of bile and efflux in isolated rat liver perfused with ^{3}H-NVB, (1, 10 and 25 µmol/l). Reprinted with permission.

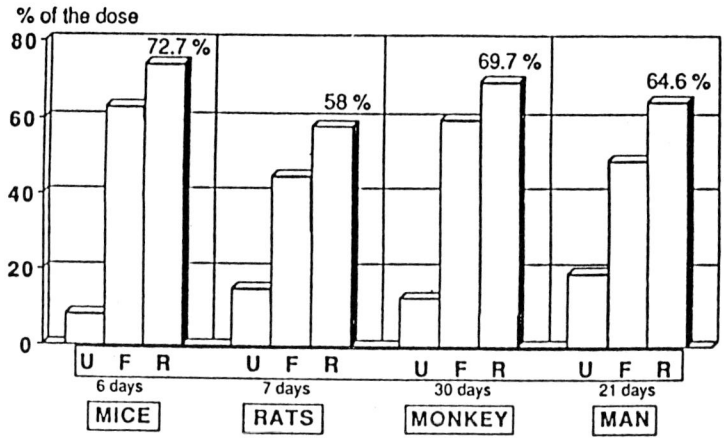

Figure 7. Elimination of ^{3}H-NVB after single iv injection. U : urine; F : feces; R : recovery.

(associated with the lower toxicity of NVB in rodents) and there are considerable similarities between monkey and man.

Conclusions

The metabolism of Navelbine® has still not been fully elucidated, even though a number of approaches have been applied to this question. Nevertheless, the studies cited above have enabled us to establish and explain certain essential aspects of the fate of Navelbine® in the body, some of which are responsible for its therapeutic activity. Pharmacokinetic studies have also represented a major determining factor in the development of the oral formulation of NVB currently undergoing therapeutic evaluation.

References

1. Rahmani R, Martin M, Barbet J et al. Radioimmunoassay and preliminary pharmacokinetic studies in rats of 5'-Noranhydrovinblastine (Navelbine®). *Cancer Res* 1984; 44 : 5609-5613.
2. Jehl F, Debs J. Determination of navelbine and desacetylnavelbine in biological fluids by high-performance liquid chromatography. *Journal of Chromatography* 1990; 525 : 225-233.

3. Nicot G, Lachatre G, Marquet P, *et al.* High performance liquid chromatographic determination of Navelbine® in human plasma and urine. Accepté par *Journal of Chromatography*.
4. Rahmani R, Bore P, Van Cantfort J, *et al.* Pharmacokinetics of a new anticancer drug, Navelbine® in patients. *Cancer Chemother Pharmacol* (in press).
5. Rahmani R *et al.* Clinical pharmacokinetics of the antitumor drug Navelbine® (5'-Noranhydrovinblastine). *Cancer Research* 1987; 47 : 5796-5799.
6. Nelson RL, Dyke RW, Root MA. Comparative pharmacokinetics of vindesine, vincristine and vinblastine in patients with cancer. *Cancer Treat Rev* 1980; 7 : 17-24 (suppl).
7. Sethi VS, Surratt P, Spurr CL. Pharmacokinetics of vincristine, vinblastine and vindesine in rhesus monkeys. *Cancer Chemother Pharmacol* 1984; 12 : 31-35.
8. Bromet N, Krikorian A, Bernouillet C. *2nd International ISSX Meeting*, Kobe, Japan, May 16-20, 1988.
9. Bromet N, Krikorian A, Bernouillet C. Study of tissue distribution of 3H Navelbine® ditartrate after oral and intravenous administration in monkey. *Deuxièmes journées de Pharmacocinétique clinique oncologique*, Lille, juin 1988.
10. Rahmani R, Bore P, Favre R, *et al.* Preliminary studies on vindesine (VDS) and Navelbine® (NVB) metabolisms using both human isolated hepatocytes and microsomal fractions. *Proceedings 5th NCI/EORTC Symposium on new drugs in cancer therapy*, Amsterdam, October 22-24, 1986 (abstr 10, 12).

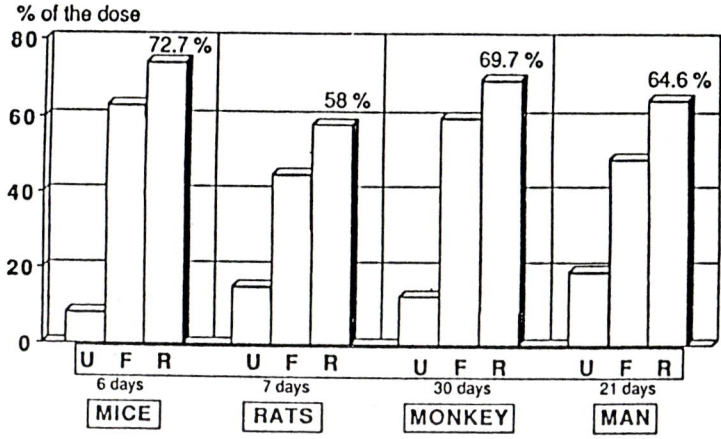

Figure 7. Elimination of ^{3}H-NVB after single iv injection. U : urine; F : feces; R : recovery.

(associated with the lower toxicity of NVB in rodents) and there are considerable similarities between monkey and man.

Conclusions

The metabolism of Navelbine® has still not been fully elucidated, even though a number of approaches have been applied to this question. Nevertheless, the studies cited above have enabled us to establish and explain certain essential aspects of the fate of Navelbine® in the body, some of which are responsible for its therapeutic activity. Pharmacokinetic studies have also represented a major determining factor in the development of the oral formulation of NVB currently undergoing therapeutic evaluation.

References

1. Rahmani R, Martin M, Barbet J et al. Radioimmunoassay and preliminary pharmacokinetic studies in rats of 5'-Noranhydrovinblastine (Navelbine®). *Cancer Res* 1984; 44 : 5609-5613.
2. Jehl F, Debs J. Determination of navelbine and desacetylnavelbine in biological fluids by high-performance liquid chromatography. *Journal of Chromatography* 1990; 525 : 225-233.

3. Nicot G, Lachatre G, Marquet P, et al. High performance liquid chromatographic determination of Navelbine® in human plasma and urine. Accepté par *Journal of Chromatography*.
4. Rahmani R, Bore P, Van Cantfort J, et al. Pharmacokinetics of a new anticancer drug, Navelbine® in patients. *Cancer Chemother Pharmacol* (in press).
5. Rahmani R et al. Clinical pharmacokinetics of the antitumor drug Navelbine® (5'-Noranhydrovinblastine). *Cancer Research* 1987; 47 : 5796-5799.
6. Nelson RL, Dyke RW, Root MA. Comparative pharmacokinetics of vindesine, vincristine and vinblastine in patients with cancer. *Cancer Treat Rev* 1980; 7 : 17-24 (suppl).
7. Sethi VS, Surratt P, Spurr CL. Pharmacokinetics of vincristine, vinblastine and vindesine in rhesus monkeys. *Cancer Chemother Pharmacol* 1984; 12 : 31-35.
8. Bromet N, Krikorian A, Bernouillet C. *2nd International ISSX Meeting*, Kobe, Japan, May 16-20, 1988.
9. Bromet N, Krikorian A, Bernouillet C. Study of tissue distribution of 3H Navelbine® ditartrate after oral and intravenous administration in monkey. *Deuxièmes journées de Pharmacocinétique clinique oncologique*, Lille, juin 1988.
10. Rahmani R, Bore P, Favre R, et al. Preliminary studies on vindesine (VDS) and Navelbine® (NVB) metabolisms using both human isolated hepatocytes and microsomal fractions. *Proceedings 5th NCI/EORTC Symposium on new drugs in cancer therapy*, Amsterdam, October 22-24, 1986 (abstr 10, 12).

PART II

Navelbine® and non small cell lung cancer

A. Non small cell lung cancer

6

Introduction

J. CHRÉTIEN

Clinique de pneumo-phtisiologie, Hôpital Laennec, 42, rue de Sèvres, 75007 Paris, France

In view of the severity of lung cancer (bronchogenic cancer developing in the lung) and the uncertainties about its evolutionary pattern and prognosis, as well as the problems of therapeutic indications under different circumstances, particular care has been given to establishing different clinico-pathological entities in this condition. It is customary to contrast small cell cancers characterized by aggressive behavior, dramatically rapid and spontaneous progress, and usually sensitive response to chemotherapy, with non small cell cancers. Progression of the latter is usually slower, and a third of them are amenable to surgical intervention with all the valid hopes this affords in the often disappointing treatment of lung cancers. This highly simplified classification, however, is far from satisfactory; it does not exactly conform to what is known about lung cancer histogenesis, it is imprecise, approximate and hardly suitable to ensure the precision called for by a concrete, refined and constructive approach aiming at a strict therapeutic evaluation and firm initial prognosis of lung cancer. It is desirable to carry out this evaluation right after the initial diagnosis, but this almost Manichean classification does not match reality, nor does it provide any formal guarantee about the medium-term prognosis of lung cancers. The experience of bronchogenic cancers and, particularly, the in-depth study of clinico-morphological correlations, does not lead us to accept such arbitrary and simplistic compartmentalization of bronchial cancers into two anatomo-clinical groups. This cancer, which occurs in direct relationship to the problem of respiratory clearance of various contaminants — with tobacco as the most evident carcinogen — often appears in its anatomo-clinical variations as a kind of continuous spectrum ranging from extensive and generally ill-differentiated forms to more differentiated, more slowly progressive forms, but there are no hard-and-fast rules available. The presence of intermediate histological forms in different areas of the same tumor, or at different stages of evolution, warrants the finer tuning of therapeutic decisions if these are to rest solely on histological data. In routine practice, characterization by small cell or non small cell histological type is based on data from light microscopy only. Its interpretation should always be complemented by supplementary details : on what sample has this schematic classification been based ? Was it based only on cytological data from aspiration ? On biopsy data from endoscopic samples ? On a surgical specimen, etc. At what evolutionary stage of the tumor can such a qualification be given ? At the first symptoms ? At the first examination ? After a likely time of evolution ? After therapeutic intervention ? What if it is a relapse ? etc. Histological interpretation and decisions about the therapeutic approach cannot be made without this information.

In any case, clinicians should not overlook the excessively schematic aspect of these morphological classifications. For example, it is too arbitrary to state dogmatically that surgery should be discarded on the sole basis of a histological label of small cell cancer. *A fortiori,* relying in such cases on chemotherapy or radiotherapy alone to afford a truly curative action and claiming it to be the only solution is a rigid standpoint which often betrays a lack of experience and knowledge of the usual clinical history of bronchopulmonary cancer.

The same can be said about the group of cancers known as "non small cell" cancers, a totally heterogeneous group which can only be identified by contrasting it with small cell cancer. In fact, it includes extraordinarily disparate entities. It is a kind of waste paper basket collecting scores of histological and evolutionary varieties. One thinks in particular of epidermoid cancers, the most frequent type, and the most related to smoking habits. They often present every grade of differentiation and all possible patterns of clinical evolution. Some spread just as rapidly as small cell cancer. This group also contains large cell cancers which are not considered unanimously to have a defined nosological significance; it also includes glandular cancers which caused much ink to flow in the past owing to the disseminated systematic aspect of their metastatic nature. They seem to be occurring with an increasing frequency. In many cases, they appear to be homogeneous, but also, often contain focal histological areas in the center of an otherwise well differentiated epidermoid cancer. If we consider the successive stages of differentiation in the histogenesis of the bronchial epithelium, these glandular forms are actually the ones considered to be the least differentiated and this may help in understanding the very poor prognoses of some of them. In fact, the prognostic implications are also controversial. Bronchiolo-alveolar cancers with a totally different histological origin can also be included in the group of non small cell cancers. However, they are only remotely related to other histological varieties. Clear cell cancers are yet another entity, and many other varieties — not to mention the mixed types or the carcinoid tumors for example — and all the various bronchogenic tumors with slow clinical evolution converge to make this term of non small cell cancers the expression of a rather indistinct, negatively defined framework which ought to be reconsidered for its practical worth.

In any case, for every single form defined by this terminology, the very first medical step is to assess the possibilities for surgical resection of the tumor. In principle, it is the only hope for cure in bronchopulmonary cancer. But when surgical management of lung cancer cannot be proposed for functional reasons, because of anatomical extension, or for reasons linked to the patient's general condition or age, the fight to be waged is a rearguard battle calling for a different arsenal. It is then best to battle without striking down the patient in trying to strike out the disease. The pulmonologist and cancer specialist should always be mindful of the patient's comfort. In non small cell cancer, talking of curing bronchopulmonary cancer through chemotherapy alone is an illusion, if not a deception. In regard to this rearguard strategy, oncologists and pulmonologists have of course always hoped to avail themselves of a truly active drug, but above all of an easily manageable, well tolerated drug which — on account of its tolerability — could also allow for complementary, in-depth, and sometimes more effective actions, such as radiotherapy and surgery. If chemotherapy can be proposed to enhance the results of prior modes of management and make them more beneficial without increasing discomfort, one can only praise the growing extent of possibilities in this field.

The introduction of vinorelbine should be viewed in the light of this search for sufficiently manageable, easily tolerable chemotherapy which would apply to common type cancers. Its palliative action has been demonstrated in non small cell lung cancers on the basis of results recorded by several research teams. Because of the absence of major side-effects and given the reversibility of the latter in all cases, this drug is more manageable than other derivatives. Prospects of oral administration are opening up its therapeutic indications, particularly as second line chemotherapy. The drug is therefore one of the major modes of treatment currently available.

All the different teams that have reported here on their results and experience acknowledge the importance of this new drug and the prospects it affords in routine pneumological practice. The data presented were rapidly obtained because of the unfortunate frequency of lung cancers — a recurring problem in the daily practice of oncology and pulmonology —, but would not have been possible without precise basic research and constant help in conducting the first trials leading up to the preparation of today's meeting, a welcome opportunity for a synthesis of the knowledge obtained so far.

As a conclusion, may I stress that it is high time that, besides the therapeutic management of lung cancer — one of the most topical and disturbing problems in carcinology — we endeavor to act effectively against its causes and that an ever greater effort be made in particular to fight the major cause of lung cancer. Such were my thoughts when I saw the persistance of smoking habits among certain attendees during the breaks, despite the fact that witnessing the hazards of tobacco should have been a daily deterrent. May they remember that they stand as an example to the public and that their statements on cancer treatment are empty words if they neglect to maximize efforts towards prevention.

7

Epidemiology and prognosis of non small cell lung cancer

B. DAUTZENBERG

Service de Pneumologie et de Réanimation Respiratoire, Groupe hospitalier Pitié-Salpêtrière, 75651 Paris Cedex 13, France

Summary

Lung cancer is diagnosed in fifteen million people throughout the world every year. Its incidence is approximately 70/100 000 males and 10/100 000 females. Although this figure is still rising in France, the incidence of lung cancer in males in the UK and USA has been falling over the past 5 years. This change in pattern follows a 10 year period during which the epidemiology of tobacco use has also been changing throughout the world. The mean age at which lung cancer is diagnosed is 61 years. Asbestos, other industrial and occupational factors, and passive smoking exert a negligible epidemiologic effect compared with active smoking. Individual prognosis depends more on the histologic type and the extension of the cancer than on a specific treatment. Resectable non small cell lung cancers (NSCLC) have a median survival time of 24 months with 5-year survival of 25 %. Nonresectable locoregional forms have a median survival time of 20 months with 5-year survival of 15 %. Patients with metastases have a median survival time of 5 months and 5-year survival of 1 %. In terms of public health provisions, a curative treatment for lung cancer has still to be found.

Lung cancer is the major cause of cancer deaths (20 000 p.a. in France and 1 500 000 worldwide). Its incidence has increased most rapidly in industrialized and developing countries while the incidence of other cancers has declined (*Figure 1*) [1].

Nevertheless, it is essentially a preventable cancer [2-3]. Success achieved in the fight against smoking in some countries, the USA and UK in particular, has resulted within a few years in a decrease in the incidence of lung cancer. For example, a

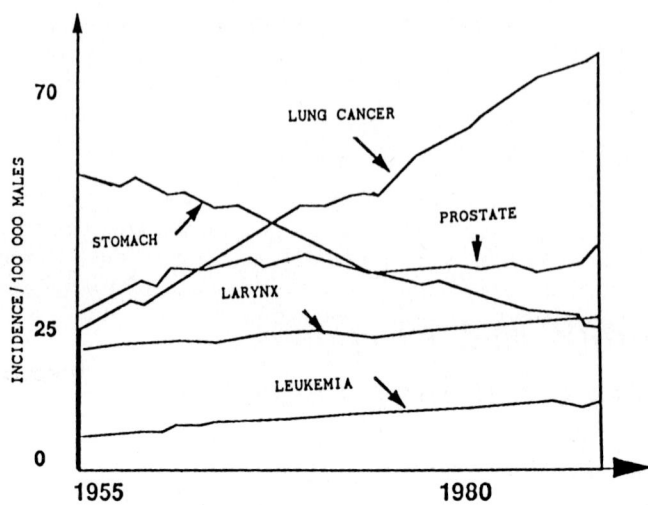

Figure 1. Changes in the incidence of lung cancer in males in the USA.

reduction in the incidence of lung cancer in British medical practitioners was noted after the incidence of smoking in this demographic category declined from 43 % to 12 % over a 20-year period, other risk factors remaining relatively constant. Nevertheless, the incidence of lung cancer in the USA and UK remains higher than in France. Within the European Community, France is only in fourth position with respect to tobacco consumption per head [4], with a significantly higher incidence of lung cancer in males (70/100 000) than in females (10/100 000).

The prognosis for lung cancer patients, despite considerable advances achieved in the medical sphere, remains bleak. In all large non-selected series, 5-year survival is approximately 8 % [5]. The future for lung cancer patients remains poor because no specific treatment has so far been developed.

NSCLC accounts for 80 % of lung cancers [6], the three major types being squamous cell carcinoma (55 %), adenocarcinoma (20 %) and large cell carcinoma (5 %). The prognosis for patients with large cell carcinoma is poorer than for those with andeno- or squamous cell carcinomas. The effects of screening programs on the prognosis for lung cancer have been studied in a large sample including more than 30 000 heavy smokers (more than 20 cigarettes/day) aged over 45. Few cases were detected and the prognosis was only modified following early detection in 1/5 cases. The cost of lung cancer screening is therefore excessively high in relation to the benefit achieved. Moreover, systematic mass screening should not be undertaken using current techniques [7].

Since lung cancer can be prevented in over 90 % of cases, risk factors should be taken into consideration to a greater extent than with any other cancer. The incidence of lung cancer in the absence of known risk factors is less than 7/100 000. Tobacco plays a fundamental role in squamous cell carcinomas. The quantity of tobacco smoked during the patient's lifetime (which can be expressed as packets/year, kilograms, quintals or the number of times a person has smoked the equivalent of his or her bodyweight in tobacco) is the main factor in calculating the risk (*Figure 2*). The risk of dying from lung cancer increases from 1 for a non-smoker to 29 for an individual smoking 40 cigarettes/day (*Table I*).

Tobacco plays a marked but less significant role in the development of adenocarcinomas. The search for a "safe" cigarette is illusory. Smokers often try to "cheat", obtaining their dose of nicotine through filters and low-tar cigarettes, the effects of which can only be analyzed accurately on experimental smoking models under certain conditions. Minimal variations in experimental conditions induce enormous changes in the composition of the smoke and increase the quantity of tar released from the combustion of a so-called "ultra-light" cigarette to the level obtained with a high tar product [8].

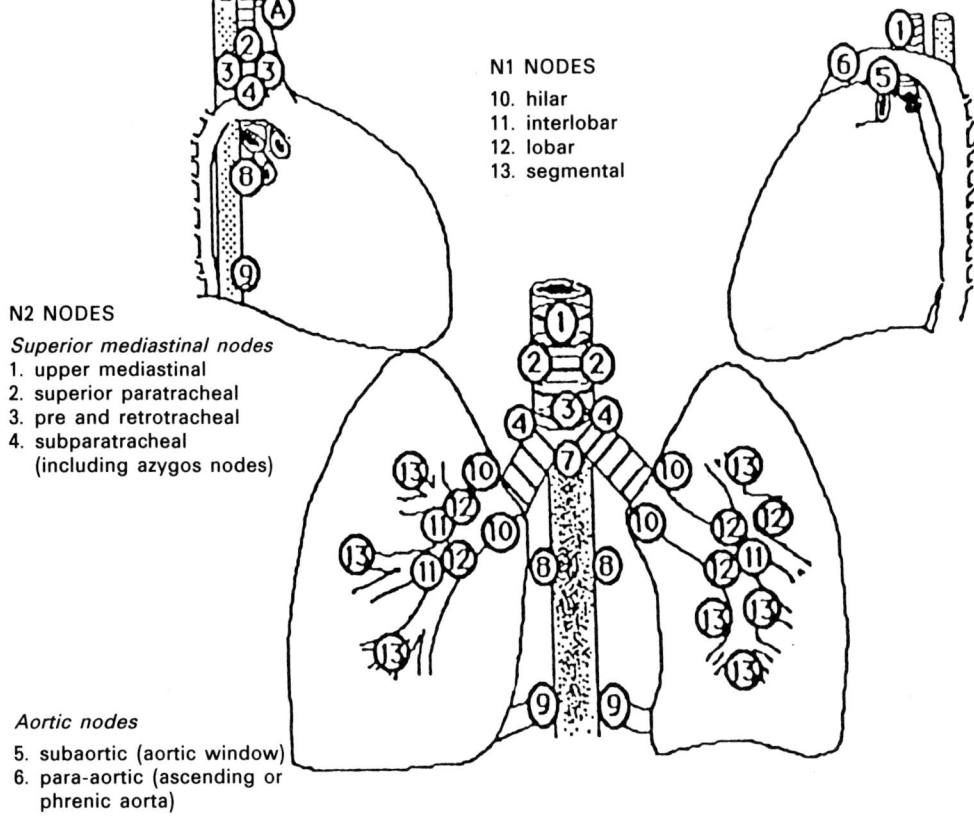

N1 NODES
10. hilar
11. interlobar
12. lobar
13. segmental

N2 NODES

Superior mediastinal nodes
1. upper mediastinal
2. superior paratracheal
3. pre and retrotracheal
4. subparatracheal
   (including azygos nodes)

Aortic nodes
5. subaortic (aortic window)
6. para-aortic (ascending or phrenic aorta)

Inferior mediastinal nodes
7. subcarinal
8. para-esophageal (below the carina)
9. triangular ligament

Figure 2. Classification of lymph node extension in lung cancer.

Table I. Multiplication of the risk of lung cancer (except for adenocarcinoma) according to tobacco use [2].

Low risk		High risk	
Situation	Risk factor	Situation	Risk factor
Nonsmoker	× 1	Smoker 40 cig/24 h	× 29
Started after age 25	× 14	Started before age 16	× 20
Smoker < 25 years	× 4	Smoker > 45 years	× 26
No inhalation	× 12	Deep inhalation	× 21
Quit within 2 years	× 4	Quit after 1-3 years	× 35

The most important of all other risk factors is asbestos. In June 1987, it was recognized in France as an agent likely to cause occupational lung cancers, quite apart from asbestosis, if the link with asbestos is "medically characterized". The role of asbestos is so crucial that it is systematically investigated by means of a detailed occupational questionnaire and analysis during bronchioalveolar lavage or through lung biopsies obtained during surgery. Another 6 other situations have been recognized in France as possible occupational causes of lung cancer (*Table II*).

Although no specific familial factors have been identified in the case of lung cancer, certain genetic features have been described. One such aspect concerns the metabolism of carcinogenic compounds. It is possible to classify individuals as slow or fast methylators on the basis of genotype. Methylation, like cytochrome P450 oxidation, is important in the detoxification of carcinogens. Studies are currently being undertaken in order to determine whether slow methylators and oxidizers show a higher risk of developing lung cancer where the use of tobacco remains constant.

Table II. Lung cancers of occupational origin identified in France (February 1988).

N°	Tumor	Compounds or processes
6	Lung carcinoma by inhalation	Ionized radiation
10[ter]	Lung carcinoma	Chromic acid, alkaline or alkaline-earth chromates, and bichromates, zinc chromate
22[bis]	Lung carcinoma	Inhalation of arsenic particles or vapor
30	Lung carcinoma (asbestos link medically characterized)	Inhalation of asbestos particles
37[ter]	Lung carcinoma	Ni_3S_2 matte roasting
43	Lung carcinoma	Inhalation of iron oxide particles or smoke (in the presence of siderosis and work in iron mining)
81	Lung carcinoma	Bis(chloromethyl)ether

Table III. TNM classification (1986).

T0		No primary tumor detected.
T1		Solitary tumor ≤ 3 cm maximum diameter, on a lobar or segmental branch.
T2		Tumor ≥ 3 cm more than 2 cm from the carina, involving the visceral pleura or inferior atelectasis in one lung.
T3		Tumor extending beyond the lung (chest wall, diaphragm, mediastinum, supraclavicular fossa, mediastinal pleura, pericardium) or tumor located less than 2 cm from, but not touching, the carina.
T4		Tumor affecting the mediastinum, heart, great vessels, trachea, esophagus, vertebrae or carina or associated with effusion (unless the effusion is confirmed as noncancerous).
N0		No histologic invasion of nodes.
N1		Tumoral invasion of peribronchial or homolateral hilar nodes, including direct extension.
N2		Ipsilateral mediastinal or subcarinal invasion of nodes.
N3		Mediastinal contralateral, scalene or subclavicular invasion of nodes.
M0		Absence of metastasis.
M1		Presence of metastases.

Genetic defects such as the deletion of the short arm of chromosome 13 and other anomalies have only been described inside the actual tumor. There is no evidence to suggest that lung cancer patients exhibit any anti-oncogen deficiency, as occurs in the case of certain other types of cancer such as retinoblastoma [9].

Prognostic factors for NSCLC have been investigated in several studies. General behavior, evaluated using the Karnofsky or WHO performance status scales, represented an excellent prognostic factor in all studies, as did simple laboratory tests, e.g. polymorphonuclear neutrophil or gamma GT levels. The main prognostic factor for NSCLC, however, is the extension of the disease at the time of diagnosis. The TNM classification was modified recently [5] and constitutes the fundamental prognostic criterion (*Table III*).

Nodal classification has been precisely defined, giving rise to the current consensus on nodal terminology and the need to remove adenopathies systematically during lung cancer surgery in order to obtain an accurate measure of the node extension [5] (*Figure 2*).

The survival of lung cancer patients and the treatment prescribed are primarily determined by the stage of the disease. Fortunately, there are no longer any groups of patients left untreated who would exhibit the natural course of the disease.

Overall 5-year survival for resected stage I, II and III lung cancer is approximately 25 % [5] (*Figure 3*). Although the prognosis is better following lobectomy than pneumonectomy, no comparative series have been published. Lobectomy is performed in the most restricted cases. Age has little influence on prognosis : the 5-year survival of patients operated over 80 years of age is 24 % [10].

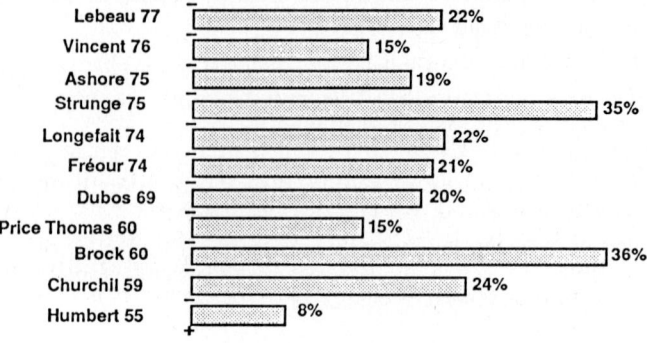

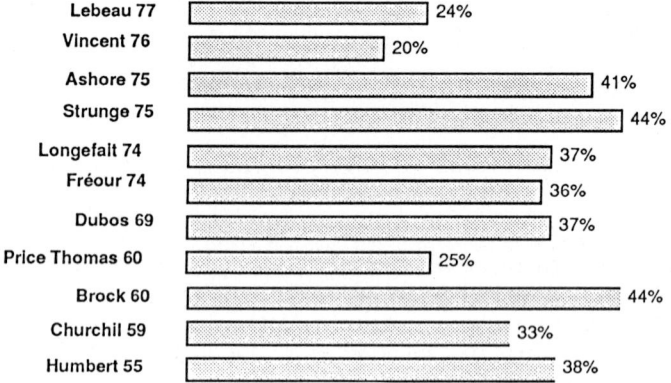

Figure 3. Prognosis for patients operated for non small cell lung cancer.

Adjuvant treatments have not demonstrated any epidemiologic benefits, although they may prove useful in certain situations. More than 90 % of comparative immunotherapy studies have produced negative results, 5 % have shown benefit from placebo and 5 % have produced results favoring immunotherapy. Standard immunotherapeutic modalities are consequently without effect. All but one [11] radiation therapy studies using 40 or 50 Gy cycles have produced negative results. While the prognosis for nonoperated but irradiated patients with localized stage IIIB and stage T4NO thoracic tumors is poorer than for operated patients, cases of survival have been documented after 5 years [5].

The prognosis for patients with metastatic carcinoma is very poor, with a 3.5 month survival time if untreated. Even with treatment, the median survival time does not exceed 6 months, notwithstanding the responses observed in 30 %-50 % of cases receiving chemotherapy and exceptional cases of recovery.

Conclusion

The treatment of lung cancer can be regarded as a preventive treatment based on abstention from tobacco use and help for smokers to give up the habit. According to current epidemiologic data, this is the only genuinely effective treatment that is able to exert a significant influence on the incidence and prognosis of NSCLC. Further therapeutic research is also required since, irrespective of the expected outcome of such preventive measures, patients suffering from lung cancer are likely to benefit from "curative" treatment.

References

1. Silverberg E, Lubera JA. Cancer Statistics. *Cancer J Clin* 1988; 38 : 5-22.
2. Minna JD, Pass H, Glatstein E, Ihde D. Etiology of lung cancer. *In* : De Vita, Hellman S, Rosenberg SA eds, *Cancer Principles & Practice of oncology,* 3rd, New York 1988 : 593-600.
3. Benhamou S, Benhamou E, Tirmarche M, *et al.* Lung cancer and use of cigarettes : A French case-control study. *J Nat Cancer Inst* 1985; 74 : 1169-1175.
4. Commissions des Communautés Européennes. *L'Europe contre le cancer.* CEE ed, Luxembourg 1989 : 2-19.
5. Mountain CF. A new international staging system for lung cancer. *Chest* 1986; 89 : 225S-232S.
6. Sanderson D, Fontana R. Results of the Mayo lung project : An interim report : Recent results. *Cancer Res* 1982, 82 : 179-186.
7. The National Cancer Institute Cooperative Early Lung Cancer Detection Program. Early lung cancer detection : Summary and conclusions. *Am Rev Respir Dis* 1984; 130 : 541-570.
8. Kozlowski LT, Rickert WS, *et al.* Estimating the yields to smokers of tar, nicotine and carbon monoxide from the lowest-yields "ventilated-filter cigarettes". *Br J Addict* 1982; 77 : 159-65.
9. Shirakusa T, Tsutsui M, Iriki N *et al.* Results of resection for bronchogenic carcinoma in patients over the age of 80. *Thorax* 1989; 44 : 189-91.
10. Lad T, Rubinstein L, Sadeghi A, for the Lung Cancer Study Group. The benefit of adjuvant treatment for resected locally advanced non-small-cell lung cancer. *J Clin Oncol* 1988; 6 : 9-17.

8

Advantages of chemotherapy in non small cell lung cancer

F. SOYEZ[1], J.-P. KLEISBAUER[2]

[1] Hôpital Salvador, 249, boulevard de Sainte-Marguerite, BP 51, 13274 Marseille Cedex 9, France
[2] Hôpital Sainte-Marguerite, 270, boulevard de Sainte-Marguerite, BP 29, 13274 Marseille Cedex 9, France

It has been demonstrated that non small cell lung cancer (NSCLC) is highly resistant to chemotherapy. It therefore seems to us important to establish the precise value of chemotherapy in the treatment of this disease and not to focus exclusively on the rates of survival observed in polymetastatic forms. We believe it would be useful to evaluate the extent to which chemotherapy can assist the surgeon (by reducing tumor size in operable patients, rendering formerly inoperable patients candidates for surgery and treating any residual carcinoma), society in general (in terms of health care costs) and, of course, the patient, by improving both quality of life and survival.

Adjuvant chemotherapy

Chemotherapy eradicates the tumor

Gralla [1] obtained 8 complete responses (CR), supported by histologic confirmation on the lung biopsy sample, in a total of 41 patients (19 %) initially staged as T1-3 N2 MO. Clavier [2] also obtained 15 % CR with cisplatin in operable patients and found that chemotherapy presented no obstacle to surgery. Similar results have been published recently by other groups : Burkes [3] and Pujol [4] (1989) report 8.6 % and 16 % CR respectively, with histopathologic confirmation on biopsy.

Many recent studies have confirmed that chemotherapy reduces tumor size in operable patients

This fact suggests that this type of chemotherapy will probably prove beneficial. For example, it would help patients previously inoperable owing to poor respiratory function to become candidates for surgery. It would decrease the surgical mortality rate and reduce the risk involved (mortality rates : 6.2 % pneumonectomy; 3 % lobectomy; 1.4 % segmentectomy) in addition to increasing the level of control over the primary tumor.

Finally, in more theoretical terms, it should be borne in mind that operated patients exhibit a marked tendency to develop a second primary lung cancer (5-10 %) [5, 6], subsequently requiring further surgery. The main reason for surgical failure is not locoregional recurrence but metastatic dissemination, usually occurring within 2 years of surgery, and therefore subclinically present at the time of resection : 80 % of recurrences are extrathoracic at stage III and 72 % and 71 % at stages I and II respectively (Mountain [7]). This kind of chemotherapy, which is in theory active against micro-metastases, is certainly very attractive.

Most of the studies published recently (*Table I*) imply that a 50 % partial response rate can be obtained by prescribing chemotherapy for patients with only limited neoplasia. It should be stressed that all authors used cisplatin-based chemotherapy. Nevertheless, these results (both partial and complete responses) should be weighed against the possibility of significant progression during chemotherapy (36 % progression > 50 % reported by Dautzenberg *et al.* [8] in a study of 13 patients receiving cisplatin/vindesine/cyclophosphamide), or even death resulting from chemotoxicity (14 % : Burkes [3], 5 % : Pujol [4], 7 % : Vokes, Bitran [9, 10]).

Table I. Chemotherapy reduces tumor mass in operable patients.

	Year	CR	PR
Bitran	1988		58 %
Clavier	1988	16 %	49 %
Gralla	1988	19 %	56 %
Dautzenberg	1988		45 %
Nishiwaki	1989		71 %
Burkes	1989	8,6 %	60 %
Elias	1989	3 %	40 %
Pujol	1989	16 %	50 %

CR : complete response; PR : partial response.

Inoperable patients may become candidates for surgery with chemotherapy

Many authors, inspired by the promising results achieved with neoadjuvant chemotherapy in ORL oncology (results which have nevertheless failed to show increased survival), have been searching for similar alternatives in the treatment of locally advanced non small cell lung cancer (NSCLC).

Takita (Cancer 1986) administered a cisplatin-based drug combination to 29 patients (5 T3N0, 2 T2N0, 14 T3N2, 7 T2N2), followed by surgery in 19 cases, and obtained 30.5-month median survival and 5-year survival of 17%. Eagan [11] reported in 1987 that 19 out of 39 (48%) initially inoperable patients (all stage III M0) were rendered operable after 51% significant responses were obtained following cisplatin-based chemotherapy. Median survival remained at 11 and 14 months for operated patients, with a 2-year survival of 10%. Vokes and Bitran, 1989 [10], examined 27 patients (stage T2-3N2-3) using systematic mediastinoscopy following 2 cycles of cisplatin-based chemotherapy. The overall response rate was 48% and 4 patients (15%) underwent surgery followed by a course of radiotherapy. Median survival remained at 8 months and 1 of the operated patients is still alive after more than 4 years.

Burkes [3] also reported that 21 of a total of 35 patients (60%) initially described as inoperable following systematic mediastinoscopy became operable. The resection was considered to be complete in 17 of the 35 cases (50%). Two post-surgical deaths occurred (9%), which approximates to the standard percentage observed. Finally, Pujol [4] enabled 55% of 18 initially inoperable patients (stage IIIa) to undergo surgery, achieving complete resection in 8 cases (44%).

It would therefore appear reasonable to state that the remission rate with neodjuvant chemotherapy is of the order of 50% for locally advanced NSCLC, with the possibility of subsequent surgery in 15% (Vokes, Bitran, 1989) to 48% (Eagan, 1987) of cases. The disparity between these figures can be explained by the differences in eligibility criteria, mediastinal evaluation and surgical indications (*Table II*).

Neoadjuvant chemotherapy does not appear to increase survival. However, in 1988, Goua and Clavier [12] published a study conducted in 21 patients initially classified as inoperable due to parietal, tracheal of mediastinal tumor extension. They received 2 or 3 cycles of cisplatin-based chemotherapy and were then operated according to the responses observed. Survival was 17 months, with 12 patients still alive after 2.5 years. Only 3 of the 9 deaths were related to local or regional tumor recurrence. Elias [13, 14] also obtained interesting results: 45% of stage IIIa and 16% of stage IIIb

Table II. Percentage of patients operated for NSCLC following first-line neoadjuvant chemotherapy.

	Year	Number of patients	% surgery	% complete resection *
Takita	1986	29	65	
Eagan	1987	39	48	
Gralla	1988	41	68	51
Bitran	1989	27	15	
Burkes	1989	35	60	50
Pujol	1989	18	55	44

* of the total number of patients included.

patients treated with neoadjuvant chemotherapy, with or without radiotherapy prior to surgery (in those not responding to chemotherapy), are still alive after 3 years.

Chemotherapy in the treatment of residual carcinoma

Lad [15] conducted a randomized study in 164 eligible patients with residual carcinoma following surgery. He found a 14 % difference in survival rates between the group treated with a combination of radiation and chemotherapy and the group receiving radiotherapy alone. This difference can be explained by the presence of a longer disease-free interval ($p = 0.04$) in the chemotherapy group. In 1985, Holmes [16] also reported benefits obtained with chemotherapy compared with immunotherapy in this type of patient. Only two histologic types were included : adenocarcinomas and large cell undifferentiated carcinomas.

These results must however be assessed in the light of the lack of any significant difference detected in other randomized studies conducted in 1988 by Dautzenberg, Feld and Imaizumi, comparing cisplatin-based chemotherapy with placebo (*Table III*).

Table III. Chemotherapy versus placebo in the treatment of residual carcinoma.

Authors	Year	Chemotherapy	Result
Thomas-Feld	1988	EDX-ADR-CDDP	Idem
Dautzenberg	1988	EDX-VDS-CDDP	Idem
Imaizumi	1988	MITO-EDX-TEGAFUS	Idem
Holmes	1986	EDX-ADR-CDDP	+
Lad	1988	EDX-ADR-CDDP	+

Chemotherapy in the treatment of diffuse cancers

Is chemotherapy beneficial in the treatment of advanced carcinomas ?

It has been established that tumor extension and changes in performance status represent the fundamental prognostic factors relating to response to treatment and survival. Consequently, mere differences in survival between responders and non-responders do not confirm the efficacy of a given chemotherapy and, when the response to chemotherapy involves improved prognosis, it is theoretically impossible to establish a direct connection. This can only be achieved by means of placebo-controlled comparative trials in patient groups with identical tumor extension and performance status. Seven such randomized studies are summarized in *Table IV*. All the studies show a longer survival time for chemotherapy patients, with a relatively low objective response rate, ranging from 22 % to 35 %.

Table IV. Result of randomized studies comparing chemotherapy with place.

Authors	Year	CT	Evaluable patients	OR (CT group)	Survival (months)		P
					Placebo	CT	
Woods [17]	1985	CDDP-VDS	103	30 %	5.25	6	NS
Celerrino [18]	1988	CTX-EPI-CDDP + MTX-VP16-CCNU	89	21 %	5	8.5	NS
Ganz [19]	1989	CDDP-VBL	48	22 %	3.4	5.1	NS
Cormier [20]	1982	MTX-ADR-EDX-CCNU	39	35 %	2.1	7.6	<0.0005
Rapp [21]	1988	CDDP-VDS (1) or ADR-EDX-CDDP (2)	233	25.3 % (1) 15.3 % (2)	4.2	8.15 (1) 6.15 (2)	0.01 0.05
Williams [22]	1987	CDDP-VDS	188	28 % Localized forms	4 6.5	5.75 10.75	NS <0.05
Quoix [23]	1988	CDDP-VDS	43	39 %	2.2	6.4	<0.01

OR = objective response.

The following studies failed to demonstrate any overall advantage :
— the Woods study [17] was never published. The findings constituted the preliminary results presented at the ASCO Congress;
— the Celerrino study [18] demonstrated a certain degree of efficacy since the chemotherapy group showed a mean progression of 4 months, compared with 2 months in the placebo group (p. < 0.01);
— the Ganz study [19] included only a small patient sample (48) and the group not receiving chemotherapy benefited from radiotherapy, which explains the 12 % objective response rate seen in this group.

The following studies demonstrated overall benefits :
— the Cormier study [20] has been criticized in several respects, including the small patient population (39) and the extremely short median survival time seen in non-treated subjects (2.1 months);
— the Rapp study [21] is without doubt one of the most complete, including 233 patients (only 14 % at stage IIIb). While the relatively complex methodology has been criticized for including three randomized groups, the study was able to demonstrate a direct relationship between objective response and survival, increasing in significance as the response improves;
— the Williams [22] study showed chemotherapy to be effective in localized forms only;
— although the Quoix study [23] is of interest because all patients were stage IV, it is inconclusive owing to the very short median survival in those not treated with chemotherapy and the small sample included.

Although the findings obtained to date have proved modest, we believe that chemotherapy exhibits a certain level of efficacy in the treatment of NSCLC. Attention is drawn to the following :
— the efficacy of chemotherapy is directly related to the extension of the disease;

Table V. Most frequently used and most effective chemotherapy regimens.

	Number of studies	Number of patients	Objective response
CISP-VP16	32	1 534	27 %
CISP-VDS	14	565	37 %
CISP-MITO-VDS	8	484	41 %
CISP-MITO-VELBE	5	301	37 %

— the younger the patient and the better his or her general health, the greater will be the response and tolerance to treatment;
— the presence of an objective response to chemotherapy represents a favorable prognostic factor.

On the basis of the above, we have formulated our current approach as follows: It would appear that, as a first-line treatment in locally advanced, non-resectable carcinoma (IIIb), chemotherapy is able to produce objective responses allowing the possibility of subsequent surgery. It can be used safely in combination with radiotherapy, an alternative indicated in the absence of surgery. It frequently improves tolerance to radiotherapy, allows the field of irradiation to be reduced and decreases the extent of local inflammation.

Chemotherapy should be used to treat disseminated (stage IV) forms in an attempt to prolong survival. The objective response rates recorded in the randomized studies mentioned above ranged from 21 % to 30 % (with the exception of the Cormier study (35 %) in which 50 % of patients were IIIb). New protocols based on the combination of CDDP/mitomycin with vindesine or vinblastine appear to demonstrate a slight therapeutic advantage with a response rate of 37 %-41 % (*Table V*). Similarly, Navelbine® has proved encouraging, with a 33 % response rate when administered alone [24]. These modest findings will probably lead to a marked improvement in the survival of these patients.

Chemotherapy and society

The connection that is frequently made between chemotherapy and reduced quality of life has prevented its systematic use. Quality of life is an elusive concept and is difficult to measure. Nevertheless, if we accept that it shows good correlation with the Karnofsky scale, then no clear benefit is seen with chemotherapy, as stated by Ganz [19]. It should be noted that the most effective current regimens (cisplatin, mitomycin and vindesine) are also the most neurotoxic and induce severe asthenia.

Conversely, when chemotherapy does prove effective, it can restore appetite and reduce dyspnea, bone pain and paraneoplastic syndromes. It also represents an important psychological tool for the physician, giving hope and motivation to patients and their families.

Table VI. Cost of chemotherapy.

Treatment	Median survival (per week)	Total cost ($ Canadian)	Cost per week of survival
CDDP-VDS	32.6	12 232	375
CDDP-ADR-EDX	24.7	7 645	309
P	17	8 595	505

In some cases, the overall cost of chemotherapy is also a decisive factor. Rapp [21] states that the cost per number of days survival is no higher than the costs incurred with palliative treatment, and may even be lower in some cases. Does this not provide an additional indicator of the efficacy of chemoterapy ? (*Table VI*). Financial considerations should not in any case present any obstacle to prescribing chemotherapy.

Conclusion

The various parameters that have been used to assess the efficacy of chemotherapy are now approaching statistical significance. We therefore believe that chemotherapy now represents a viable indication for the treatment of stage IIIb and IV patients, particularly in the light of the 40 % objective response rates obtained with the newer drug combinations. We are also in agreement, however, with the general view that treatment should be discontinued if no objective response is observed after 2 treatment cycles. Finally, we think it desirable, even obligatory, at present to include patients in therapeutic protocols, and particularly those including neoadjuvant chemotherapy.

References

1. Gralla RJ, Kris MG, Martini N. A trial of preoperative chemotherapy in NSCLC with Mitomycin + Vinca Alkaloid + Cisplatin chemotherapy in patients with clinically apparent ipsilateral mediastinal lymph node involvement. *Memorial Sloan-Kettering Cancer Center*, New York NY USA, abstract de la réunion de chimiothérapie néo-adjuvante, Paris, février 1988, N3.

2. Clavier J, Zabbe Cl, Nouvet G, et al. The results at 5 years of preoperative chemotherapy in squamous cell carcinoma of lung. *Abstract de la réunion de chimiothérapie néo-adjuvante,* Paris, février 1988, n8.
3. Burkes R, Ginsberg R, Shepheard F, et al. Neo adjuvant trial with MVP chemotherapy for stage III (T_{1-3}, N_2, M_0) unresectable non small cell lung cancer. Proceeding of American Society of Clinical Oncology. *Twenty fifth Annuel Meeting,* San Francisco, Californie 1989, N° 860.
4. Pujol JL, Rossi JF, Pujol H, et al. Etude pilote sur la chimiothérapie néoadjuvante des cancers bronchiques non à petites cellules au stade IIIa. *Abstract des Journées Annuelles de la Société de Pneumologie de Langue Française,* Paris, 1989, R170.
5. Gail MH, Fagan RT, Feld R, et al. Prognostic factors in patients with resected stage 1 non SCLC. A report from the Lung Cancer Study Group. *Cancer* 1984; 54 : 1802-13.
6. Jensik RJ, Faber LP, Kittle CF, et al. Survival following resection for second primary bronchogenic carcinoma. *J. Thorac Cardiovasc Surg* 1981; 82 : 658-68.
7. Mountain C. Surgery of lung cancer including adjunctive therapy. *In* : Hansen HH, Rorth M (eds), Amsterdam, Excerpta Medica, *Lung Cancer* 1980; 71-92.
8. Dautzenberg B, Chastang Cl, Lebeau B, et al. and the GETCB. A randomized Phase II trial of neoadjuvant chemotherapy in resectable bronchogenic non small cell carcinoma. *Abstract de la réunion de chimiothérapie néoadjuvante,* Paris, février 1988, N2.
9. Vokes EE, Bitran JD, Hoffman PC, et al. Neoadjuvant chemotherapy for locoregionally advanced NSCLC. *Abstract de la réunion de chimiothérapie néoadjuvante,* Paris, février 1988, N5.
10. Vokes EE, Jacob D, Bitran JD, et al. Neoadjuvant Vindesine Etoposide and Cisplatin for locally advanced non small cell lung cancer. Final report of a phase 2 study. *Chest* 1989; 96 : 110-13.
11. Eagan RT, Ruud C, Lee RE, et al. Pilot study of induction therapy cyclophosphamide, doxorubicin and Cisplatin and chest irradiation prior to thoracotomy in initially inoperable stage III M_0 non SNLC. *Cancer Treat Rep* 1987; 71 : 895-900.
12. Goua S, Zabbe Cl, Lemarie E, et al. Preoperative chemotherapy in patients with initially unresectable lung cancer. *Abstract de la réunion de chimiothérapie néoadjuvante,* Paris, février 1988, N4.
13. Elias AD, Skarin AT, Socinski MA, et al. Neoadjuvant therapy for stage IIIa non small cell lung cancer. *Proceedings of American Society of Clinical Oncology. Twenty Fifth Annual Meeting,* San Francisco, Californie, 1989, N° 941.
14. Elias AD, Skarin AT, Socinski MA, et al. Neoadjuvant therapy for unresectable stage IIIb non small cell lung cancer. *Proceedings of American Society of Clinical Oncology. Twenty Fifth Annual Meeting,* San Francisco, Californie 1989, N° 942.
15. Lad T, Rubinstein L, Sadeghi A. The benefit of adjuvant treatment for resected locally advanced non small cell lung cancer. *J Clin Oncol* 1988; 64 : 9-17.
16. Homes EC, Hill LD, Gail M. A randomized comparison of the effects of adjuvant therapy on resected stages II and III NSCLC. *Ann Surg* 1985; 203/3 : 335-41.
17. Woods RL, Levi JA, Page J, et al. Non small cell lung cancer : a randomized comparison of chemotherapy with no chemotherapy. *Proc 21st Meeting ASCO,* Houston (USA) 1985; 177 : C691.
18. Celerrino R, Tummarello P, Porfiri F, et al. Non small cell lung cancer. A prospective randomized trial with alternating chemotherapy CEP/MEC versus no treatment. *Eur J Cancer Clin Oncol* 1988; 24112 : 1839-43.
19. Ganz PA, Figlin RA, Haskell CM, et al. Supportive care versus supportive care and combination chemotherapy in metastastic non small cell lung cancer. *Cancer* 1989; 63 : 1271-78.
20. Cormier Y, Bergeron D, La Forge J, et al. Benefits of polychemotherapy in advanced non small cell bronchogenic carcinoma. *Cancer* 1982; 50 : 845-49.

21. Rapp E, Pater JL, William A, *et al.* Chemotherapy can prolong survival in patients with advanced non small cell lung cancer. *J Clin Oncol* 1988; 633-41.
22. Williams CG, Woods R, Levi J, *et al.* Randomized trial comparing cisplatine-vindesine with no chemotherapy in unresectable non small cell lung cancer. *Abstract de la 4e Conférence Européenne d'Oncologie Clinique (ESMO),* Madrid 1987, N° 49.
23. Quoix E, Dietemann A, Charbonneau J, *et al.* Disseminated non small cell lung cancer : a randomized trial of chemotherapy versus palliative care. *Abstract of Fifth World Conference on Lung Cancer,* Interlaken (Suisse) 1988, A127.
24. Depierre A, Garnier G, Dubiez A, *et al.* Etude de Phase II de la Navelbine. *Abstract de la réunion de cancérologie pulmonaire,* Marseille 23-24 octobre 1987.

9

Combined radiotherapy and chemotherapy in non small cell lung cancer

R. ARRIAGADA, B. PELLAE-COSSET, E. NASR, P. BERTHAUD, T. LE CHEVALIER

Comité de Pathologie Thoracique, Institut Gustave-Roussy, 39, rue Camille-Desmoulins, 94805 Villejuif Cedex, France

Surgery represents the treatment of choice in non small cell lung cancer (NSCLC). When tumors cannot be resected because of significant thoracic extension or distant metastasis, survival rates are very low. While radiotherapy, alone or combined with chemotherapy, can play an important role in the treatment of such tumors, the main reason for therapeutic failure in partially resected tumors is the development of resistance to radiation and/or cytotoxic drugs. The theoretical advantages of combining radiotherapy and chemotherapy are: 1) spatial cooperation between local irradiation and local and systemic chemotherapeutic effects and 2) prevention of the development of resistance to treatment.

Drug combinations can be used in order to prevent chemoresistance. If the drugs are not cross-resistant and are comparable in overall safety, the risk of resistant cell proliferation is greatly reduced. Although this effect has been demonstrated in clinical practice, for example, with the use of MOPP in the treatment of Hodgkin's disease, such therapeutic combinations are often difficult to administer owing to increased and unacceptable global toxicity. A number of theoretical and experimental models have been developed [1, 2] in an attempt to optimize procedures and prevent the proliferation of resistant cell clones. These models have highlighted the importance of the initial chemotherapeutic cycles and the value of a high "dose intensity". Alternating between different modalities such as radiotherapy and chemotherapy may also prove beneficial, always provided that the means selected are not cross-resistant. Even though examples of cross-resistance between radiotherapy and chemotherapy have been cited by some authors, they are comparatively rare and the radiosensitivity of most chemoresistant tumor populations remains unchanged. Moreover, since the toxic effects differ according to tissue type, it is possible to avoid any need for a dose reduction in either chemotherapy or radiotherapy.

The prognosis for locally advanced lung cancer (LALC) remains poor. In view of the high rate of metastases, studies combining chemotherapy and locoregional treatment have been carried out. Unfortunately, most have been phase II, and any phase III studies have included few patients. The global results have not therefore given rise to any conclusions as to the effectiveness of such combinations.

For the sake of simplicity, we shall concern ourselves with just two subjects : 1) the combination of chemotherapy and locoregional treatments in resectable or partially resectable lung cancer; 2) the combination of chemotherapy and radiotherapy in LALC.

Chemotherapy, surgery and radiotherapy in resectable NSCLC

Postoperative chemotherapy and radiotherapy

Postoperative chemotherapy was recently tested in two randomized studies, the results of which are summarized in *Table I*. The French GETCB trial (which included nearly twice as many patients as the American trial) did not demonstrate any significant chemotherapeutic effect. More data are required for the role of such adjuvant treatment to be evaluated. In general terms, it would appear logical to combine an effective locoregional treatment with some other general therapeutic effect in an attempt to reduce the rate of distant metastasis since thes latter represents the main reason for failure of treatment in more than 50 % of cases. The fundamental problem involved is the low activity exhibited by current chemotherapy regimens in these

Table I. Postoperative chemotherapy and radiotherapy in resectable lung cancer (Phase III studies).

Group	n	CT	Postop RT	MS (months)	1-year S (%)
LCSG (3)	78	CAP × 6	20 Gy/5 sessions × 2	20	68 p<0.05
	86	---	Id	13	54
GETCB (4)	138	COPAC × 3	60 Gy/24 sessions	15	67 NS
	130	---	Id	15	58

CT : chemotherapy; RT : radiotherapy; MS : median survival; S : survival; CAP : cyclophosphamide, doxorubicin, cisplatin; COPAC : CAP, vincristine, CCNU; NS : not significant.

histological types of lung cancer. Theoretically, a regimen would require an objective response rate (correctly evaluated) of more than 50 % for there to be any expectation of a moderate increase in survival. At present, such combinations are still being investigated.

Preoperative chemotherapy and radiotherapy

Recent pilot studies have used combined chemo-radiotherapy in an attempt to allow nonresectable patients become candidates for surgery. The apparent resectability rate obtained with such sequential [5, 6] or concurrent [7-9] combinations is approximately 50 % *(Table II)*. It appears that a similar rate was obtained in studies using preoperative chemotherapy only. Although these results are of considerable interest, the follow up was too short in most cases and the eligibility criteria for nonresectable patients and the definition of resectability often too vague. A randomized study comparing combined chemotherapy and surgery with immediate surgery is required if a precise assessment of the impact of initial chemotherapy on resectability and survival is to be obtained. Such a study is now being organized in France by the National Federation of Centers for the Fight against Cancer and is to start in early 1990. Patients with tumors defined as marginally resectable are eligible for inclusion.

Two treatment groups will be established :
1) 3 preoperative chemotherapeutic cycles (ifosfamide, VP16-213, cisplatin) followed by surgery and postoperative radiotherapy;
2) surgery followed by postoperative radiotherapy.

Table II. Preoperative chemotherapy and radiotherapy in lung cancer with limited resectability (Phase II studies).

Authors	n	CT	RT	% Resectability
Komaki [5]	38	VLB, CDDP, Mito C	Not stated	45
Strauss [6]	22	VDS, CDDP	Continuous 30 Gy	59
Bonomi [7]	32	VP16, CDDP, 5FU	Split-course 40 Gy (10 Gy/ 5 sessions every 21 days)	33
Rusch [8]	95	CDDP, 5FU	Continuous 30 Gy	49
Taylor [9]	66	CDDP, 5FU	Split-course 40 Gy (10 Gy/ 5 sessions every 9 days)	61

CT : chemotherapy; RT : radiotherapy; VLB : vinblastine; CDDP : cisplatin; Mito C : mitomycin; VDS : vindesine; VP16 : etoposide; 5FU : 5-fluorouracil.

Combined chemo- and radiotherapy in LALC

The generally poor prognosis in LALC justifies the attempt to isolate a group of apparently non-metastatic patients, for whom there is low probability of cure (5-year survival approximately 5 %). The attitude that full dose radiotherapy may be regarded as the standard treatment for this type of cancer has recently been subject to dispute [10] : studies comparing radiotherapy alone with symptomatic medical treatment have included very few patients. The current pragmatic approach is to try to select patients who might benefit from such treatment; correctly executed studies would enable optimal doses and treatment intervals to be defined.

Appropriately indicated and correctly administered radiotherapy should produce the following results when used alone [11, 12] : a) approximately 30 % complete remission, b) 1 and 2-year survival of 45 % and 25 % respectively and c) 5-year survival of just 5 %.

The very same arguments discussed above in respect of resectable tumors also apply to combined chemo/radiotherapy. Several pilot studies have given encouraging results [13] but confirmation is required by randomized studies. A French study comparing combined radiotherapy and VCPC (vindesine, cyclophosphamide, cisplatin, CCNU) with radiotherapy alone was completed in February 1989. This type of study should be promoted because only with combined chemo- and radiotherapy (provided that the former proves active) is there any hope of decreasing distant metastasis and perhaps even improving the locoregional effects of radiotherapy.

Non-randomized studies including small patient populations have been carried out, combining "split-course" (two series) or standard radiotherapy at doses of 40-65 Gy with chemotherapeutic combinations of various drugs (usually alkylating agents, alkaloids, anthracyclines, cisplatin and etoposide). Reported median survival was only 9-13 months [14, 15]. At the Gustave-Roussy Institute, combined VCPC-radiotherapy (60-65 Gy) was tested in 75 patients [13]. Median survival was 13.5 months : the major problem remained the lack of local control (85 % at 3 years).

Numerous randomized studies in more than 1 000 patients have been conducted comparing radiotherapy alone with treatment combining chemotherapy before and after radiotherapy. *Table III* summarizes the results of studies including over 100 patients. Only in one of these [16] showed chemotherapy to have a significant effect. Only 130 of the total 180 randomized subjects were evaluable and survival was "estimated" at 1 year. Unfortunately, the study was discontinued prematurely.

Radiotherapy and chemotherapy can also be combined concurrently. Such combinations have been tested on several occasions [22-27] without demonstrating any significant improvement in survival, despite increased toxicity in many cases, proving a major problem in some studies : gastrointestinal toxicity (25) and cardiac toxicity (2 deaths out of a total of 43 patients) [25] with doxurubicin and unacceptable pulmonary toxicity with bleomycin. Two deaths and 7 pneumopathies were reported in the Miyamoto study [27] and 3 deaths in the Wedleigh study [26] from bleomycin-related pulmonary toxicity.

Three studies [28-30] compared the benefit of either a weekly dose of cisplatin alone (15-20 mg/m^2/week) or a daily dose (6 mg/m^2/day) concurrent with thoracic radiotherapy. Lapukins [28] reported survival rates of 42 % at 2 years and 21 % at 3 years in 28 patients (significantly higher than the results obtained with a classical

Table III. Combinations of radiotherapy and chemotherapy in LALC : RT alone versus RT-CT (Phase III studies including more than 100 patients).

Authors	CT	RT	n	P
Dillman [16]	CDDP, VLB	Continuous 60 Gy	180	0.003 in favor of RT-CT
Jett [17]	MTX, DOXO, CPM, CCNU	Continuous 60 Gy	197	NS
Johnson [18]	VDS	Continuous 60 Gy	319	NS
White [19]	DOXO	Split-course 55-60 Gy	107	NS
Mattson [20]	CPM, DOXO, CDDP	Split-course 55 Gy	238	NS
Trovo [21]	CPM, DOXO, MTX, CDDP	Continuous 45 Gy	111	NS

CT : chemotherapy; RT : radiotherapy; DOXO : doxorubicin, MTX : methotrexate, CDDP : cisplatin; CCNU : lomustine, CPM : cyclophosphamide; VDS : vindesine; VLB : vinblastine; NS : not significant.

series receiving radiotherapy alone at a total dose of 50 Gy). Two randomized studies are summarized in *Table IV*. Soresi [30], in a study conducted in 95 patients, observed a significant decrease in local relapse rate (24 % compared with 43 % with radiotherapy alone : p = 0.01). Median survival was 16 months in the treatment group receiving radiotherapy alone (total dose 50 Gy, continuous : p = 0.06). The EORTC phase II randomized study [29], which included 100 patients, demonstrated improved

Table IV. Concurrent combination of radiotherapy + cisplatin (Phase III study : RT alone versus RT-CT).

Authors	CT	RT	n	P (for survival)
Schaake-Koning [29]	CDDP weekly (3 mg/m^2)	Split-course	100	NS
	CDDP daily (6 mg/m^2)	55 Gy		
Soresi [30]	CDDP (15 mg/m^2)	Continuous 50 Gy	103	NS

CT : chemotherapy; RT : radiotherapy; CDDP : cisplatin.

results in terms of rates and time of appearance of local relapses with the concurrent combination of daily CDDP and radiotherapy compared with radiotherapy alone (split-course, 30 Gy for 10 sessions followed by 25 Gy for 10 sessions). Severe toxicity was however observed : GI toxicity : > 38 %, severe pulmonary fibrosis : 48 % (radiotherapy/chemotherapy group) although the latter may have been related to the fractionation used (3 Gy/session). The follow-up is too short to confirm any genuine long-term survival benefit, but the concurrent combination of high dose radiotherapy and daily or weekly doses of cisplatin does appear highly promising.

Evaluation of results

Overall analysis of the results highlights one fundamental problem which entails three major aspects : a) many of the phase II studies report encouraging results; b) there are few phase III studies and they generally include few patients; c) the results of several phase III studies appear contradictory.

a) The promising results obtained in phase II studies generally vanish because 1) the analyses are repeated with longer follow up data and the final results are then rarely published; 2) more patients are included, thus reducing the statistical variance; 3) the results are not confirmed by a phase III study.

Phase II studies are crucial for opening up new avenues of therapeutic research. They are intended to confirm the feasibility of a given treatment and give an approximate idea of its efficacy. They are very popular because they are relatively straightforward, with a short inclusion period and few patients. Results can often be obtained very quickly and thus give rise to a higher number of publications. One disadvantage is the fact that they are unable to provide an accurate evaluation of the treatment since no control group is included. Comparison with classical series, even where appropriate, involves too high a degree of bias for any conclusions to be drawn and this type of study can only give an indication of a given therapeutic effect. A good phase II study with encouraging results should, of course, be followed by a phase III study. However, many of those who promote phase II studies soon become "specialists" in such studies and do not even follow up and verify their own preliminary data. A prime example is that of preoperative chemotherapy, for which hundreds of patients have been included in phase II studies. How long shall we have to wait for the first phase III studies to start ?

b) The statistical power of phase III studies is a problem. The word "randomization" is not a magic wand that is able to solve all of the problems encountered in the field of therapeutic evaluation. Phase III studies are based on a precise methodology that must be respected if studies of any value are desired. It is essential to ensure that sufficient patients have been entered in order to decrease the risk or false positive (alpha risk) or false negative (beta risk) results.

For example, among 6 studies [31-36] including fewer than 100 patients comparing radiotherapy alone with combined radio/chemotherapy in the treatment of LALC, 2 [32, 36] demonstrated significant effects. These studies included 81 and 33 patients respectively: the statistical variance in both studies was enormous and probably induced wrong conclusions. Furthermore, the long-term results have neither been published nor confirmed by similar studies.

The effects of adjuvant treatments in solid tumors are generally only moderate; long-term survival gains exceeding 10 % are unlikely, usually falling between 5 % and 10 %. However, though moderate, such gains should not be disregarded, especially when very frequent tumors are concerned. In such cases, very small therapeutic gains would involve many patients. It is therefore important to establish whether this actually exists and, if so, to quantify it. These answers will be obtained in phase III studies including a large number of patients.

c) The contradictory results obtained in some phase III studies can cause the clinician to choose one particular study or group of studies, but on which objective criteria should this choice be based ? Should a study be selected from among the "negatives" or the "positives" ? The subjective nature of this choice renders it wide open to criticism. If the objective is to seek an objective answer, it would be better, and less biased, to take into account all data obtained from previous studies concerned with the same question : radiotherapy/no radiotherapy, chemotherapy/no chemotherapy, etc. A systematic review of the literature and careful analysis of results can produce a conclusion or even the absence of a conclusion (where the data are insufficient for any answer). The latter is currently the most frequent with this pathology. How can this be related directly to individual patients ? Should we offer them hypothetical assurances based on insufficient data ? The only certainty we have today is the value of surgery in resectable tumors. But we know very little about adjuvant treatments. In France, about 25 000 new cases of lung cancer are reported every year and fewer than 3 % are included in randomized studies. One might not be excused for thinking that all the questions have already been answered. Shouldn't we now resolve to offer patients opinions based on accurate information in the future ? Advances in the treatment of lung cancer will surely follow, and many of our future patients will most certainly expect this of us.

References

1. Goldie JH, Coldman AJ, NG V, et al. A mathematical and computer-based model of alternating chemotherapy and radiation therapy in experimental neoplasms. in : Arriagada R, Le Chevalier T, *Treatment Modalities in lung Cancer.* Karger 1. *Antibiot Chemother.* 1988; 41 : 11-20.
2. Looney WB. Special lecture : alternating chemotherapy and radiotherapy. *NCI Monogr.* 1988; 6 : 85-94.
3. Lad T, Rubinstein L, Sadeghi A. For the Lung Cancer Study Group. The benefit of adjuvant treatment for resected advanced non-small-cell lung cancer. *J. Clin Oncol* 1988; 6 : 9-17.
4. Chastang C, Arriagada R, Dautzenberg B, et al. the GETCB. Post-operative chemotherapy in resected bronchogenic carcinoma (stage II and III) second interim analysis of a clinical trial (268 patients). *Lung Cancer* 1988; (4 Suppl) : A163.
5. Komaki R, Schultz C, Cox JD, et al. Pre-operative neoadjuvant combination chemotherapy and radiation therapy for non small carcinoma of the lung. *Lung Cancer* 1988; 4 : A162.

6. Strauss G, Sherman D, Schwartz J, et al. Combined modality therapy for regionally advanced stage III non small cell carcinoma of the lung employing neodjuvant chemotherapy, radiotherapy and surgery. *Proc Amer Soc Clin Oncol* 1986; 5 : A675.
7. Bonomi P, Rowland KM, Taylor SG, et al. Phase II trial of therapy with Etoposide, 5-Fluorouracil by continuous infusion, Cisplatin, and simultaneous split-course radiation in stage III non-small cell bronchogenic carcinoma. *NCI Monogr* 1988; 6 : 331-334.
8. Rusch V, Weiden P, Hill L. Patterns of relapse following neodjuvant therapy for regionally inoperable small cell lung cancer. *Lung Cancer* 1988; 4 : A161.
9. Taylor SG, Murthy AK, Bonomi P, et al. Concomitant therapy with infusion of Cisplatin and 5-Fluorouracil plus radiation in stage III non-small cell lung-cancer. *NCI Monogr* 1988; 6 : 327-329.
10. Payne DG. Non-small-cell lung cancer : should unresectable stage III patients routinely receive high dose radiation therapy ? *J Clin Oncol* 1988; 6 : 552-558.
11. Holsti LR, Mattson K. A randomized study of split-course radiotherapy of lung cancer : long term results. *Int J. Radiat Oncol Bio Phys* 1980; 6 : 977-981.
12. Perez CA, Stanley K, Grundy G, et al. Impact of irradiation technique and tumor extent in tumor control and survival of patients with unresectable non small cell carcinoma of the lung. *Cancer* 1982; 50 : 1091-1099.
13. Le Chevalier T, Arriagada R, Baldeyrou P, et al. Combined chemotherapy (vindesine, lomustine, cisplatin and cyclophosphamide) and radical radiotherapy in inoperable non metastatic squamous cell carcinoma of the lung. *Cancer treat Rep* 1985; 69 : 469-472.
14. Fram R, Skarin A, Balikian J, et al. Combination chemotherapy followed by radiation therapy in patients with regional stage III unresectable non-small cell lung cancer. *Cancer Treat Rep* 1985; 69 : 587-590.
15. Osoba D, Rusthoven JJ, Evans WK, Turnbull KA. Combined chemotherapy and radiation therapy for non-small cell lung cancer. *Semin Oncol* 1986; 13 : 121-124.
16. Dillman RO, Seagren SL, Propert K, et al. Protochemotherapy improves survival in regional non small cell lung cancer (Abstract). *Proc Amer Soc Clin Oncol* 1988; 7 : 195.
17. Jett J, Morton R, Maher L, Therneau T. Randomized trial of thoracic radiation (TRT) with or without chemotherapy for locally unresectable non small cell lung cancer (NSCLC). *Lung Cancer* 1988; 4 : A162.
18. Johnson DH, Einhorn LH, Birch R, et al. Is immediate thoracic radiotherapy indicated in operable, non metastatic non small cell lung cancer ? *Proc Amer Soc Clin Oncol* 1989; 873.
19. White JE, Chen T, Reed R, et al. Limited squamous cell carcinoma of the lung : a Southwest Oncology Group randomized study of radiation with or without doxorubicin chemotherapy and with or without levamisole immunotherapy. *Cancer Treat Rep* 1982; 66 : 1113-1120.
20. Mattson K, Holsti LR, Holst P, et al. Inoperable non small cell lung cancer : radiation with or without chemotherapy. *Eur. J Clin Oncol* 1988; 24 : 477-482.
21. Trovo MG, Veronesi A, Bortolus R, et al. Is chemotherapy necessary in the management of unresectable nonmetastatic non-small cell lung cancer ? *In* : Arriagada R, Le Chevalier T, Eds, *Treatment Modalities in Lung Cancer.* Karger 1988; 126-130.
22. Byfield JE, Stanton W, Sharp TR, et al. Phase I-II study of 120 hour infused 5-FU and split course. Radiation therapy in localized non small cell lung cancer. *Cancer Treat Rep* 1983; 67 : 933-935.
23. Friess GG, Baikadi M, Harvey WH. Concurrent cisplatin and etoposide with radiotherapy in locally advanced non-small cell lung cancer. *Cancer Treat Rep* 1987; 71 : 681-684.
24. Gordon W, Stanberry PK, Weiss GB. Concurrent chemotherapy and radiation therapy for limited unresectable non-small cell carcinoma of the lung. A phase I study. *Amer J Clin Oncol* 1988; 11 : 119-121.

25. Umsawasdi T, Valdivieso M, Barkley HT Jr, *et al.* Combined chemoradiotherapy in limited-disease, inoperable non-small cell lung cancer. *Int J Radiat Oncol Biol Phys* 1988; 14 : 43-48.
26. Wedleigh RG, Lunzer S, Krasnow SH, *et al.* Simultaneous chemotherapy and radiotherapy for squamous cell lung cancer. *Amer J Clin Oncol* 1988; 11 : 122-125.
27. Miyamoto. Acute squamous metaplasia of the whole lung after combined radiation and chemotherapy in advanced lung cancer. *Gan No Rinsho* 1987; 33 : 89-96.
28. Lapukins Z, Lietz-Scholten Ckober B. Interim results of combined chemotherapy and irradiation for inoperable squamous cell carcinoma of the lung, compared to a historic control group of patients treated with irradiation alone. *Lung Cancer* 1988; 4 : A162.
29. Schaake-Koning C, Bartelink H. Radiotherapy and cisdiammine dichloro-platinum as a combined treatment modality in patients with inoperable non-small cell lung cancer. A randomized phase II study. *Lung Cancer* 1988; 4 : A 161.
30. Soresi E, Clerici M, Grilli R, *et al.* A randomized trial comparing radiation therapy versus radiation therapy plus cis-dichloro-diammine platinum (II) in the treatment of locally advanced non small cell lung cancer. *Sem Oncol* 1988; 15 : 20-25.
31. Alberti W, Niederle N, Stuschke M, *et al.* Prospective randomized study comparing immediate radiotherapy, combined chemo- and radiotherapy and delayed radiotherapy. *Lung Cancer* 1988; 4 : A167.
32. Anderson G, Deeley TJ, Jani J. Comparison of radiotherapy alone and radiotherapy with chemotherapy using adriamycin and 5-fluorouracil in bronchongenic carcinoma. *Thorax* 1981; 36 : 190-193.
33. Crino L; Marazano E, Corgna E, *et al.* Combined modality treatment for locally advanced non small cell lung cancer. A randomized trial. *Lung cancer* 1988; 4 : A164.
34. Landgren RC, Hussey DH, Samuels ML, Leary WV. A randomized study comparing irradiation alone to irradiation plus procarbazine in inoperable bronchogenic carcinoma. *Radiology* 1973; 108 : 403-406.
35. Van Houtte P, Klasterky J, Renaud A, *et al.* Induction chemotherapy with cisplatin, etoposide and vindesine before radiation therapy fon non-small cell lung cancer. A randomized study. In : Arriagada R, Le Chevalier T, Eds. *Treatment Modalities in Lung Cancer.* Karger (Basel). *Antibiot Chemother* 1988 41 : 131-137.
36. Wils JA, Utama I, Naus A, Verschueren TA. Phase II randomized trial of radiotherapy alone versus the sequential use of chemotherapy and radiotherapy in stage III non-small cell lung cancer. Phase II trial of chemotherapy alone in stage IV non-small cell lung cancer. *Eur. J Cancer Clin Oncol* 1984; 20 : 911-914.

10

Biological contribution to the study of lung cancer

M.F. POUPON[1], F. ARVELO[4], M. JACROT[2]
with the collaboration of Y. Bourgeois[1], Y. Rolland[1],
P. Baldeyrou[3], R. Arriagada[3], T. Le Chevalier[3], A.F. Goguel[1]

[1] *Biologie des métastases, CNRS, 7, rue Guy-Mocquet, BP 8, 94802 Villejuif Cedex, France*
[2] *Cytogénétique, Faculté de Médecine de Grenoble, Domaine de la Merci, 38700 La Tronche, France*
[3] *Institut Gustave-Roussy, rue Camille-Desmoulins, 94805 Villejuif, France*
[4] *Université de Caracas, Venezuela.*

The prognosis of lung cancer has remained particularly bleak despite the efforts made to improve its treatment over the last decades. Small cell lung cancer (SCLC) is a clear example in this regard. The diverse combinations of chemotherapeutic agents, with or without radiotherapy, are remarkably active in first line treatment. Relapse, however, is rapid except in a small fraction of patients with this form of cancer, which corresponds to 25 % of all lung cancers. The basic research data are plentiful and a large literature is currently available. A recent review, written by F. Thomas, in the *Revue de Maladies Respiratoires* makes a good point of the large amount of publications.

SCLC is very interesting from a biological point of view. It constitutes a model for studying the evolution of cancers with a constant increase malignancy which is marked by an early onset potential of widespread metastases, and the transition from chemosensitivity to chemoresistance.

The interests of biological researchers sometimes differ from those of clinicians. We asked ourselves the question, what are the results, out of the mass of available biological data, that might be useful in obtaining an improved prognosis in the treatment of SCLC ? What can be learned from a biological standpoint about this pathological entity ? And among the currently available parameters which should we choose ? Are biological models relevant, are the ones we have selected and applied in the study of SCLC valid, and can they be used for other types of tumor localization ?

These were the objectives we set ourselves in our biological laboratory studies of SCLC.

Since the early beginnings of our studies, we have tried to define the importance of numerous factors pertinent to the biology of SCLC with regard to clinical, diagnostic, pronostic or therapeutic objectives :

• *Histological studies* distinguish two types of tumors : classical and variant. The former, comprised of "oat cells", will have a better prognosis than the latter, which differs histologically by the greater amount of cytoplasm found in the neoplastic cells. Our studies do not show such a relationship. At most, in the only case where we were able to obtain a tumor before and after treatment, the frequency of large cells in the relapsing tumor biopsy characteristic of the variant type was higher than in the original biopsy. Furthermore, among our series of 20 tumors studied so far, the only patient who is still alive, after eight years, had a classic type SCLC (this tumor was among those obtained in the series by M. Jacrot, from patients treated in Grenoble, France by Pr C. Brambilla). Nevertheless, nine tumors out of seventeen were of the classic type and had an unfavorable evolution.

• *Electronic microscopy* provides important elements, showing the neuroendocrine differentiation of these tumors and thus clarifying diagnosis in difficult cases. These results help establish the diagnosis, but they do not have prognostic value.

• The "biology", in other words *the cytologic or enzymatic markers,* bombesin or L-dopadecarboxylase for example, can, like electronic microscopy, strengthen an uncertain diagnosis and confirm the neuroendocrine origin of the tumor cells. Enolase, or NSE (Neuron Specific Enolase), is interesting: its detection in the patient's blood allows the evaluation of the volume of neoplastic tissue. The increase in its concentration in the blood, particularly in the initial phase of treatment, reflects the destruction of tumor tissue with liberation of this intracellular enzyme into the circulation. Immunological determinants, found on the cellular surface using monoclonal antibodies, are of diagnostic interest, but do not provide any prognostic information on the cancer evolution.

• *Cytogenetic analysis* proves that there is a very large number of rearrangements, gene deletions, or duplication of chromosomes. The loss of a fragment of the chromosome 3p is especially common. However, it is not specific for this pathology: it is also found in the tumor tissue of secondary lung metastasis, as well as in renal tumors. More specific is the increased frequency of abnormalities, the origin of which is still unclear, but which reflect an instability of the chromosomic structure itself, and is certainly dependent on a basic genetic disruption of these cells. The cytogenetic study of our SCLC tumor biopsy series is currently under way.

• *The research of genomic amplification,* namely of oncogenes, seemed to hold particular interest, to the extent that it could provide a basis for prognosis.

Among the likely candidates, it has been proven that the amplification of the *myc family* oncogenes, especially L-myc, was relatively frequent in SCLC. This has been demonstrated in cell lines derived from tumor biopsies. Gene amplification, however, is more difficult to detect (when it exists at low level) than the overexpression of the same genes, revealed by the level of RNA transcripts which we have researched.

Research on overexpression of other genes coding for growth factors, such as gastro-releasing peptide (GRP), a precursor of *bombesin* utilized by tumor cells to sustain their proliferation, may also have prognostic and possibly therapeutic interest, when bombesin antagonists can be produced on a large scale.

The research of an overexpression of genes coding for the molecules responsible for multidrug chemoresistance seems to be essential, because prognosis is strictly linked to a response to treatment.

Two mechanisms of resistance have recently been defined. One is determined by the MDR1 gene, coding for a membrane glycoprotein with a molecular weight of 170 kd, the role of which is the prompt extrusion of drugs such as adriamycin and vinblastine which penetrate the cell passively. This limits the exposure of the tumor cells to the antineoplastic effects of drugs which enter the cells in this way. Certain agents, such as verapamil (Isoptin), more known for its inhibiting effect on calcium ion exchange through membrane channels (notably in myocardial cells), are capable of blocking the action of this P-glycoprotein. The advantage of detecting overexpressions of these resistance genes clearly rests in the possibility of using agents such as verapamil in therapeutic combinations which are capable of preventing or counteracting chemoresistance. Multidrug resistance is detectable either by probing the amplification of the MDR1 gene (which is difficult since the gene is not easily detectable at low level even though it may be highly active), or by identifying overexpression of the gene through an evalutation either of (RNA) transcript level or of protein detected by specific antibodies in histological sections. In this way a diagnosis of resistance may be made, and a new element in the treatment armamentarium provided.

A second, well defined mechanism of chemoresistance operates through glutathione S-transferase, which allows the detoxification of numerous antineoplastic agents. The overexpression of gene transcripts coded by glutathione S-transferase (π) is detectable by a molecular (GTS) probe, or by antibodies specific to the molecule coded by this gene. Here again, it is possible to envision the utilization of glutathione S-transferase inhibitors in order to sensitize the tumors to chemotherapy.

Even though fundamental studies have enabled us to define these genes and their function in single cell suspensions in culture, we still do not know if we can use them as prognostic markers or as targets for therapy in SCLC patients. After considering these points, the objective of our study was to answer the following questions:

1) Is there a relationship between response to chemotherapy and the expression of resistance genes ?

2) Is there a relationship between the resistance to chemotherapy and biological characteristics such as the expression of oncogenes, or genes coded by growth factors ?

3) Is it possible to reproduce artificially the evolution of SCLC under chemotherapy and to try to circumvent chemoresistance, for example by adding verapamil to the chemotherapy ?

Practical application of an experimental model

Biopsies of tumor tissue, when they are resected from the primary tumor or from a metastasis, are usually of very small volume, which impedes any exhaustive study. We therefore decided to transplant such tumor tissues in athymic nude mice. The frequency with which we can obtain tumor growth is only 10 % with bronchial biopsies (because of frequent necrosis, or crushing of the biopsy tissue), but is 80 % with surgical or tru-cut biopsies (higher quality tissue). Twenty tumors were obtained in this manner, and currently nine of them were the subject of a completed study. The histological study of these tumors before and after transplantation allowed us to verify the absence of any modifications that might have been caused by the transplantation. The karyotype, which was systematically performed, showed the human origin of these tumors. The utilization of the DNA typing technique for the detection of repeated sequences of DNA, as used in criminology, provided confirmation of the individual origins of these tumor transplants.

Experimental study of SCLC response to chemotherapy

Response was evaluated in each patient during the course of treatment. We tried to reproduce this response in the laboratory by treating nude mice with a chemotherapeutic treatment that was as close as possible to that administered in man. The chemotherapy given to the patients at the Institut Gustave-Roussy is a combination of four agents: adriamycin (ADR), cisplatin (CDDP), cyclophosphamide (CPA) and VP16. The doses given to the mice were defined as a function of the maximum tolerated doses: ADR 6 mg/kg, CDDP 3 mg/kg, CPA 50 mg/kg, VP16 8 mg/kg. Higher dosage was tested, and caused an increase of mortality up to 30 % using ADR 10 mg/kg, CDDP 6.4 mg/kg, VP16 24 mg/kg, CPA 200 mg/kg. The drugs were administered over five days, according to the IGR protocol. Twice daily rehydration was necessary. The treatment cycle was done consecutively over five days, and it was given when the tumor implants reach a volume of 100 mm^3. The antitumoral effect is expressed by the percentage of growth inhibition in the treated tumors, relative to

---

Figure 1. Response of the SCLC-6M tumor to different antitumor agents, constituents of the "4-D" protocol, alone or in combination. A: Antitumor effect of the combination of four drugs: ADR, CDDP, VP16 and (CPA), designated as "4D". B: Comparison of the antitumor effect of the 4D combination with the combination of CDDP and VP16. C: Antitumor effect of CDDP compared to that of the 4D protocol. D: Comparison of the effect of VP16 alone or in combination with CDDP. E: Absence of an antitumor effect with the combination of ADR and VP16. F: Absence of an antitumor effect with ADR administered alone as a single dose. G: The loss of chemosensitivity of SCLC-6M tumors after 9 cycles of treatment. Chemosensitizing effect of the combination of verapamil with the "4-D" combination.

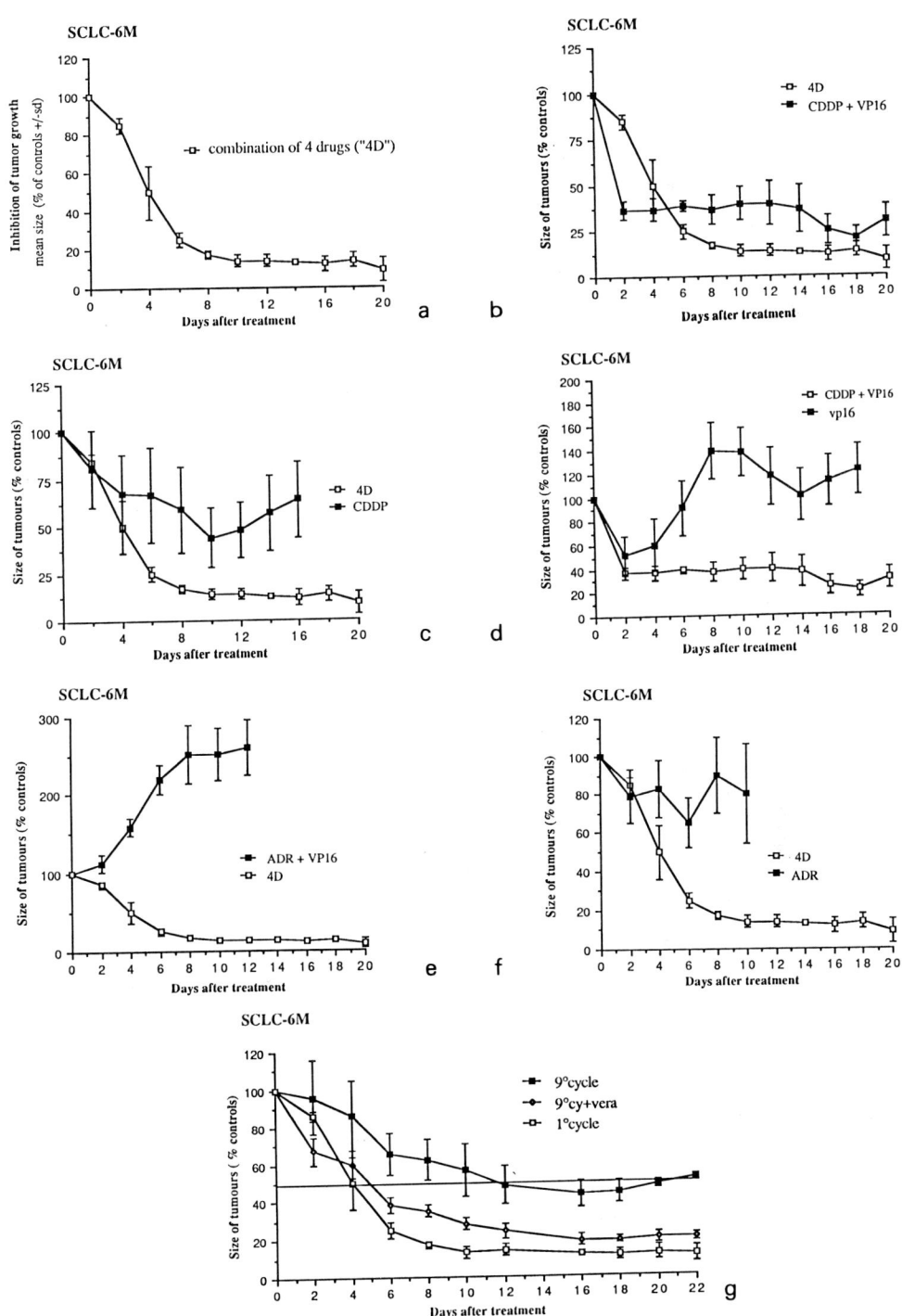

the growth in untreated tumors. The different groups have five mice each, treated identically.

The antitumoral effect of the combination of the four drugs (4-D) was compared to that of each drug separately, given in one dose of 10 mg/kg. A combination of CDDP and VP16, which was chosen as the reference combination, was also tested. These studies were conducted on tumor transplants of the variant type of SCLC taken from an untreated patient. This tumor (SCLC-6M) had a rapid doubling time (4 days), expresses the c-myc oncogene strongly, and does not express any of the two chemoresistance genes. The results are reported in *Figures 1, A, B, C, D, E, F* and *G*. They clearly demonstrate the efficacy of the 4-D treatment on the growth of the SCLC-6M tumor *(Figure 1A)*. Increase in dose did not provide any extra benefit. The CDDP and VP16 combination is also very active *(Figure 1B)*. Alone, VP16 is inactive *(Figure 1D)*, but CDDP given in monotherapy produced significant growth inhibition *(Figure 1C)*. The adriamycin and VP16 combination enhanced consistently and dangerously stimulates the growth of these tumors *(Figure 1E)*. ADR alone shows little efficacy *(Figure 1F)*.

The antitumoral effect is characterized both by its intensity, in that an 80-90% inhibition is obtained, and by its transient and partial characteristics. The tumor can be reduced but it does not disappear under treatment. No complete regressions were observed. The patient tumor progressed in a comparable fashion: complete regression followed by relapse. The tumor treated in the nude mice was transplanted and retreated in order to reproduce the effects of the repeated cycles of treatment given to patients. *Figure 1G* shows that after nine cycles of treatment the tumor loses chemosensitivity, inhibition being 50% compared to 85% after the first cycle.

Following the same protocol of the 4-D treatment, nine tumors have currently been tested. Three of them (SCLC-10M, SCLC-61M and SCLC-82M) were cured by this treatment: all the tumor transplants from each of these three tumors disappeared

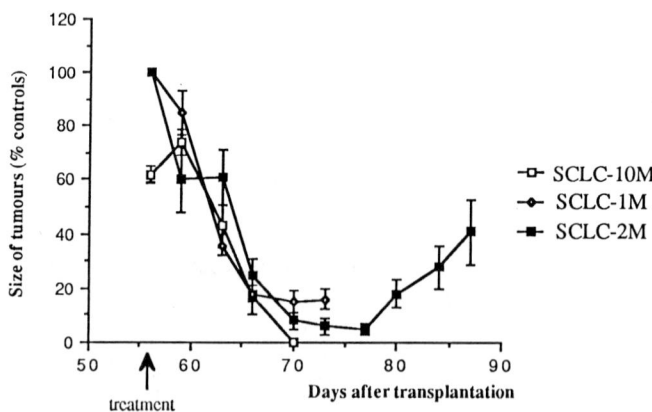

Figure 2. Antitumor effect of the "4-D" protocol in the tumors from three different patients. The SCLC-10 tumor removed from a patient with a remission for a number of years, chemocurable when it is transplanted and treated in nude mice.

completely under treatment. Only one of the three patients is alive at the present time. *Figure 2* shows the growth inhibition curves of SCLC-10M (curable), compared with those of SCLC-2M and SCLC-1M, where growth reappears after an initial strong growth inhibition. The tumor SCLC-41M is also very chemosensitive, but not chemocurable: this transplanted tumor acquires an evident chemoresistance after the fifth cycle of treatment *(Figure 4)*. The SCLC-75M *(Figure 3A)* tumor was chemosensitive, but presented an initial stimulation of volume growth, reproducible and unexpected. After the sixth transplant, this tumor became completely chemoresistant. The donor of this tumor had a very similar course: a remarkable effect after the first treatment, then relapse and rapid death. The last study was done on tumors from the

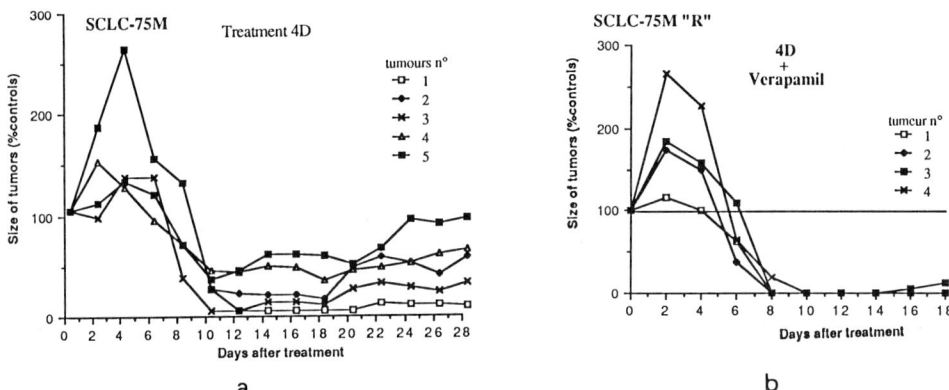

Figure 3. Above: The antitumor effect of the "4-D" protocol on the SCLC-75M tumor, preceded by an initially stimulating effect. Below: The combination with verapamil allowing complete regression in the mice.

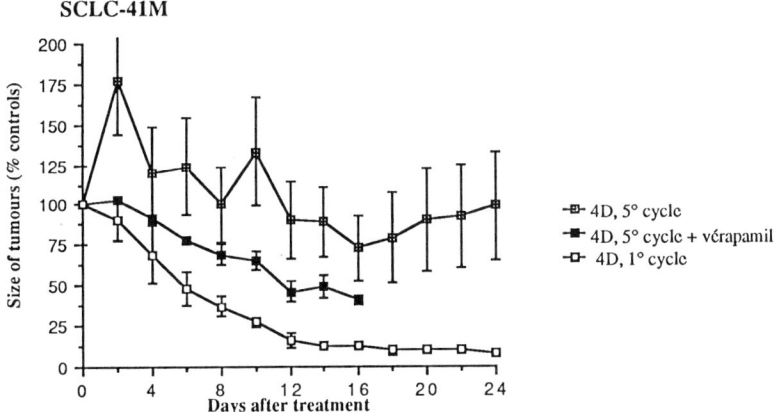

Figure 4. The antitumor effect of the "4-D" protocol in the SCLC-41 tumor, after one or five cycles of treatment. The combination of four drugs with verapamil gives an improvement of antitumor response.

same patient, removed before (-S) and after chemotherapy (-R). The SCLC-74-SM tumor is more chemosensitive that the SCLC-74-RM tumor *(Figure 5)*.

Overall this study shows that the SCLC transplants are effectively chemosensitive, as reported in the patient donors of the tumors. Some are curable with a combination of drugs as used at the Institut Gustave-Roussy. Chemoresistance appeared during the evolution of these tumors, observed either spontaneously or as a result of repeated treatments.

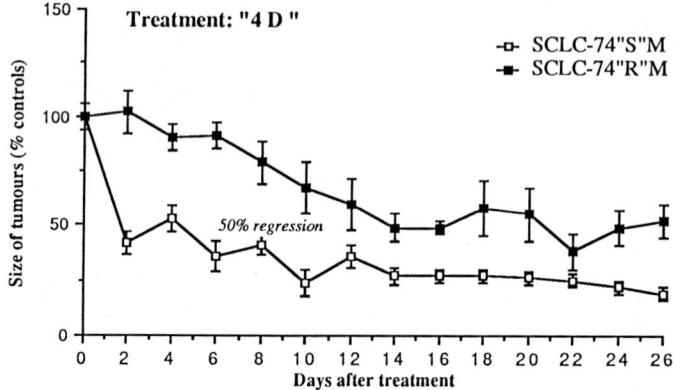

Figure 5. The comparison of the chemosensitivity of the SCLC-74 tumor removed from the same patient, and transplanted before (S) and after (R) chemotherapy.

Table I. Expression of genes and oncogenes in SCLC (semiquantitative evaluation of the amount of RNA transcripts).

	c-myc	L-myc	N-myc	Ha-ras	Ki-ras	GRP	MDR1	GST
SCLC-1M	0	0	0	0	+	0	0	0
SCLC-2M	0	0	0	+	++	+	0	+
SCLC-6M	+++	0	0	+	+++	0	0(+)[3]	+
SCLC-10M[1]	0	0	+	+	++	+	0	0
SCLC-41M	0	0	+	+++	+++	+++	0(+)	0
SCLC-61M	0	0	+	+++	+	0	0	0
SCLC-74«S»M	0	+++	0	0	+++	0	0(+)[3]	+
SCLC-74«R»M[2]	0	++	0	0	++	0	+	++
SCLC-75M	0	0	0	+	+++	++	+++++++	

[1] patient in remission, [2] treated patient, [3] in parentheses, rate expressed after various treatment cycles. 0 = non expressed, + expressed, + + + + overexpressed rate of expression of the transcripts in the total RNA extracted from tumors removed from different patients and transplanted in nude mice.

Expression of oncogenes and genes

Table I shows the level of RNA transcripts detected after extraction from the RNA of transplanted tumors. The genes belonging the myc family, c-, L- and N-, are overexpressed in four of the nine tumors. In a larger study, 11 out of 20 tumors overexpress one of these three genes. L-myc is overexpressed most often. Ki-ras and N-ras are also frequently overexpressed. An activation of the GRP gene, coding for bombesin, is common (5/9). An activation of the MDR1 gene was discovered in 2/9 tumors, one of which was SCLC-75M.

In a larger series, an increase in the rate of the MDR1 transcript was noted in 5/20 tumors. The GST gene is frequently but not intensely activated.

Study of the reversion of the multidrug chemoresistance

Numerous agents have the capacity to block the pump function of the membrane P-glycoprotein coded by the MDR1 gene. A review of these different agents is published in "les Cahiers de Cancérologie" by Chevillard *et al*. Verapamil was chosen for use in our experiments. It is administered at doses of 25 mg/kg, daily, 24 hours before the first administration of antitumor agents, and is used in combination with them. This combination is relatively toxic, and we registered a mortality of approximately 30 %. Despite this toxicity, the results clearly demonstrated that this is a promising approach. *Figure 2* shows the antineoplastic effect of this combination in the growth of the SCLC-6M tumor which became resistant after nine cycles of treatment. A

Table II. Study of the correlation between different parameters, linked to the malignancy of SCLC.

	Histology	Clinical evolution	Chemo-sensitivity	myc or GRP	mdr or GST
SCLC-1M	classic	slow	partial	0	0
SCLC-2M	variant	slow	partial	0	0
SCLC-6M	variant	intermediate	partial	+++	0 (+)[3]
SCLC-10M[1]	classic	surviving	complete	+	0
SCLC-41M	classic	-	partial	+++	0 (+)[3]
SCLC-61M	classic	slow	complete	+	0
SCLC-74«S»M	variant	rapid	weak	++	++
SCLC-74«S»M[2]	variant	rapid	none	+++	+++
SCLC-75M	classic	rapid	partial to none	+++	+++

[1] patient in remission, [2] treated patient, [3] in parentheses, rate expressed after various treatment cycles. 0 = non expressed, + expressed, ++++ overexpressed rate of expression of the transcripts in the total RNA extracted from tumors removed from different patients and transplanted in nude mice.

comparable effect was obtained in using the SCLC-41M tumor. The effect of the verapamil and the "4-D" combination on the growth of the SCLC-75M tumor — MDR1 — is remarkably positive, since we obtained complete remissions. On the other hand the SCLC-74RM tumor, obtained after the treatment of the patient, was not sensitive to this combination (results not presented).

Conclusions

The first conclusions that can be drawn from this study, which is still to be completed, are the following:
Considering the malignancy of the tumors studied, as judged by the outcome in patients treated by chemotherapy, radiotherapy and sometimes surgery, we can distinguish three different phenotypes. These appear to correspond to the different stages of disease, rather than to three types of disease: the first phenotype, the least common, is represented by the SCLC10-M tumor. It combines classical type histology, complete experimental chemosensitivity, no expression of multidrug resistance genes and a weak expression of genes involved in proliferation and represented in this tumor by the N-myc gene. A second phenotype, particularly threatening, of which the SCLC-74M tumor is representative, shows rapid progression in the patient, variant type histology, multidrug chemoresistance determined by at least two mechanisms and a very active expression of proliferation genes. A third, intermediate phenotype, is the most common in our series since we have primarily studied tumor in patients before treatment. This is represented by the SCLC-6M or 41M tumors and foreshadows what could be an evolutionary stage of SCLC: unfavorable prognosis, classical or variable histology, remarkable but partial and transient chemosensitivity and the possibility of the selection of resistant cells after treatment. One interesting phenomenon, which could herald the transition to a highly threatening phenotype, is the overexpression of genes or oncogenes coding for proteins involved in proliferation, such as the myc oncogenes or the GRP gene. From a biological point of view this relationship between a proliferative potential and an increased malignancy, linked to the acquisition of resistance to treatment, poses an interesting question. It suggests that the parental cells of the resistant variants are recruited belatedly and in response to an acceleration of cell proliferation. From a clinical standpoint, our results suggest that these SCLC tumors are the candidates of choice for an attempt to test chemosensitizers such as verapamil. As far as experimental chemotherapeutic studies are able to predict, these tumors, which have the capacity of developing multidrug resistance, can be completely eradicated by a chemotherapeutic combination of such agents.

References

1. Arriagada R, De Thé H, Le Chevalier T, *et al.* Limited small cell lung cancer : possible prognostic impact of initial chemotherapy doses. *Bull. Cancer* 1989; 76 : 605-615.
2. Brambilla E, Jacrot M, Batandier C, *et al.* Heterotransplantation of small cell lung carcinoma into nude mice. *Cancer* 1989; 64 : 1238-1247.
3. Awasthi YC, Singh SV, Ahmad H, Moller PC, Gupta V. Expression of glutathione S-transferase isoenzymes in human small cell lung cancer cell lines. *Carcinogenesis* 1988, 9 : 89-93.
4. Moody TW, Pert CB, Gazdar AF, Carney DN, Minna JD. High levels of intracellular bombesin characterize human small-cell lung carcinoma. *Science* 1981, 214 : 1246-1248.
5. Little CD, Nau MM, Carney DN, Gazdar AF, Minna JD. Amplification and expression of the c-myc oncogene in human lung cancer cell lines. *Nature* 1983; 306 : 194-196.
6. Lai S-L, Goldstein LJ, Gottesman MM. *et al.* MDR1 gene expression in lung cancer. *J Natl Cancer Inst* 1989; 81 : 1144-1150.
7. Shorthouse AJ, Peckham MJ, Smyth JF, Steel GG. The therapeutic response of bronchial carcinoma xenografts : a direct patient-xenograft comparison. *Br J Cancer* 1980; 41 : 142-145.
8. Takahashi T, Obata Y, Sekido T, *et al.* Expression and amplification of myc gene family in small cell lung cancer and its relation to biological characteristics. *Cancer Res* 1989, 49 : 2683-2688.
9. Brambilla E, Brambilla Ch. Hétérogénéité des tumeurs bronchiques malignes. *Rev Mal Resp* 1986; 3 : 235-245.
10. Chauvin C, Jacrot M, Riondel J, *et al.* Amplification of oncogenes in lung carcinoma grafted in nude mice. *Anticancer Res* 1989, 9 : 449-452.
11. Thomas F, Arriagada R, Le Chevalier T, Poupon MF. Progrès récents dans la biologie du carcinome bronchique à petites cellules. *Rev Mal Resp* 1988; 5 : 451-461.
12. Radice PA, Matthews MJ, Ihde DC, *et al.* The clinical behavior of « mixed » small cell/large cell bronchogenic carcinoma compared to « pure » small cell subtypes. *Cancer* 1982; 50 : 2894-2902.
13. Gazdar AF, Helman LJ, Israel MA, *et al.* Expression of neuroendocrine cell markers L-dopa decarboxylase, chromogranin A, and dense core granules in human tumors of endocrine and nonendocrine origin. *Cancer Res* 1988, 48 : 4078-4082.
14. Tsuruo T. Mechanisms of multidrug resistance and implications for therapy. *Jpn J Cancer Res* (Gann) 1988; 79 : 285-296.
15. Graziano SL, Cowan BY, Carney DN, *et al.* Small cell lung cancer cell line derived from a primary tumor with a characteristic deletion of 3 pl. *Cancer Res* 1987, 47, 2148-2155.
16. Mori N, Yokota J, Oshimura M, *et al.* Concordant deletions of chromosome 3p and loss of heterozygosity for chromosomes 13 and 17 in small cell lung carcinoma. *Cancer Res* 1989; 49 : 5130-5135.
17. Kartner N, Riordan J, Ling V. Cell surface P-glycoprotein associated with multidrug resistance in mammalian cell lines. *Science* 1983; 221 : 1285-1288.

11

Design and analysis of phase II cancer clinical trials. Interest of the triangular test, a group sequential method

E. BELLISSANT, J. BENICHOU, Cl. CHASTANG

Département de Biostatistique et Informatique Médicale, Formation Associée Claude-Bernard « Biostatistique et Recherche Clinique », Hôpital Saint-Louis, 1, avenue Claude-Vellefaux, 75475 Paris Cedex 10, France

Summary

In cancer, the purpose of phase II studies is to determine whether the response rate p to a new treatment is greater than a prespecified value p_o, defined as the largest response rate for which phase III studies are not worthwhile. It concerns, for example, determining whether the response rate to a new drug is greater than 20 %. The main problem is in decision making, and amounts to the comparison of an observed percentage with a theoretical percentage. One way of resolving it is to perform a single statistical analysis after the inclusion of a predetermined number of patients N, but it is not always possible because of excessively high N values. Furthermore, this approach presents ethical problems when elements in favor of inefficacy or efficacy are available early in the trial. For these reasons, several authors have developed methods which allow to perform repeated analyses and possibly to reach an early conclusion of the study : two-stage, multistage, sequential and group sequential methods.

This article considers the main decision making methods proposed in the literature for phase II studies in oncology. The bibliographic study, which highlights the interest of using group sequential methods, and especially the Triangular Test, is confirmed by a comparative study of the statistical properties of the different methods. In the final section, we discuss the practical problems arising in the design and analysis of a study using the Triangular Test.

Introduction

In cancer, phase II clinical trials are most of the time non comparative trials and aim at determining whether the efficacy of a new treatment is sufficient to warrant further studies in phase III [1, 2]. The usual endpoint in these trials is the response rate p (i.e. the success rate), estimated by the ratio of the number of observed successes S to the number of included patients N [3]. The study should be able to determine if p is greater than a prespecified value p_o, defined as the largest response rate for which the investigators consider that phase III studies are not worthwile. For example, the problem is to determine whether the response rate to a new chemotherapy is greater than 20 %. In statistical terms, the problem, of a decision-making nature, amounts to the comparison of an observed percentage (p) with a theoretical percentage (p_o), and can be expressed by the test of the null hypothesis H_o given by $p \leq p_o$ (inefficacy hypothesis) against the alternative hypothesis H_a given by $p > p_o$ (efficacy hypothesis).

To work out this problem, the simplest method consists in performing a single statistical analysis after the inclusion of a predetermined number of patients N. N is calculated by choosing p_o and the value of the type I error rate α, and by specifying the alternative hypothesis, that is by choosing the threshold response rate p_a above which the investigators consider that phase III studies are absolutely necessary (p_a corresponds to the minimum clinically interesting benefit when compared with p_o), and the value of the type II error rate ß under this particular hypothesis $p = p_a$. In practice, this single-stage design is difficult to implement due to recruitment-related (N is usually too large) and ethical problems (impossibility of stopping an ongoing study when the drug appears clearly ineffective or effective). Thus, many other methods which allow repeated analyses to be performed have been developed, their goal being the ability to stop early ongoing studies when the preliminary results show either evident inefficacy and/or efficacy. At the end of each analysis, it is possible to determine whether the study should be continued or interrupted. Some methods foresee only two stages (Gehan [4], Staquet and Sylvester [5], Sylvester and Staquet [6], Lee et al. [7]), whereas some others do not make theoretical limitations on the number of analyses (Herson [8], Fleming [9]). In these multistage methods, the number of analyses k is chosen at the beginning of the study (generally k = 2 to 4) and the required number of subjects N is divided into k groups which may be or not of equal sizes. Finally, some other methods, termed sequential methods, plan for a new analysis each time an included patient is evaluated (strictly sequential methods such as Wald's continuous Sequential Probability Ratio Test [10] or Anderson's Triangular Test [11]), or each time a sample of n included patients is evaluated (group sequential methods such as the discrete Sequential Probability Ratio Test or the Triangular Test [12]) without predetermining a maximum number of analyses.

The purpose of this article is, in the first section, to describe the main methods proposed in the literature for phase II trials in oncology, and then, in the second section, to compare their statistical properties. The third section focuses on the more practical problems that arise during the design and analysis of a phase II trial when using the method which appears to be the most interesting, namely the Triangular Test.

Main methods proposed for phase II studies in oncology : principle, advantages and disadvantages

The single stage design

This is the reference method, deduced from the 'dogma' of the analysis of a clinical trial, which allows to perform only one analysis when the predetermined number of patients have been evaluated.

Principle

As described in the introduction, it is possible, from a given set of p_o, p_a, α and β values, to calculate the required number of subjects N and the number of successes C corresponding to the decision threshold. At the end of the inclusion of N patients, the drug under study is classified as either ineffective or effective according to the observed number of responses S : if $S \leq C$, the conclusion is that the null hypothesis cannot be rejected, signifying that the response rate is not shown to be superior to p_o, and therefore that phase III studies should not be undertaken; if $S > C$, the conclusion is that the null hypothesis is rejected, signifying that the response rate is superior to p_o, and therefore that phase III studies should be considered.

Advantages

This method is easy to implement and its statistical analysis is simple to perform. In addition, it takes the predetermined type I and II error rates into account, since exact values for N and C can be calculated using the binomial distribution (S follows a binomial distribution with parameters N and p).

Disadvantages

This method is, most of the time, impossible to implement because of too high values for N : for example if $p_o = 0.20$, $p_a = 0.40$, $\alpha = \beta = 0.05$, the required number of subjects is $N = 60$. It also poses ethical and economic problems when there are early arguments in favor of inefficacy or efficacy, since it requires the inclusion of a predetermined number of patients before a conclusion can be made. For these two reasons, a great number of authors have proposed multistage methods which aim at allowing a more rapid conclusion and, consequently, a reduction in the required number of subjects.

The two-stage method proposed by Gehan (1961) [4]

This method gives an estimate of the response rate in two stages, allowing early stopping when there is a high probability that the response rate will be inferior to a predefined value. It combines testing (at the first stage) and estimation (at the second stage).

Principle

At the end of the first stage, in which n_1 subjects have been included, the decision is taken to continue or to stop the study according to the observed number of responses S : if S = 0 (no response was observed), the study is stopped and the drug is abandoned; if S > 0 (at least one response was observed), the study continues with the inclusion of n_2 subjects, this number being determined in order to estimate the success rate p with a predefined precision. The calculation of n_1 relies on the choices of the value of p_a and of the corresponding type II error rate β : n_1 is equal to the minimum number of subjects required in order that the probability of observing no success will be lower than the prespecified value β if the response rate p to the new drug is equal to p_a. For example, if the value of p_a is chosen at 20 % and β at 5 %, n_1 equals 14. The calculation of n_2 depends on the choice of a value for σ which is the standard error corresponding to the desired precision in the estimation of p : n_2 is the number of subjects to add to n_1 to estimate the response rate p with a 95 % confidence interval of width 4σ. In the former example, if the value of the observed number of responses S is equal to 2 and σ is 5 %, n_2 equals 63.

Advantages

The major advantage of this method is the simplicity of its implementation; it allows early stopping if the drug shows very poor efficacy.

Disadvantages

The major disadvantage of this method is the selection of a large number of ineffective drugs for the second stage (since type I error rate α is not taken into account) and it leads to high sample sizes if one wants to estimate p with a good precision : in the former example, if the real response rate of the drug is 5 %, the probability of making a second stage is 0.51, and the inclusion of 77 patients is required to estimate p with a precision corresponding to a standard-error σ = 5 %, that is to say a 95 % confidence interval with a width of 20 %. Furthermore, if this method gives a precise estimation of p, it does not allow (except when there is no response in the first stage) to decide whether the development of the drug must be abandoned or continued in phase III.

The multistage method proposed by Herson (1979) [8]

This is a multistage procedure (2, 3, 4 or more stages) the purpose of which is to allow early stopping when preliminary results show evident inefficacy. Herson does not consider an early stopping rule when there is a high probability of efficacy, because he believes that, in this case, it is preferable to include the entire predetermined sample N, in order to obtain a more precise estimate of the response rate and to simultaneously study the toxicity of the drug.

Principle

Given the values of p_o, p_a, α and β, the required number of patients N is calculated (the same as for the standard single stage design) and then the number of stages and the number of patients to be included at each stage are chosen. At the end of each stage, a statistical analysis is performed and the trial can be stopped. At stage g, the decision depends upon the number of responses S observed since the beginning of the trial : if $S \leq C_g$ (the threshold value at the end of stage g), the study is stopped and the drug is abandoned; if $S > C_g$, the study continues to the next stage. This procedure is repeated until the final stage k, in which $C_k = C$ (the threshold value for a single stage design including $N_k = N$ patients). The determination of the threshold value C_g is based on the calculation of the probability of observing, at the end of the trial, at most C responses on N patients when S_g responses on N_g patients (S_g and N_g being respectively the cumulated numbers of observed responses and included patients) have been observed at the end of stage g. This probability is called predictive : when it is greater than a threshold value P_o to be determined (0.85 for example), it means that there is a high probability that the number of responses at the end of the study will be inferior or equal to the final threshold value C, and that it is then possible to stop the study at this stage.

Advantages

This procedure allows early stopping if the drug under study shows evident inefficacy. When the response rate is inferior to p_a, the procedure usually requires fewer patients than the corresponding single stage design.

Disadvantages

Planning is relatively difficult, and a computer is needed to calculate C_g. Furthermore, this method takes into account various interrelated parameters and thus generates, for certain choices of p_o, p_a, α and β, cases for which it is impossible to calculate, for some given values of k and N_g, values of C_g which allow to obtain a predictive probability that is greater than or equal to the chosen threshold value P_o. Finally, the alternative possibility of early stopping when the drug shows evident efficacy is not considered.

The multistage method proposed by Fleming (1982) [9]

This is a multistage procedure (2, 3, 4 or more stages) the purpose of which is to allow early stopping when preliminary results show either evident inefficacy or efficacy.

Principle

Given the values of p_o, p_a, α and β, the required number of patients N is calculated (Fleming uses the normal approximation of the binomial distribution) and then the number of stages and the number of patients to be included at each stage are chosen as in the method proposed by Herson [8]. At the end of each stage, a statistical analysis is performed and the trial can be stopped. At stage g, the drug is classified as ineffective or effective according to the number of responses S obtained since the beginning of the trial compared with two critical values a_g and r_g ($a_g < r_g$) : if $S \leq a_g$, the study is stopped and the drug is abandoned; if $S \geq r_g$, the study is stopped and the drug is selected for phase III studies; and if $a_g < S < r_g$, the study continues until the next stage. This procedure is repeated until the final stage k where $a_k = r_k - 1$, and a decision concerning the inefficacy or the efficacy of the drug is necessarily taken. The threshold values a_g and r_g of each stage g are calculated from the standard normal approximation of the binomial distribution of the number of responses to theoretically guarantee type I and II error rates α and β for the chosen values of p_o and p_a.

Advantages

This procedure allows early stopping if the drug under study shows either evident inefficacy or efficacy.

Disadvantages

The normal approximation of the binomial distribution leads to a slight underestimation of N, and Fleming, in order to obtain a conservative enough test (i.e. a test which respect the type I error rate α) has to increase the inferior threshold values a_g. The consequence is a reduction of power, that is of the probability of detecting the efficacy of a drug whose response rate is greater than p_o.

The sequential probability ratio test (SPRT) of Wald (1947) [10]

This is the first sequential method planning a statistical analysis after each patient's inclusion. It relies on the use of a sequential plan defined by a system of orthogonal axes in which the X-axis represents the number of included patients and the Y-axis represents the number of observed responses. Two other straight parallel lines called the boundaries of the sequential plan, separate the continuation region (situated in between these lines) from the regions of non-rejection of the null hypothesis (situated below the bottom line) and of rejection of the null hypothesis (situated above the top line) *(Figure 1)*.

Principle

A statistical analysis is performed after the evaluation of each new included patient and allows to decide if the trial must be continued or stopped. The method consists in determining the coordinates of a point on the sequential plan from the numbers of included patients and observed responses since the beginning of the study.

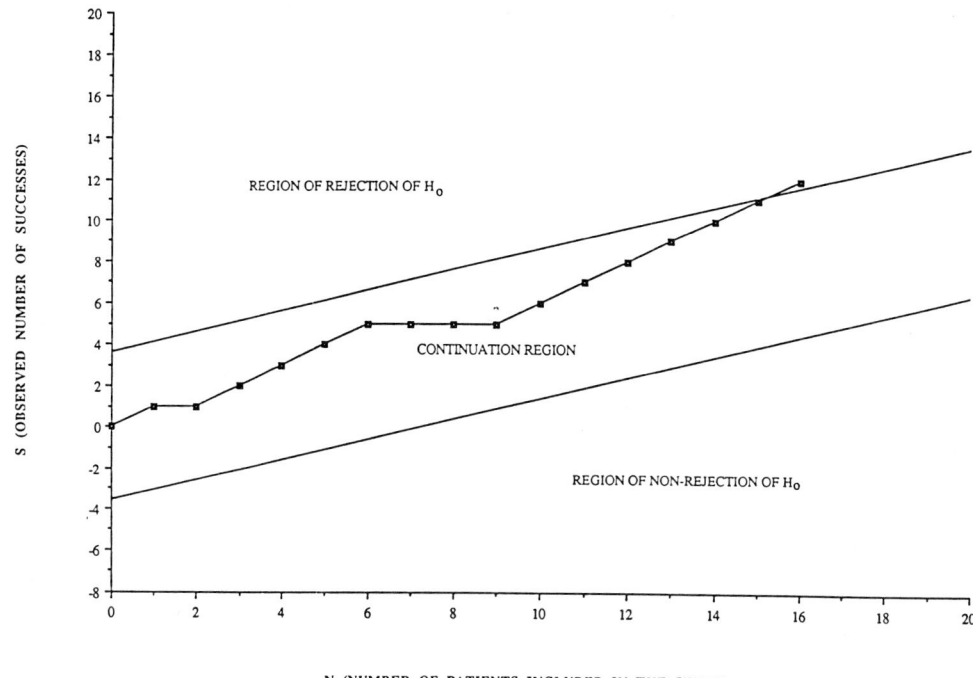

Figure 1. Wald's sequential probability ratio test : $p_o = 0.40$, $p_a = 0.60$, $\alpha = \beta = 0.05$, simulated data.

Successive points determine a sample path. As long as the path stays within the two boundary lines, the study is continued and another patient is included. When the path crosses either one of the boundaries, the study is stopped and the conclusion is obtained : crossing the bottom boundary determines that the null hypothesis should not be rejected; crossing the top boundary determines that the null hypothesis should be rejected. The equations for the boundaries depend on the values chosen for p_o, p_a, α and β. *Figure 1* shows, for example, the sequential plan obtained for $p_o = 0.40$, $p_a = 0.60$, $\alpha = 0.05$ and $\beta = 0.05$ and a path, obtained from simulated data, which leads to reject the null hypothesis after the 16th inclusion.

Advantages

This method is interesting from an ethical point of view because it allows early stopping if the drug under study shows either evident inefficacy or efficacy. Furthermore, it leads, most of the time, to an important reduction in the sample size, generally more important than those obtained with the multistage designs, while guaranteeing type I and II errors rates α and β [12].

Disadvantages

This method becomes less interesting when recruitment is rapid as compared to the delay required for obtaining responses. Furthermore, an open plan being used (the boundaries are parallel), the number of patients who can be included is potentially infinite. Moreover, in some cases, when the response rate of the drug is situated between p_o and p_a, the average sample number of patients can be greater than that of the corresponding single stage design. Finally, the likely reason this method is rarely used in practice is the difficulties of its implementation, particularly when the study is multicentric, since the analyses are extremely frequent (one after each patient).

The Triangular Test (TT) of Anderson (1960) [11]

This is a modification of Wald's SPRT presenting optimal properties, i.e. which allows the most important reduction in the average sample number of patients when p is between p_o and p_a, while guaranteeing type I and II error rates α and β. It uses a sequential plan defined by two orthogonal axes, but in which the boundaries of non rejection and of rejection of the null hypothesis converge and define, with the Y-axis, a continuation region with a triangular shape. As with the SPRT, the X-axis represents the number of included patients, the Y-axis represents the number of observed responses, the lower boundary delimits the region of non rejection of the null hypothesis, whereas the upper boundary delimits the region of rejection of this hypothesis.

Principle

An analysis is performed after each new included patient evaluation in the same way as for Wald's SPRT. The study is continued as long as the sample path remains inside the continuation region.

Advantages

The Triangular Test is a sequential method and presents the same ethical advantage as the SPRT of Wald. It has good statistical properties, and as compared to the SPRT, allows a reduction in the average sample size for the values of p situated between p_o and p_a, but this benefit is counterbalanced by a slight increase in the average sample size for the extreme values of p, inferior to p_o or superior to p_a.

Disadvantages

If the potential disadvantage of a prolonged inclusion is solved by choosing a closed continuation region, analyses should always be performed after the evaluation of each new included patient and the difficulties of implementation described previously for the SPRT, remain.

The Group sequential methods : The discrete Sequential Probability Ratio Test and the discrete Triangular Test [12]

Two sequential methods have been proposed by Jones and Whitehead in 1979 [13-16] for the analysis of comparative phase III studies, and we have extended them to the comparison of an observed percentage with a theoretical percentage (as in the non comparative phase II studies in oncology) [12]. These methods, which use the principles of Wald's Sequential Probability Ratio test and Anderson's Triangular Test respectively, do not require to perform an analysis after the evaluation of each new included patient but do allow analyses to be done after the evaluation of groups of n subjects. They use a sequential plan defined by two orthogonal axes where the X-axis represents a statistic, V, and the Y-axis, another statistic, Z. In the case of the comparison between an observed percentage and a theoretical percentage we have demonstrated [12] that these two statistics have simple expressions : $V = N p_o (1 - p_o)$ and $Z = S - Np_o$. Their interpretation is easy : Z corresponds to the difference between the number of observed responses S and the number of expected responses Np_o under the null hypothesis after the inclusion of N patients, and V represents the variance of Z under the null hypothesis. *Figure 2* is a diagram of the discrete Triangular Test.

Principle

In practice, at the end of the inclusion of a group of n patients, the two statistics Z and V are calculated from all the data collected since the beginning of the study. The point so defined is reported on the sequential plan. As soon as the sample path formed by the successive points crosses one of the boundaries of the test, the conclusion is obtained and the study is stopped. For both methods, the equations of the straight line stopping boundaries depend on the chosen values of p_o, p_a, α, β and n (which determine the frequency of analyses). *Figure 2*, displays, for example, the sequential plan obtained with the Triangular Test where $p_o = 0.40$, $p_a = 0.60$, $\alpha = 0.05$, $\beta = 0.05$ and $n = 3$ and the path obtained from the analysis of the preceding simulated data, which leads to reject the null hypothesis at the end of the sixth analysis (18th inclusion).

Advantages

The group sequential procedures keep the ethical advantages of strictly sequential methods. The study of their statistical properties shows that they have nominal type I and II error rates α and β, and they allow important reductions in the required sample size [12]. These points are discussed in greater details in the following section.

Disadvantages

As with Wald's SPRT, the discrete SPRT has the disadvantage of a potentially infinite number of analyses (open plan), which is not the case with the TT (closed plan).

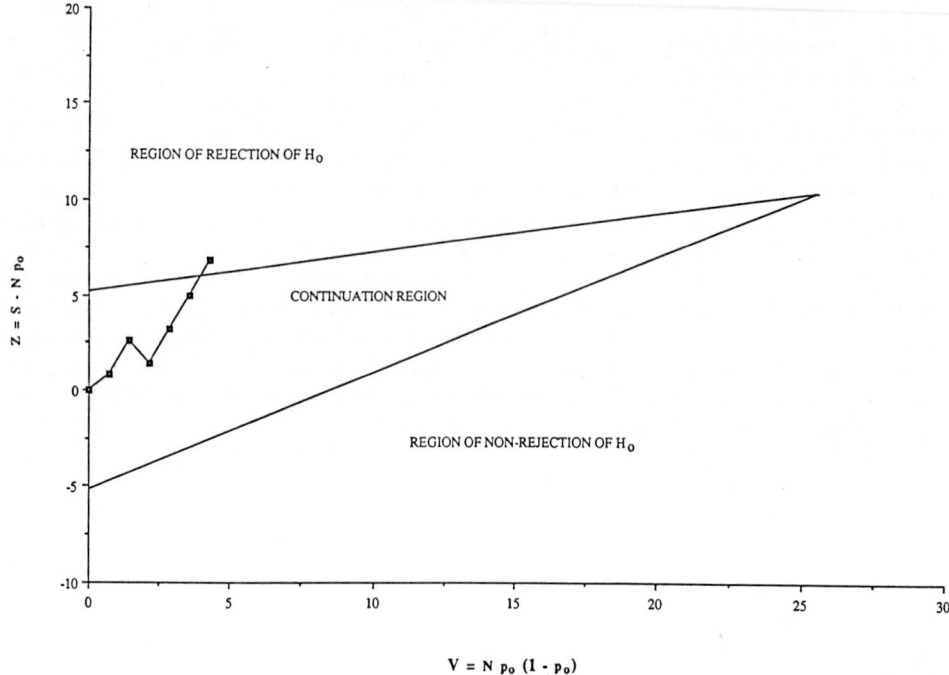

Figure 2. Triangular test : $p_o = 0.40$, $p_a = 0.60$, $\alpha = \beta = 0.05$, n = 3, simulated data.

Comparison of the statistical properties of the different methods

Methodology

In order to determine the specific advantages and disadvantages of the main methods proposed in the literature for phase II cancer clinical trials, it is necessary to compare their statistical properties in a wide range of situations. We have retained all the methods previously described with the exception of Gehan's method [4] because of its lack of decisional character and Anderson's Triangular Test [11] due to its non-utilization in oncology. Therefore, the single stage design (chosen as the reference method), the multistage designs of Herson [8] and Fleming [9], the Sequential Probability Ratio Test of Wald [10] and the group sequential methods (discrete SPRT and TT) [12] were compared. The single stage and multistage designs were studied from an analytical approach (exact calculations were made from Schultz's formulas [17]). Sequential methods were studied using simulations which led, for each studied case, to generate 30,000 phase II independent studies in which each patient could be classified as a responder (with a probability p) or a non-responder (with a probability 1-p).

In order to compare some statistical methods allowing to perform an hypothesis test, it is first necessary to verify if these methods guarantee the chosen type I and II error rates α and β, and then to study the average sample number (ASN) of patients required to reach a conclusion. The simulation study [12] allowed to estimate both the type I and II error rates α and β, and the ASN for different values of p, in different cases defined by their values of p_o, p_a, α, β and n. We have selected nine cases for p_o and p_a : (I) 0.05/0.20, (II) 0.10/0.30, (III) 0.20/0.40, (IV) 0.30/0.50, (V) 0.40/0.60, (VI) 0.50/0.70, (VII) 0.60/0.80, (VIII) 0.70/0.90 and (IX) 0.80/0.95. Concerning the type I and II error rates, we have chosen four different values for α (0.05, 0.10, 0.15 and 0.20) and only one for β because we consider, as Sylvester and Staquet [6] or Lee et al. [7], that the most important error which can occur in phase II is the inability of the study to detect an effective treatment. For each case, different values of the response rate p have been successively studied (21 values from 0.0 to 1.0 by a 0.05 step). Furthermore, the influence of the frequency of the analyses was studied considering, for multistage methods different numbers of stages (k = 2, 3 and 4), and for group sequential methods all the odd values of n between 1 and 15.

Results

Type I error rate α and power 1-β

Tables I and II, respectively, give the estimated values of the type I error rate α and the power 1-β obtained for five of the nine studied plans (I, III, V, VII, IX), and for the six methods previously presented. The k (maximum number of analyses) and n (number of subjects included at each analysis) values respectively retained for the presentation of the results of the multistage and of the group sequential methods (TT and discrete SPRT), are equal to 3 and 7, which corresponds to the intermediate values among the studied cases. The results concerning the other k and n studied values are similar and will be discussed later in the study of the influence of frequency of analyses (final subsection in this section).

For the three sequential methods (continuous SPRT of Wald, discrete SPRT and TT) and the single-stage design, the type I error rate α is always close to the target value, for each of the four studied values of α (0.05, 0.10, 0.15 and 0.20). For the only studied value of β (0.05), the power 1-β under the alternative hypothesis (p = p_a) is always close to 0.95. For Herson's multistage method, the type I error rate α is sometimes superior to the target value — for example in case VII, for a target value equal to 0.05, the observed value is 0.18 — whereas the power is always close to 0.95. For Fleming's multistage method, the type I error rate α is always inferior to the target value (due to the method of calculation used by Fleming to determine the thresholds), but the power is generally inferior to 0.95 : for example in case V, with α chosen equal to 0.05, the real power is 0.76 (or a type II error rate β of 0.24).

For the group sequential methods, we observe that the statistical properties (type I error rate α and power 1-β) of the TT and SPRT are identical to the target values for plan V (0.40/0.60). Type I error rate α and power 1-β tend to increase when p_o/p_a decreases : the type I error rate is approximately 0.07/0.06 (for a target value of 0.05) and the power is approximately 0.99/0.98 for plans I (0.05/0.20) and II (0.10/0.30) respectively. On the other hand, these probabilities tend to decrease when p_o/p_a

Table I. Type error α for the single stage design, the multi-stage designs of Herson and Fleming (k = 3), the group sequential methods (n = 7), and Wald's sequential probability ratio test.

p_o/p_a	α	Single stage	Herson (k = 3)	Fleming (k = 3)	SPRT (n = 7)	TT (n = 7)	Wald
0.05/0.20	0.05	0.04	0.03	0.03	0.09	0.07	0.03
(I)	0.10	0.07	0.06	0.07	0.13	0.12	0.06
	0.15	0.11	0.09	0.10	0.18	0.15	0.08
	0.20	0.19	0.14	0.13	0.17	0.18	0.10
0.20/0.40	0.05	0.04	0.04	0.05	0.05	0.06	0.04
(III)	0.10	0.10	0.09	0.08	0.13	0.11	0.08
	0.15	0.14	0.13	0.08	0.16	0.16	0.11
	0.20	0.17	0.16	0.12	0.18	0.21	0.15
0.40/0.60	0.05	0.05	0.09	0.04	0.06	0.05	0.04
(V)	0.10	0.08	0.15	0.09	0.10	0.10	0.08
	0.15	0.14	0.15	0.12	0.17	0.14	0.13
	0.20	0.20	0.20	0.13	0.19	0.22	0.19
0.60/0.80	0.05	0.04	0.18	0.03	0.03	0.05	0.04
(VII)	0.10	0.10	0.26	0.08	0.10	0.09	0.09
	0.15	0.13	0.26	0.10	0.13	0.16	0.13
	0.20	0.20	0.41	0.14	0.20	0.22	0.18
0.80/0.95	0.05	0.05	0.12	0.03	0.01	0.03	0.05
(IX)	0.10	0.10	0.19	0.08	0.06	0.10	0.09
	0.15	0.14	0.24	0.12	0.10	0.09	0.14
	0.20	0.18	0.35	0.09	0.25	0.24	0.17

increases : the type I error rate is approximately 0.04/0.03 (still for a target value of 0.05) and the power is approximately 0.90/0.85 for plans VIII (0.70/0.90) and IX (0.80/0.95) respectively. These small variations between the target and the observed values are related to the approximation of the normal distribution of Z (Z ~ $N(\theta V, V)$, [15]) which is less accurate when p_o and p_a move away from 0.50. Nevertheless, the differences between the observed and target values are acceptable in practice for α and β, since very low values of p_o and p_a (as in plans I and II) or very high values (as in plans VIII and IX) are rarely used in phase II cancer clinical trials.

The group sequential methods — and especially the TT — are thus methods which allow repeated analyses with good statistical properties (neither an increase of the type I error rate nor a loss of power).

Table II. Power 1-β under the alternative hypothesis (p = p_a) for the single stage design, the multi-stage designs of Herson and Fleming (k = 3), the group sequential methods (n = 7), and Wald's sequential probability ratio test.

p_o/p_a	α	Single stage	Herson (k = 3)	Fleming (k = 3)	SPRT (n = 7)	TT (n = 7)	Wald
0.05/0.20	0.05	0.95	0.93	0.92	0.99	0.99	0.85
(I)	0.10	0.96	0.94	0.92	0.98	0.99	0.82
	0.15	0.96	0.91	0.90	0.98	0.98	0.82
	0.20	0.96	0.87	0.90	0.95	0.98	0.81
0.20/0.40	0.05	0.96	0.94	0.85	0.97	0.98	0.94
(III)	0.10	0.96	0.93	0.84	0.97	0.97	0.94
	0.15	0.95	0.94	0.83	0.95	0.97	0.94
	0.20	0.96	0.94	0.80	0.94	0.97	0.94
0.40/0.60	0.05	0.95	0.94	0.76	0.95	0.95	0.96
(V)	0.10	0.95	0.95	0.81	0.94	0.95	0.96
	0.15	0.95	0.93	0.84	0.95	0.95	0.94
	0.20	0.96	0.95	0.82	0.94	0.95	0.95
0.60/0.80	0.05	0.96	0.96	0.79	0.95	0.93	0.96
(VII)	0.10	0.96	0.95	0.82	0.92	0.93	0.95
	0.15	0.96	0.94	0.85	0.92	0.93	0.96
	0.20	0.97	0.96	0.83	0.93	0.91	0.96
0.80/0.95	0.05	0.96	0.93	0.89	0.81	0.77	0.97
(IX)	0.10	0.96	0.95	0.93	0.87	0.85	0.92
	0.15	0.97	0.96	0.95	0.91	0.85	0.93
	0.20	0.96	0.93	0.85	0.93	0.91	0.92

Average sample number (ASN)

For the single stage design, the sample size depends only on p_o, p_a, α and β, whereas for the multistage and the sequential methods, it also depends on the value of the response rate p. Table III shows the ASN required to reach a conclusion under both H_o and H_a for the five plans already presented, and the six studied methods. The k and n values are not modified (k = 3 and n = 7).

As compared with the single stage design, the Triangular Test allows large decreases in the sample size which are similar to those obtained with the SPRT of Wald. Under the null (p = p_o) and the alternative (p = p_a) hypotheses, the discrete SPRT allows the same reductions as the TT. The reductions obtained with the group sequential methods are approximately of 50 % : for example, for p_o = 0.20, p_a = 0.40, α = 0.05 and β = 0.05, the single stage design requires 60 subjects whereas an average

Table III. Average sample number (ASN) under the null (p = p₀) and alternative (p = pₐ) hypotheses for the single stage design, the multi-stage designs of Herson and Fleming (k = 3), the group sequential methods (n = 7), and Wald's sequential probability ratio test.

p_o/p_a	α	Single stage	Herson (k = 3)	Fleming (k = 3)	SPRT (n = 7)	TT (n = 7)	Wald
0.05/0.20	0.05	50	31-49	34-28	41-21	47-28	20-19
(I)	0.10	44	29-43	30-25	35-18	38-20	17-14
	0.15	37	22-36	21-20	32-16	36-20	16-12
	0.20	30	18-28	20-19	26-15	30-16	15-11
0.20/0.40	0.05	60	37-59	25-28	34-28	38-32	29-27
(III)	0.10	45	29-44	20-21	31-20	31-25	26-21
	0.15	39	28-38	19-21	26-18	29-21	24-17
	0.20	36	27-35	15-15	23-17	27-18	22-15
0.40/0.60	0.05	67	37-65	25-31	34-33	38-37	37-37
(V)	0.10	56	36-55	20-25	29-26	32-29	34-27
	0.15	45	29-44	20-21	27-21	28-25	27-22
	0.20	42	30-41	17-19	24-19	26-20	24-17
0.60/0.80	0.05	60	32-59	22-30	29-34	28-31	27-31
(VII)	0.10	47	28-46	18-24	21-22	24-25	25-24
	0.15	40	24-39	18-21	20-19	20-18	23-19
	0.20	35	24-34	14-17	18-16	15-15	21-16
0.80/0.95	0.05	50	24-48	23-36	16-39	18-26	22-30
(IX)	0.10	38	22-37	22-30	16-24	14-18	18-22
	0.15	35	21-34	21-27	16-20	14-18	16-17
	0.20	27	16-26	15-21	12-12	12-14	15-15

of 38 is required under the null hypothesis (p = p₀) and 32 under the alternative hypothesis (p = pₐ) with the TT when an analysis is performed every 7 subjects. For identical values of p_o, p_a, α and β, the continuous SPRT of Wald requires respectively an average of 29 and 27 subjects under the same hypotheses. The multistage method of Herson enables under the null hypothesis similar reductions to those obtained with the group sequential methods. On the other hand, it requires under the alternative hypothesis a sample size close to that of the single stage design. In the multistage method of Fleming, reductions in the ASN under both the null and alternative hypotheses are as important as those obtained with the group sequential methods. This is, however, in part a consequence of the underestimation in the calculation of N (which leads to decrease the number of subjects included at each stage) and is obtained at the price of an important loss of power.

Figure 3 represents the ASN as a function of the value of p in case V (p_o = 0.40, p_a = 0.60) for α = β = 0.05.

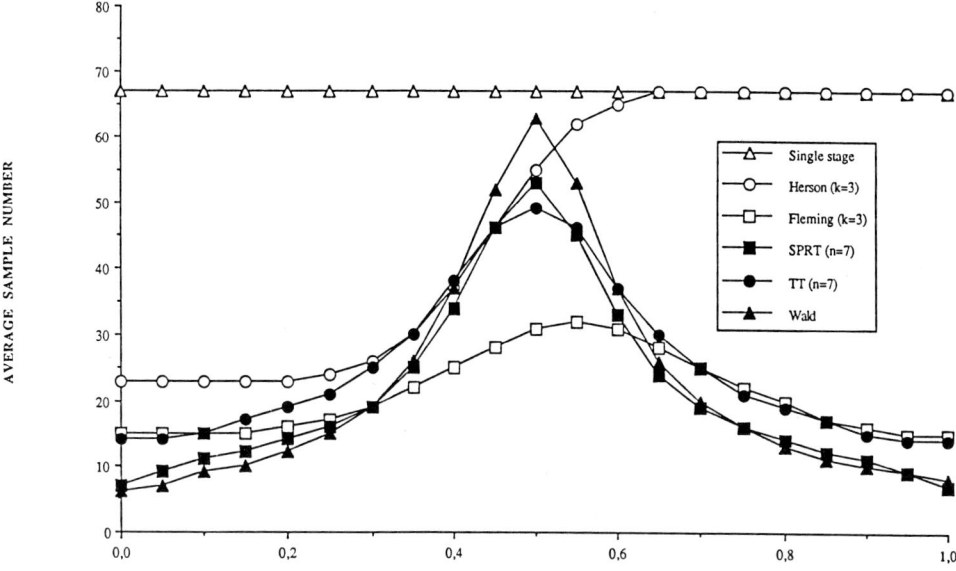

Figure 3. Average sample number (ASN) as a function of the response rate p for the single stage design, the multi-stage designs of Herson and Fleming (k = 3), the group sequential methods (n = 7), and Wald's sequential probability ratio test. Case V : $p_o/p_a = 0.40/0.60$, $\alpha = \beta = 0.05$.

For the three sequential methods the curves are symmetrical with respect to a maximal value situated between p_o and p_a. The ASN is minimal for the extreme values of p (close to 0 or 1) and increases to a reach a maximum for p = 0.50. Between p_o and p_a, the ASN is greater with the SPRT of Wald (maximum 63) and the discrete SPRT (maximum 53) than with the TT (maximum 49). However, for the values of p much lower than p_o or much higher than p_a, the SPRT allows larger reductions in the ASN. This is a classical feature of the TT [11, 16], linked to the modification of the SPRT from which it originates : the boundaries of the TT are optimal in the sense that they minimize the value of the maximal ASN (which lies between p_o and p_a). This is achieved at the cost of a small increase in the ASN on the extremities of the curve, in other words, when p is inferior to p_o or superior to p_a, since for the low values of V, the continuation region of the TT is broader than that corresponding to the SPRT. In Herson's multistage method, the decrease obtained is as high as with the sequential methods for the values of p between 0 and $(p_o + p_a)/2$. For the high values of p (p ≥ p_a), the ASN tends to be the same as the value required by the corresponding single stage design. In Fleming's multistage method, the decreases in the ASN are equal to (for the values of p inferior to p_o or superior to p_a) or larger (between p_o and p_a) than with the group sequential methods, but this is achieved at the cost of a decrease of power.

Influence of the frequency of analyses

To study the influence of the frequency of analyses on the properties of the multistage and group sequential methods, we have studied type I and II error rates α and β and the ASN under both the null ($p = p_o$) and alternative ($p = p_a$) hypotheses for different values of k and n.

Tables IV and V, respectively, present the results for the type I error rate α, the power 1-β, and the ASN under the null and alternative hypotheses for the three k (k = 2, 3 and 4) and four of the eight n (n = 1, 5, 9 and 15) studied values for case V (0.40/0.60)

For Herson's multistage method, the increase in the number of stages leads to a rise in type I error rate α, especially evident when there are more than three stages, but without any concomitant variation in the power. The ASN under H_o ($p = p_o$) is reduced when the number of stages increases, whereas it remains constant under H_a ($p = p_a$). For Fleming's multistage method, the increase in the number of stages does not lead to any variation in type I error rate α, but the power, already small, decreases with the number of stages. The ASN under H_o and H_a are inversely related to the number of stages.

For the group sequential methods, the type I error rate α and the power 1-β are not modified by the frequency of analyses (at least for $n \leq 15$). The ASN under H_o

Table IV. Type I error α, power 1-β, and average sample number (ASN) under the null ($p = p_o$) and alternative ($p = p_a$) hypotheses as functions of the number of stages for the multi-stage methods of Herson and Fleming. Case V : $p_o/p_a = 0.40/0.60$.

	α	Fleming (k = 2)	Fleming (k = 3)	Fleming (k = 4)	Herson (k = 2)	Herson (k = 3)	Herson (k = 4)
α	0.05	0.03	0.04	0.03	0.04	0.09	0.20
	0.10	0.08	0.09	0.08	0.08	0.15	0.23
	0.15	0.12	0.12	0.12	0.14	0.15	0.28
	0.20	0.14	0.13	0.17	0.18	0.20	0.37
1 - β	0.05	0.74	0.76	0.74	0.93	0.94	0.94
	0.10	0.84	0.81	0.80	0.94	0.95	0.93
	0.15	0.84	0.84	0.84	0.94	0.93	0.92
	0.20	0.86	0.82	0.83	0.94	0.95	0.96
ASN under H_o	0.05	27	25	24	44	37	35
	0.10	25	20	20	41	36	29
	0.15	22	20	19	35	29	25
	0.20	22	17	16	31	30	29
ASN under H_a	0.05	35	31	31	66	65	65
	0.10	28	25	24	55	55	53
	0.15	24	21	21	45	44	43
	0.20	22	19	16	41	41	41

Table V. Type I error α, power 1-β, and average sample number (ASN) under the null ($p = p_o$) and alternative ($p = p_a$) hypotheses as functions of the frequency of the analyses for the group sequential methods. Case V : $p_o/p_a = 0.40/0.60$.

	α	TT (n = 1)	TT (n = 5)	TT (n = 9)	TT (n = 15)	SPRT (n = 1)	SPRT (n = 5)	SPRT (n = 9)	SPRT (n = 15)
α	0.05	0.05	0.05	0.05	0.05	0.05	0.06	0.05	0.07
	0.10	0.10	0.10	0.10	0.10	0.11	0.11	0.11	0.10
	0.15	0.16	0.15	0.17	0.16	0.15	0.16	0.15	0.17
	0.20	0.21	0.19	0.18	0.20	0.20	0.20	0.21	0.18
1 - β	0.05	0.96	0.96	0.96	0.96	0.95	0.96	0.95	0.96
	0.10	0.95	0.95	0.95	0.95	0.94	0.95	0.94	0.95
	0.15	0.95	0.95	0.95	0.95	0.94	0.94	0.94	0.95
	0.20	0.95	0.95	0.93	0.95	0.93	0.94	0.95	0.95
ASN under H_o	0.05	36	38	39	42	32	35	35	38
	0.10	30	31	33	34	28	30	29	33
	0.15	26	28	28	32	24	27	28	30
	0.20	24	25	25	27	21	23	25	29
ASN under H_a	0.05	35	37	37	41	31	32	35	34
	0.10	27	28	29	32	24	25	25	29
	0.15	22	23	22	27	19	21	23	23
	0.20	18	20	21	22	16	18	19	23

and H_a increase when the frequency of analyses decreases. In practice, the impact is moderate : for example in case V ($p_o = 0.40$, $p_a = 0.60$) with $\alpha = \beta = 0.05$, the ASN under the null hypothesis is equal to 36 for n = 1, increases to 38 for n = 7 and 42 for n = 15. The results are similar for the other studied plans.

Reduction of the frequency of analyses has no influence on type I and II error rates α and β (until n = 15) and leads to a relatively small increase in the ASN. The advantage of the group sequential methods, namely the possibility of making analyses every n subjects, is not obtained at the expense of the statistical properties and thus it is unnecessary to make too many analyses. Nevertheless, we have to emphasize the fact that the ASN represents an average over simulations and that, in practice, conclusions can only be obtained for an exact multiple of n. For example, for $p_o = 0.40$, $p_a = 0.60$, $\alpha = 0.05$, $\beta = 0.05$ and n = 9, the ASN under H_o is equal to 39, but the study cannot be stopped under this hypothesis unless the number of subjects is a multiple of 9, most likely 36 or 45. Therefore, it is necessary, in order to keep the benefit of the sequential approach, not to choose too high values for n.

This comparative study of the statistical properties of the main decision making methods proposed in the literature for phase II studies makes clear the practical advantages of the sequential methods : these statistical methods, conceived with the idea of repeated analyses, are among the only methods studied which allow large reductions in the ASN with type I and II error rates close to their target values. Among them, in comparison with strictly sequential methods, the group sequential methods have the advantage of an easier implementation since it is possible to analyze the data after each group of n evaluated patients. In addition, it is preferable to use the TT because it is a closed plan with therefore a limited number of analyses.

Design and analysis of a phase II trial with the Triangular Test

Given the interest of the Triangular Test, this last section aims at helping investigators in the design and analysis of phase II trials with this method.

Design

This part of the study, which rests on the determination of the values of p_o, p_a, α, β and n, should be conducted with a particular care since it conditions the feasibility of the study, its implementation, and the results. It should be done by clinicians and biostatisticians together.

The determination of the values of the study parameters

The choice of p_o : first, we have to determine the largest response rate for which it is considered that further investigations in phase III are not worthwile. This should be done very carefully because it affects the final results of the study. As a matter of fact, whatever the method used, the statistical test can only answer one question : is p inferior or equal to p_o (non rejection of the null hypothesis) or is p superior to p_o (rejection of the null hypothesis) ? If p_o is too small, there is a risk of selecting an insufficiently effective drug for phase III studies. Conversely, if p_o is too high, there is a risk of abandoning a sufficiently effective drug. Therefore p_o should be chosen based on an in-depth knowledge of the bibliography and on a good clinical experience.

The choice of p_a : secondly, we have to determine the lowest benefit or gain clinically interesting in comparison with p_o, in other words the response rate for which investigators consider that phase III studies are absolutely necessary. This choice should also be made very carefully because it affects the required number of subjects and the probabilities of rejecting the hypothesis of inefficacy for the values of p greater than p_o : this number will be higher when the advantage the investigators want to detect is small. If p_a is too small, there is a chance of a useless increase in the required number of subjects. On the other hand, if p_a is too high, there is a chance of not detecting effective drugs with a response rate slightly superior to p_o. Then, as for p_o, the choice of p_a should be based on good clinical and bibliographic knowledge, but it is also necessary, at this stage, to consider the possibilities of recruitment.

The choices of α and β : thirdly, we have to choose the probabilities of declaring effective a drug whose response rate is equal to p_o (type I error rate α) and declaring ineffective a drug whose response rate is equal to p_a (type II error rate β). Ideally these probabilities should be as small as possible, but it is necessary to choose them so they do not affect statistical requirements and recruitment constraints. In practice there are few possibilities, the choices being usually made between 0.05 and 0.10. Error probabilities less than 5% often imply too high sample sizes, and error probabilities over 10% are too elevated and should be avoided. When two different values are chosen for α and β, it is often preferable, contrary to the rule admitted for phase III studies, to privilege β, that is to choose $\alpha > \beta$, in order to favor the probability of detecting an active drug. In practice, the choice is often $\alpha = 0.10$ and $\beta = 0.05$.

The choice of n : finally we have to define the number of subjects to be included at each stage. The higher this number, the less chance there will be of obtaining early stopping using sequential methods (a conclusion is inevitably obtained for a number of subjects that is always a multiple of n), but the simpler will be the implementation. Therefore, a compromise must be found. One solution generally acceptable for determining n is to consider the required ASN under the null hypothesis, and to divide it by 6 or 7, which usually leads to reach the conclusion with a number of analyses between 4 and 10.

When clinicians and biostatisticians have chosen values for p_o, p_a, α, β and n, which are compatible with the scientific question, the possibilities of recruitment and the implementation of the study, the calculations of the boundaries equations of the continuation region of the sequential plan can be made. The choices made during the planning phase are decisive since they have an influence both on the duration of the study and on the conclusion obtained at the end of the trial.

The determination of the boundaries equations

The boundaries, defined to warrant a type I error α and a power $1-\alpha$ (type I and II error rates both equal to α) are given by [16]:

$$Z = a + \lambda V \text{ and } Z = -a + \mu V$$

in which:

$$a = a' - 0.583\sqrt{I},$$

$$a' = \frac{2}{\theta_a} \log\left(\frac{1}{2\alpha}\right), \quad \lambda = \frac{1}{4}\theta_a \text{ and } \mu = \frac{3}{4}\theta_a,$$

$$\text{with } \theta_a = \log\left\{\frac{p_a(1 - p_o)}{p_o(1 - p_a)}\right\}.$$

The term $0.583\sqrt{I}$ is a correction to take into account the group character of the data analysis [18], I corresponding to the increase in V between two analyses for analyses performed every n patients, namely $I = n\, p_o(1 - p_o)$.

When the value chosen for β differs from the value chosen for α, it is necessary to introduce a corrected value, θ'_a given by:

$$\theta'_a = \theta_a [2\Phi^{-1}(1 - \alpha)/\{\Phi^{-1}(1 - \alpha) + \Phi^{-1}(1 - \beta)\}]$$

in which $\Phi(x)$ is the distribution function of the standardized normal distribution, namely :

$$\Phi(x) = P(X \leq x) = \int_0^x f(x)\, dx$$

where X is a random variable following the standardized normal distribution.

The correction for θ_a proceeds from the fact that Z follows asymptotically a normal distribution with mean θV and variance V. Therefore, the boundaries are calculated to guarantee a type I error rate α and power $1-\alpha$ for $\theta = \theta'_a$.

We recall that the equations of the discrete SPRT are given by :

$$Z = a + bV \text{ and } Z = -a + bV$$

in which :

$$a = a' - 0.583 \sqrt{I},$$

$$a' = \frac{1}{\theta_a} \log\left(\frac{1-\alpha}{\alpha}\right) \text{ and } b = \frac{1}{2}\theta_a,$$

with :

$$\theta_a = \log\left\{\frac{p_a(1-p_o)}{p_o(1-p_a)}\right\}.$$

Example of application

Suppose that one wants to design a phase II trial to study the effects of a new polychemotherapy treatment in lung cancer. Considering the response rates currently reported in this cancer, a response rate inferior or equal to 20 % is insufficient and justifies stopping the studies ($p_o = 0.20$). A response rate equal to 40 % constitutes an interesting advance and must be absolutely detected if true ($p_a = 0.40$), for example with a 95 % probability ($\beta = 0.05$). The required power being high, in order to limit the number of subjects, a type I error rate α superior to 5 % can be chosen, for example 10 % ($\alpha = 0.10$). Analyses can be made frequently without any difficulty, and to keep all the advantages of the sequential approach, n is chosen equal to 5. Finally, among the two group sequential methods, the Triangular Test is chosen.

The following calculations concern the determination of the boundaries of the TT where $p_o = 0.20$, $p_a = 0.40$, $\alpha = 0.10$, $\beta = 0.05$ and $n = 5$.

The calculations proceed as follows :

$\theta_a = \log\{[0.40 \times (1 - 0.20)] / [0.20 \times (1 - 0.40)]\} = \log\{0.32 / 0.12\} = 0.98$

$\theta'_a = 0.98 \times ([2 \times 1.282] / [1.282 + 1.645]) = 0.98 \times (2.56 / 2.93) = 0.98 \times 0.88 = 0.86$

$\lambda = 0.86 / 4 = 0.22$

Triangular test, sequential method

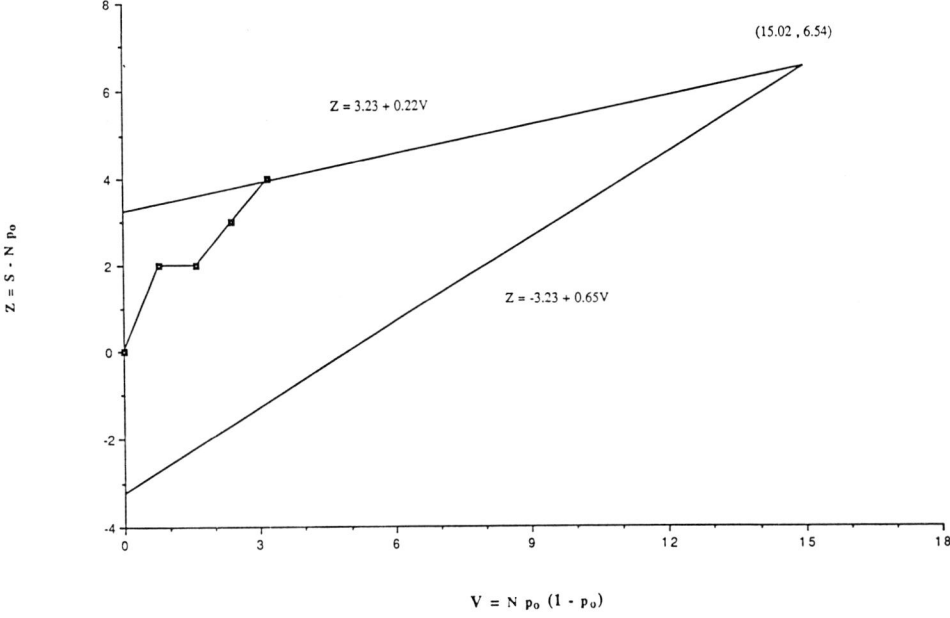

Figure 4. Example of analysis of simulated data (p = 0.35) with the triangular test : $p_o = 0.20$, $p_a = 0.40$, $\alpha = \beta = 0.05$, n = 5.

μ = [3 × 0.86] / 4 = 0.65

a' = (2 / 0.86) log { 1 / [2 × 0.10] } = 2.33 × 1.61 = 3.75

I = 5 × 0.20 × (1 − 0.20) = 0.80

a = 3.75 − 0.583 $\sqrt{0.80}$ = 3.75 − 0.52 = 3.23

Thus, we obtain the following equations for the boundaries of the sequential plan :
— for the lower boundary of non rejection of H_o : Z = − 3.23 + 0.65V
— for the upper boundary of rejection of H_o : Z = 3.23 + 0.22V

The coordinates of the point of intersection of the two axes (point of the triangle) are obtained by resolving the system based on the two preceding equations. In this case we obtain : V = 15.02 and Z = 6.54.

The corresponding sequential plan is displayed in *Figure 4*

The next phase is the inclusion and evaluation of the first five patients which enables the first analysis to be performed.

Analysis

An analysis is made each time a new group of n patients has been evaluated. It consists in determining the total number of observed responses S since the beginning of the study (after the inclusion of the first N patients) and then calculating the corresponding V and Z values according to the following formulas :

$$V = N p_o (1 - p_o)$$
$$Z = S - N p_o$$

We have simulated some data which could correspond to the preceding example (Triangular Test where $p_o = 0.20$, $p_a = 0.40$, $\alpha = 0.10$, $\beta = 0.05$, and $n = 5$). We chose the actual response rate to be 0.35 (corresponding to an effective treatment).

Table VI. Simulated data obtained with a response rate p of 0.35 : numbers of subjects included (n) and observed successes (s) at each stage and corresponding values of N, S, Z, and V.

Analysis	n	s	N	S	V	Z
1	5	3	5	3	0.80	2.00
2	5	1	10	4	1.60	2.00
3	5	2	15	6	2.40	3.00
4	5	2	20	8	3.20	4.00

Table VI presents the successive results of this simulation and V and Z values calculated at each analysis. The corresponding sample path on the sequential plan is represented on figure 4.

At the first analysis three responses were observed in five patients :

$$V = 5 \times 0.20 \times 0.80 = 0.8$$
$$Z = 3 - (5 \times 0.20) = 2$$

Since the point obtained is situated inside the continuation region, the study is continued with the inclusion of five additional patients. At the end of the second and third analyses, the path is still inside the continuation region and the study is continued. When the fourth analysis is performed, the path crosses the upper boundary and the study is stopped with the rejection of the null hypothesis.

Then, we can conclude that the chemotherapy under study displays an activity superior to 20 %. This conclusion is obtained with 20 patients whereas 45 would have been necessary with a classical single stage design. This simulation illustrates the fact that, despite an actual response rate between p_o and p_a, an important reduction in the number of subjects required to reach the conclusion is obtained by using the Triangular Test.

Development of a software for the design and analysis

We are currently developing a computer program which allows one to perform both the design and analysis of phase II studies with the Triangular Test. Based on the values chosen for the different parameters p_o, p_a, α, β and n, the option 'Design' allows to obtain, by simulation, the statistical properties of the test (i.e. the values of the type I and II error rates α and β, more generally the probability of accepting the hypothesis of inefficacy for all the values of the response rate p between 0 and 1 and multiple of 0.05) as well as the average sample number required to reach the conclusion (under both the null and the alternative hypotheses, and for all of the preceding values of p). So, this option gives a complete theoretical knowledge of the properties of the test in the cases of interest and facilitates the choice of the best compromise between the statistical constraints and the recruitment possibilities. The option 'Analysis', based on the result of each evaluated patient, allows one to calculate the values of V and Z for each analysis, and plots the sequential plan and the path from the beginning of the study to the conclusion.

Conclusion

Phase II studies in oncology whose aim is to select sufficiently effective drugs to justify further studies in phase III, lead, from a statistical point of view, to the comparison between observed and theoretical percentages. In these studies, the required number of subjects with the single stage design, calculated from the chosen values of the parameters p_o, p_a, α and β is often too high. Furthermore, it is advisable, for ethical reasons, that studies can be stopped early when the drug appears clearly ineffective or effective. To obtain a more rapid conclusion, various methods have been proposed.

Multistage methods constitute a first approach. We have shown that the method proposed by Fleming (1982) leads to important reductions in the sample size, but that this advantage is accompanied by a power much lower than expected. This makes the detection of active drugs more difficult. The bayesian method proposed by Herson (1979) also has the advantage of decreasing the sample size, but, only when the response rate to treatment is inferior to the threshold value of efficacy. When the drug has superior activity, the required number of subjects increases quickly towards the calculated value for the corresponding single stage design. In addition, the probability of concluding falsely to the efficacy of an inactive drug (type I error rate α) increases with the number of stages, particularly for three or four stages and for values of p_o/p_a superior to 0.20/0.40.

Sequential methods, and more recently, group sequential methods developed for comparative phase III trials, which we have adapted to phase II cancer clinical trials, constitute a second approach. These methods (discrete SPRT and TT), allowing analyses every n subjects to be performed, present good statistical properties (for all the studied situations, the results obtained show that type I and II error rates α and β are close to the target values) and the conclusion can be reached with a large reduction in the sample size as compared with that of the corresponding single stage design. The frequency of analyses does not affect the statistical properties, and the average sample number increases slightly when the frequency decreases ($n \leq 15$). The development of a computer program for planning and analysing phase II studies with the Triangular Test must make the use of this method easier.

Therefore, when planning a non-comparative phase II trial, there are numerous arguments in favor of using a group sequential method such as the Triangular Test:

1) It meets the need (derived from ethical considerations) of repeated analyses during the study;

2) It has good statistical properties (type I and II error rates α and β are close to their target values) and allows to reach, as compared to the single-stage design, the conclusion earlier, thus with a decrease in the sample size;

3) It is simple to implement: the boundaries of the sequential plan are easy to calculate from the values attributed to p_o, p_a, α, β and n, and the values of V and Z obtained at each analysis are easily calculated from the total number of patients included in the study and the number of corresponding observed responses; interpretation is also very straightforward;

4) Inclusion cannot be delayed indefinitely due to the closed character of the sequential plan;

5) The possibility of not performing an analysis after each patient, as with the SPRT of Wald, allows to avoid the necessity of obtaining the response quickly relative to the rate of inclusion in the study, and facilitates the implementation of the study (possibility of multicentric studies);

6) The existence of a computer program allowing both planning and analysis of these studies should also facilitate their implementation.

Due to these advantageous properties, research should be continued to find solutions to unresolved problems, namely: the calculation of the significance level, the unbiased estimation of the response rate p and of its confidence interval taking into consideration the sequential character of the analysis, and the possibility of considering covariables in the analysis.

Acknowledgements

This work was supported by grants from the ARC (Association pour la Recherche contre le Cancer) and Fondation de France.

References

1. Carter SK. Clinical Trials in Cancer Chemotherapy. *Cancer* 1977; 40 : 544-557.
2. Williams CJ, Carter SK. Management of Trials in the Development of Cancer Chemotherapy. *British Journal Cancer*, 1978; 37 : 434-447.
3. Herson J. Statistical Aspects in the Design and Analysis of Phase II Clinical Trials. *In* : Buyse ME, Staquet MJ, Sylvester RJ (Eds). *Cancer Clinical Trials : Methods and Pratice.* Oxford University Press, Oxford, England; 1984 : 239-257.
4. Gehan EA. The Determination of the Number of Patients Required in a Preliminary and a Follow-up Trial of a New Chemotherapeutic Agent. *Journal of Chronic Diseases,* 1961; 13 : 346-353.
5. Staquet M, Sylvester, R. A Decision Theory Approach to Phase II Clinical Trials. *Biomedicine,* 1977; 26 : 262-266.
6. Sylvester RJ, Staquet MJ. An Application of Decision Theory to Phase II Clinical Trials in Cancer. *In* : Tagnon HJ, Staquet MJ (Eds). *Recent Advances in Cancer Treatment.* Raven Press, New York, 1977; 1-11.
7. Lee YJ, Staquet M, Simon R, *et al.* Two-Stage Plans for Patient Accrual in Phase II Cancer Clinical Trials. *Cancer Treatment Reports,* 1979; 63 : 1721-1726.
8. Herson J. Predictive Probability Early Termination Plans for Phase II Clinical Trials. *Biometrics,* 1979; 35 : 775-783.
9. Fleming TR. One-Sample Multiple Testing Procedure for Phase II Clinical Trials. *Biometrics,* 1982; 38 : 143-151.
10. Wald A. *Sequential Analysis.* Wiley, New York 1947.
11. Anderson TW. A Modification of the Sequential Probability Ratio Test to Reduce the Sample Size. *Annals of Mathematical Statistics,* 1960; 31 : 165-197.
12. Bellissant E, Bénichou J, Chastang C. Application of the Triangular Test to Phase II Cancer Clinical Trials. *Statistics in Medicine,* 1990; 9 : 907-917.
13. Jones DR, Whitehead J. Sequential Forms of the Logrank and Modified Wilcoxon Tests for Censored Data. *Biometrika,* 1979; 66 : 105-113.
14. Whitehead J, Jones DR. The Analysis of Sequential Clinical Trials. *Biometrika,* 1979; 66 : 443-452.
15. Whitehead J. *The Design and Analysis of Sequential Clinical Trials.* Ellis Horwood, Chichester 1983.
16. Whitehead J, Stratton I. Group Sequential Clinical Trials with Triangular Continuation Regions. *Biometrics,* 1983; 39 : 227-236.
17. Schultz JR, Nichol FR, Elfring GL, Weed SD. Multiple-Stage Procedures for Drug Screening. *Biometrics,* 1973; 29 : 293-300.
18. Siegmund D. Corrected Diffusion Approximations in Certain Random Walk Problems. *Advances in Applied Probability,* 1979; 11 : 701-719.

B. Navelbine® : clinical results in non small cell lung cancer

12

Navelbine® and non small cell lung cancer. Some general remarks

R.A. JOSS

*Division of Medical Oncology, Department of Medicine
Kantonspital, Luzern, Switzerland*

Nothing in modern medical history is more tragic than the almost exponential increase in mortality from lung cancer which has occurred over the last fifty years. Almost unknown at the turn of this century, lung cancer is now the number one killer among malignant tumors in males and may soon become the most frequent form of cancer in women. This pandemic of lung cancer is a monstrous by-product of our modern society and life-style. Overwhelming evidence links the majority of lung cancers to cigarette smoking, but despite this well established association, the production and consumption of tobacco continues to increase. Every effort must be made to win the battle against tobacco, and physicians should play a leading role in this fight. But even if our preventive efforts are ultimately successful, we shall have to care for patients suffering from lung cancer over the next decades.

At the time of diagnosis the majority of patients with non small cell lung cancer will have either micrometastases not detectable by conventional diagnostic procedures or clinically manifest macrometastases. The improvement of current treatment results will therefore depend upon the development of active systemic treatments. For non small cell lung cancer this process has been frustrating. Probably in no other tumor type has single agent chemotherapy been evaluated more extensively than in non small cell lung cancer. An extensive review of single agent chemotherapy of lung cancer was published in 1979 by Cohen and Perevodchikova and we have updated this review in 1984 [1, 2].

These reviews can be summarized as follows :
— Among more than 50 agents tested only ifosfamide, mitomycin-C, fractionated vinblastine, vindesine, etoposide and cisplatin have clear-cut single agent activity. A number of other drugs have shown promising preliminary activity such as carbo-

platin [3], 10-EDAM [4] and lonidamine [5], but these results have to be confirmed by independent investigators.

— Methodological factors and patient characteristics can affect the results of phase II trials. Some of these factors, such as performance status, extent of disease, weight loss and prior cytostatic treatment, are well known. Others, such as the institution where the patient receives his treatment, are less obvious.

— Important biases can be introduced by excluding "inevaluable" cases and patients who die early in the study. In most instances, early non-toxic deaths are due to rapid disease progression and reflect the inefficacy of a given treatment.

In order to increase the efficacy of systemic treatment of non small cell lung cancer a large number of combination chemotherapy regimens have been tested in the past and only recently — with the introduction of cisplatin-based combination therapies — has there been some progress. The CAP regimen (cyclophosphamide + adriamycin + cisplatin), the combination of mitomycin-C + cisplatin + any of the vinca alkaloids (MiViP), and the combination of cisplatin + a vinca alkaloid or etoposide (ViP or VP) have led to consistent and reproducible response rates of about 30-40 % [6]. When looking at individual trials one should take into account patient characteristics, which can profoundly influence the outcome of a study. In a recently completed study of the Swiss Group for Clinical Cancer Research SAKK with the combination of mitomycin/vindesine/cisplatin a response rate of 42 % was observed in 176 evaluable patients [7]. The multivariate analysis revealed as the most important prognostic factors for response the participating institution, the number of initially involved organ sites, and weight loss. Patients with metastatic deposits in multiple organ sites had a significantly lower response rate compared to patients with locoregional disease or only one metastatic organ site (48 % for locoregional disease or one organ site versus 13 % for ≥ 2 organ sites, $p < 0.0013$). These prognostic factors were also valid for survival, together with performance status and prior radiotherapy. These results suggest that prognostic factors and the institution where the trial has been conducted can profoundly influence the outcome of a phase II trial. These factors should be taken into account when a new agent is reported to be effective in non small cell lung cancer.

Despite the improvements in response rates with newer combination chemotherapy regimens the question remains as to whether these tumor regressions will ultimately benefit the patient, i.e. lead to a better quality of life for the patient receiving treatment and/or to a prolongation of survival. Several randomized trials have recently been reported comparing best supportive care to chemotherapy. These trials are summarized in *Table I*. A consistent — albeit small — survival advantage has been observed for the chemotherapy-treated group in these trials and the differences have been statistically significant in at least two trials [9, 10]. Among the negative trials the study by the Australian Group is often cited [12]. One should note that this study had a rather critical inbalance between the 2 treatment arms with 28 % versus 11 % of the patients with multiple sites of metastatic disease in the treatment versus no-treatment group respectively. This difference may well explain the lack of a statistically significant difference between the two treatment arms. Finally one should note that in many large series a very small number of patients has enjoyed prolonged disease-free survival after cessation of chemotherapy [14].

As the development of effective combination chemotherapy regimens depends primarily on the individual activity of its components, careful clinical screening of

Table I. Chemotherapy versus best supportive care in non small cell lung cancer. Results of prospective randomised trials.

Regimen	% remissions (RC + RP)	Median survival (weeks) Chemotherapy		Control	Author (Reference)
CAMP	44 %	28	n.s.	25	Lad [8]
MACC	35 %	31	s.s.	19	Cormier [9]
CAP	15 %	25	s.s.	17	Rapp [10]
VDS/DDP	25 %	33	s.s.	17	Rapp [10]
VDS/DDP	30 %	20	n.s.	21	Ganz [11]
VDS/DDP	28 %	23	n.s.	16	Williams, Woods [12]
CEP/MEC	21 %	34	n.s.	20	Cellerino [13]

CAMP = Cyclophosphamide/Adriamycin/Methotrexate/Procarbazine
MACC = Methotrexate/Adriamycin/Cyclophosphamide/CCNU
CAP = Cyclophosphamide/Adriamycin/Cisplatin
VDS/DDP = Vindesine/Cisplatin
CEP/MEC = Cyclophosphamide/Epirubicin/Cisplatin alternating with Methrotrexate/Etoposide/CCNU

new, hopefully more active agents deserves high priority. Vinorelbine (5'-Noranhydro-vinblastine, Navelbine®) is a new semisynthetic vinca alkaloid [15]. This new agent is an attractive compound for the clinician for several reasons. First, the preliminary results suggest that vinorelbine is a highly active compound in several tumor types including non small cell lung cancer [16]. If the initial published results are confirmed, vinorelbine will belong to the most active single agents in non small cell lung cancer. Second, the side-effects are manageable and reversible. Finally, this drug is well absorbed and will be the first vinca-alkaloid which can be given orally [17], thus hopefully providing the clinician with a simple and effective outpatient treatment for the patient with non small cell lung cancer.

References

1. Cohen MH, Perevodchikova NI. Single agent chemotherapy of lung cancer. In : Muggia F, Rozencweig M. (eds). *Lung cancer : Progress in therapeutic research*. New York, Raven Press 1979 : 343-374.
2. Joss RA, Cavalli F, Goldhirsch A. et al. : New agents in non-small cell lung cancer. *Cancer Treatment Reviews* 1984; 11 : 205-236.
3. Gatzemeier U, Heckmayr M, Hossfeld DK, et al. Carboplatin in the treatment of non-small cell lung cancer. A Phase II Trial. *Contrib Oncol* 1989; 37 : 191-200.
4. Shum KY, Kris MG, Gralla ERJ, et al. Phase II study of 10-Ethyl-10-Deaza-Aminopterin in patients with stage III and IV non-small-cell lung cancer. *J. Clin Oncol* 1988; 6 : 446-450.
5. DeGregorio M, Kokron O, Scheiner W. Phase II study of Ionidamine in inoperable non-small cell lung cancer. *Proceedings of the 13th International Congress of Chemotherapy*, Vienna 1983; 248 : 97-99.

6. Joss RA, Brunner KW. Die Chemotherapie der nicht-kleinzelligen Bronchuskarzinome. *In* : Seeber S, Niederle N (eds). *Interdisziplinäre Therapie des Bronchialkarzinoms.* Berlin, Heidelberg, New York, Tokyo, Springer Verlag, 1985; 75-93.
7. Joss RA, Bürki K, Dalquen P, *et al.* Combination chemotherapy of non-small cell lung cancer with mitomycin, vindesine and cisplatin. Association of antitumor activity with initial tumor burden and treatment center. 1990; 65 : 2426-2434.
8. Lad TE, Nelson RB, Kiekamp U, *et al.* Immediate versus postponed combination chemotherapy (CAMP) for unresectable non-small cell lung cancer : a randomized trial. *Cancer Treat Rep* 1981; 65 : 973-978.
9. Cormier Y, Bergerson D, LaForge J. Benefits of polychemotherapy in advanced non-small cell bronchogenic carcinoma. *Cancer* 1982; 50 : 845-849.
10. Rapp E, Pater JL, Willan A, *et al.* Chemotherapy can prolong survival in patients with advanced non-small cell lung cancer — Report of a Canadian multicenter randomized trial. *J. Clin Oncol* 1988; 6 : 633-641.
11. Ganz PA, Figlin RA, Haskell CM, *et al.* For the UCLA Solid Tumor Study Group : Supportive care versus supportive care plus chemotherapy in advanced metastatic lung cancer : response, survival and quality of life. *Proc Am Soc Clin Oncol* 1987; 6 : 171.
12. Williams CJ, Woods R, Levi J, Page J. Chemotherapy for non-small cell lung cancer : a randomized trial of cisplatin/vindesine v no chemotherapy. *Sem Oncol* 1988; 15 (Suppl. 7) : 58-61.
13. Cellerino R, Tummarello D, Porfiri E, *et al.* Non small cell lung cancer (NSCLC). A prospective randomized trial with alternating chemotherapy CEP/MEC' versus no treatment. *Eur J. Cancer Clin Oncol* 1988; 24 : 1839-1843.
14. Finkelstein DM, Ettinger DS, Ruckdeschel JC. Long-term survivors in metastatic non-small cell lung cancer : an Eastern Cooperative Oncology Group Study. *J. Clin Oncol* 1986; 4 : 702-709.
15. Potier P. The synthesis of Navelbine® Prototype of a new series of vinblastine derivatives. *Sem Oncol* 1989; 16 (Suppl 4) : 2-4.
16. Depierre A, Lemaire E, Dabouis G, *et al.* Efficacy of Navelbine® (NVB) in non-small cell lung cancer (NSCLC). *Sem Oncol* 1989; 16 (Suppl. 4) : 26-29.
17. **Favre R, Delgado M, Rahmani R,** *et al.* **A phase I study on oral Navelbine® (NVB)** : pharmacokinetics and clinical results. Abstract O-0133, *5th European Conference on Clinical Oncology,* London, 1989.

13

Efficacy of Navelbine® and vinca alkaloids in the treatment of non small cell lung cancer (NSCLC)

A. DEPIERRE, P. JACOULET, G. GARNIER

Service de Pneumologie, CHR de Besançon, 25000 Besançon, France

Summary

Vinorelbine (NVB) was recently identified as the fourth member of the vinca alkaloids. This class of drugs exhibits notable activity in non small cell lung cancer (NSCLC), with objective response rates of 27 % (vinblastine), 12 % (vincristine), 15 % (vindesine) and 33 % (NVB : (23/78 responses) in non-pretreated patients. These agents can also be combined with cisplatin (CDDP) and response rates of 17 % and 17-46 % have been achieved with CDDP and VND-CDDP respectively. The NVB-CDDP combination is currently being investigated.

Introduction

The prognosis for NSCLC is poor in the case of nonresectable tumors, which account for 75 % of NSCLC. Patients with such tumors are usually offered systemic treatment only. Of the few active drugs known, the vinca alkaloids constitute one of the most effective classes : vinblastine (VB, Velbe®), vincristine (VCR, Oncovin®), vindesine (VND, Eldisine®) and the most recent addition, vinorelbine (NVB, Navelbine®).

Phase II studies

Vinblastine : Three phase II studies. Only the Schulman study [1] included patients with no prior treatment. Twenty-two patients were treated, 75 % with adenocarcinoma. The objective response rate was 27 % (6/22) (95 % CI : 11-50 %), with a median response duration of 22 weeks.

Vincristine : Two phase II studies. One was conducted at a single center (Brugarolas [2]), and the other by the European Organization for Research on Treatment of Cancer (EORTC). An overall response rate of 12 % (95 % CI : 5-23 %) was obtained in 65 patients, none of whom had received prior treatment.

Vindesine : Discovered in 1978, this drug has been investigated more intensively. The first study (Gralla [3]) used a dose of 3 mg/m^2/week in 46 patients, 10 of whom had received no prior treatment, and 22 % response rate was obtained. In 1987, Sorenson [4] reviewed 10 phase II studies : virtually all used a weekly regimen and 108 of the 344 patients had not been pretreated. The objective response rate was 15 % (95 % CI : 12-19 %) and the median response duration was 8-20 weeks. The only study in previously untreated patients achieved an 8 % response rate (3/37 patients).

Navelbine® : A phase II study has been conducted at 3 centers using NVB in the treatment of NSCLC. Patients with no prior treatment and no formal evidence of locoregional treatment were given 30 mg/m^2/week [5].

Of the 78 patients treated, 9 could not be evaluated for the following reasons : violation of the protocol (n = 1), early death (n = 3), loss to follow up (n = 1) and premature interruption of treatment (n = 4). 23 of the 69 patients evaluated presented a partial response. The response rates obtained were 33.3 % (95 % CI : 22-44 %) for those evaluated and 29.5 % overall. The highest response rate was seen in squamous cell carcinoma (34.7 %), although the result lacked statistical significance, nor was there any difference in response according to the stage of the disease (26.3 % for stage IV patients). The objective median response duration was 34 weeks, exceeding 1 year in 8 cases, and 18 months in 4.

Randomized studies

Of all randomized studies conducted with VLB, only that reported by Kris [6] permitted an evaluation of its efficacy. This study compared cisplatin (CDDP), combined with either VLB or VND, and gave response rates of 17 % and 20 %, response durations of 34 and 22 weeks, and 38 and 53 weeks median survival. In other words, both combinations were comparable.

Several randomized studies have included VCR in chemotherapeutic combinations without producing any clear definition of its possible benefits. Jewkes [7] compared VCR and VND and found that only VND achieved partial responses (5/35 : 14 %). However, this difference did not reach statistical significance and median survival was comparable between the two treatment groups (16 and 13 weeks respectively). In addition to these two studies, VND has also been used in various other randomized studies. Elliot [8] and Hong [9] have compared VND and CDDP. In the first study, the response rates [7 % and 33 %] and median survivals (16 and 44 weeks) differed significantly (p <-0.01). However, in the second study, response rates (3/14 : 21 % and 4/13 : 31 %) and response durations (10 and 30 weeks) showed no difference.

Shinkai [10] compared VND-MMC (mitomycin C) and VND-CDDP combinations. While the response rates obtained were significantly better with VND-CDDP (43 % vs 10 %), median survival was identical. The Memorial Sloan-Kettering Center [11] compared VND-CDDP combinations containing two different doses of CDDP (120 mg/m^2 vs 60 mg/m^2). Although response rates were similar (40 % and 46 %), the response duration with the high dose (48 weeks) was significantly higher (p < 0.02) than with the low dose (22 weeks). VND-CDDP has been compared with VLB-CDDP [12] and CDDP-VP16 (etoposide) [13], but no clear advantage has been identified for any combination. It is evident that only the VND-CDDP combination represents a significant improvement over monotherapy. Moreover, the response duration is prolonged by the inclusion of high doses of CDDP.

NVB is a relatively novel compound and it is still too soon to expect randomized studies. The first series of phase II pilot studies combining NVB and known active agents was conducted at 25 French centers under a multicenter protocol. NVB was used in combination with CDDP, ifosfamide, epirubicin, mitomycin C or etoposide. Three of these studies are reported elsewhere in this publication. The CDDP and mitomycin C combinations gave encouraging results and provide grounds for future phase III randomized studies. Two multicenter phase III randomized studies are already under way, comparing NVB alone with the NVB-CDDP combination. The first of these, conducted by T. Le Chevalier, is using a high dose of CDDP (120 mg/m^2) and gives preference to the administration of this high dose over the weekly administration of NVB. The study also contains an additional treatment group, VND-CDDP, for the purposes of comparison. The results of the preliminary feasibility study using NVB-CDDP (120 mg/m^2) are presented herein. The second study, coordinated by one of the present authors, uses a standard dose of CDDP (75 mg/m^2) in order to be able to sustain, as far as possible, the regular weekly administration of NVB.

The combination of NVB-CDDP-VP16 would appear to be of considerable interest in the light of the laboratory findings presented by S. Cros. Two similar pilot studies have been presented by Breau *et al.* and Jacoulet *et al.* and also show promising results.

Conclusion

The vinca alkaloids comprise a group of 4 active antitumor agents, the roles of which have been studied extensively in NSCLC. Among the vinca alkaloids, Navelbine® has aroused most interest owing to its higher response rates and longer response duration.

These findings provide an argument in favor of the phase III studies currently in progress.

References

1. Schulman P, Budman DR, Vinciguerra V, et al. Phase II study of divided-dose vinblastine in non-small cell bronchogenic carcinoma. *Cancer Treat Rep* 1982; 66 : 171-172.
2. Brugarolas A, Lagave AJ, Ribas A, Miralles MTG. Vincristine (NSC 67574) in non-small cell bronchogenic carcinoma. Results of a phase II clinical study. *Eur J Cancer* 1978; 14 : 501-505.
3. Gralla RJ, Raphael BG, Golbey RB, Young CW. Phase II evaluation of vindesine in patients with non-small cell carcinoma of the lung. *Cancer Treat Rep* 1979; 63 : 1343-1346.
4. Sorensen JB, Osterlind K, Hansen HH. Vinca alkaloids in the treatment of non-small cell lung cancer. *Cancer Treatment Rev* 1987; 14 : 29-51.
5. Depierre A, Lemarie E, Dabouis G, et al. Efficacy of Navelbine® (NVB) in Non-Small Cell Lung Cancer (NSCLC). *Seminars in Oncology* 1989; 16 (2), suppl. 4 (April) : 26-29.
6. Kris MG, Gralla RJ, Kalman LA, et al. Randomized trial comparing vindesine plus cisplatin with vinblastine plus cisplatin in patients with non-small cell lung cancer, with an analysis of methods of response assessment. *Cancer Treat Rep* 1985; 69 : 387-395.
7. Jewkes J, Harper PG, Tobias JS, et al. Comparison of vincristine and vindesine in the treatment of inoperable non-small cell bronchial carcinoma. *Cancer Treat Rep* 1983; 67 : 1119-1121.
8. Elliott JA, Ahmedzai S, Hole D, et al. Vindesine and cisplatin combination chemotherapy compared with vindesine as a single agent in the management of non-small cell lung cancer : a randomized study. *Eur J Cancer Clin Oncol* 1984; 20 : 1 025-1 032.
9. Hong WK, Pennacchio J, Pugatch R, et al. Vindesine versus vindesine with cis-platinum in metastatic non-small cell lung cancer. Proceedings of the international vinca alkaloid symposium — vindesine. Basel, Karger S, 1981.
10. Shinkai T, Saijo N, Tominaga K, et al. Comparison of vindesine plus cisplatin or vindesine plus mitomycin in the treatment of advanced non-small cell lung cancer. *Cancer Treat Rep* 1985; 69 : 945-951.
11. Gralla RJ, Casper ES, Kelsen DP, et al. Cisplatin and vindesine combination chemotherapy for advanced carcinoma of the lung : a randomized trial investigating two dosage schedules. *Ann Intern Med* 1981; 95 : 414-420.
12. Kris MG, Gralla RJ, Kelsen DP, et al. Randomized trial comparing vindesine plus cisplatin with vinblastine plus cisplatin in patients with non small cell lung cancer, with an analysis of methods of response assessement. *Cancer Treat Rep* 1985; 69 : 387-395.
13. Dhingra HM, Valdivieso M, Carr DT, et al. Randomized trial of three combinations of cisplatin with vindesine and/or VP-16-213 in the treatment of advanced non-small cell lung cancer. *J Clin Oncol* 1985; 3 : 176-183.

14

Presentation of Navelbine® combinations in the treatment of non small cell lung cancer

P. CARLES[1], E. QUOIX[2], J.-C. GUERIN[3], A.-B. TONNEL[4], F. BONNAUD[5], G. NOUVET[6], D. COETMEUR[7]

[1] CHR Purpan, Place du Dr-Baylac, 31059 Toulouse Cedex, France
[2] CHU, 1, place de l'Hôpital, 67000 Strasbourg, France
[3] Hôpital de la Croix-Rousse, 93, Grand Rue Croix-Rousse, 69004 Lyon, France
[4] Hôpital Albert-Calmette, boulevard Leclerc, 59037 Lille, France
[5] CHRU, 2, avenue Alexis-Carrel, 87000 Limoges, France
[6] Hôpital Charles-Nicolle, 1, rue Germont, 76031 Rouen, France
[7] Centre hospitalier, 17, rue des Capucins, 22023 St-Brieuc, France

Phase I studies (Ribaud and Mathe [2]) and phase II studies (Depierre *et al.* [3]) of the treatment of non small cell lung cancer (NSCLC) have provided clinical confirmation that the activity of Navelbine® (NVB) on tubulin is at least equal to that of vinblastine and vincristine [1], in addition to the low toxicity of the drug. Depierre *et al.* [3] have reported a 33 % response rate with NVB. Consequently, the combination of NVB with other drugs known to be active in NSCLC would seem valid. Several teams have used NVB in individual combinations with 6 other drugs in an attempt to find the most effective and best tolerated combination (that is, giving better results than with NVB alone).

The objectives of this study were :
1) to determine whether any NVB combination with another drug active in NSCLC [3, 4] is more active that NVB alone;
2) to establish the clinical and biological safety of such a combination.

Materials and methods

All patients included had nonresectable locally advanced or metastatic NSCLC and had received no prior chemotherapy. The eligibility criteria required the patient to be under 75 years of age, with at least one measurable or evaluable tumor, no brain metastasis and a performance status of 2 or less (WHO scale : 0 : normal, 1 : subnormal, 2 : 50 % active during waking hours, 3 : confined to bed or chair during more than 50 % of waking hours, 4 : completely disabled).

The present study was carried out with the collaboration of 25 pneumology centers. A weekly dose of NVB ($25\ mg/m^2$) was administered in combination with 1 of the following 6 drugs :
- cisplatin, 80 mg/m^2 every 3 weeks;
- epirubicin, 70 mg/m^2 every 3 weeks;
- actinomycin D, 0.4 mg/m^2, 3 days every 3 weeks;
- mitomycin C, 6 mg/m^2 every 3 weeks;
- etoposide, 80 mg/m^2, 3 days every 3 weeks;
- ifosfamide, 2 000 mg/m^2 every 3 weeks.

Individual results from each case file were entered into a Minitel computer database and were evaluated by the study coordinators according to the inclusion criteria. Computerized data processing and storage was also used to provide patient follow up, with laboratory data entered every week and radioscopic and endoscopic findings added as indicated under the protocol. This data collection method was employed in order to achieve more rapid analysis and speed communications between the investigators and coordinators involved.

Results

A total of 163 patients were included over a 1 year period and were grouped as follows :
- Navelbine® + cisplatin : 33 patients;
- Navelbine® + mitomycin C : 25 patients;
- Navelbine® + etoposide : 24 patients;
- Navelbine® + epirubicin : 26 patients;
- Navelbine® + ifosfamide : 31 patients;
- Navelbine® + actinomycin D : 24 patients.

Navelbine® + cisplatin, Navelbine® + mitomycin and Navelbine® + etoposide will be discussed elsewhere. The following preliminary results are available for epirubicin, ifosfamide and actinomycin D :

— Owing to the marked myelotoxicity and aplasia observed with epirubicin, it proved impossible to continue with weekly NVB administration, even after an epirubicin dose reduction.

— The dose of ifosfamide selected was too low, as was evident from the absence of both toxicity and efficacy. This finding justifies a further study using the same combination with different modalities and doses.
— Severe gastrointestinal intolerance was seen with actinomycin C, which caused vomiting and gastritis, even when the initial dose was rapidly reduced. This combination also caused severe hematologic toxicity, with one drug-related death.

Discussion

Epirubicin was selected on the basis of the following two criteria :
— the results obtained with adriamycin = 12 % of the response seen with the drug alone;
— cardiac toxicity was less than with adriamycin.

Although no conclusions as to the efficacy of this drug combination can yet be reached, the cumulative myelotoxicity of epirubicin and NVB soon proved to be excessively severe.

The initial doses of ifosfamide selected were too low to provide any indication of its activity in combination with NVB.

While, *in vitro*, the actinomycin D + NVB combination has been shown to be synergistic in mice with non small cell lung cancer xenografts (Roussakis, unpublished data), these experimental findings have not been confirmed in man.

The Minitel computer program used for data processing, storage and transfer exhibited the following advantages :
— rapid verification of patient inclusion criteria ;
— sustained contact between coordinators and investigators;
— updated record of number of inclusions;
— automatic grading of biological toxicity using the WHO scale.

It also suffered from the following drawbacks :
— prolonged transmission (owing to broken communications) and slow print-out of data sheets;
— data had to be re-entered every week;
— some teams failed to use the system correctly.

References

1. Cros S, Takoudju M, Schaepelynck-Lataste H, *et al.* Comparative *in vitro* and *in vivo* Study of Navelbine Ditartrate (Nor-5'-anhydrovinblastine) with the Two Antitumor Compounds Vinblastine and Vincristine Proceedings of the 14th International Congress of Chemotherapy, Kyoto. Recent Advances in Chemotherapy. *Anticancer Section* 1985; 1 : 477-478.

2. Ribaud P, Gouveia J, Maral R, *et al.* Phase-I study of 5'Noranhydrovinblastine (Navelbine®, NVB). *Proceedings of the 72nd International Congress of American Association for Cancer Research* 1981; Vol 22 : 368.
3. Joss RA, Cavalli F, Goldhirsh A, *et al.* New agents in non small cell lung cancer. *Cancer Treat Rev.* 1984; 11 : 205-236.
4. Lyss AP. Treatment of disseminated non-small cell lung cancer. Guidelines for the practising physician. *Postgrad* Med 1986; 80 : 119-127.

15

Phase II study of Navelbine®-cisplatin in non small cell lung cancer (NSCLC)

B. LEBEAU[1], J. CLAVIER[2], J.-P. KLEISBAUER[3], J.-L. REBISHUNG[4],
J.-F. MUIR[5], J.-M. BRECHOT[6], A. DEPIERRE[7]

[1] Hôpital Saint-Antoine, 184, faubourg Saint-Antoine, 75571 Paris Cedex 12, France
[2] CHU, 5, avenue Foch, 29285 Brest Cedex, France
[3] Hôpital Sainte-Marguerite, 270, boulevard de Sainte-Marguerite, 13009 Marseille, France
[4] Hôpital Saint-Joseph, 7, rue Pierre-Larousse, 75674 Paris, Cedex 14, France
[5] CHU Rouen, 76000 Rouen, France
[6] Hôtel-Dieu, 1, place du Parvis-Notre-Dame, 75181 Paris Cedex 04, France
[7] CHU, 2, place Saint-Jacques, 25000 Besançon, France

Summary

The combination of Navelbine® (NVB) 25 mg/m² once a week and cisplatin (CDDP) 80 mg/m² every three weeks has been used in a phase II multicenter trial. Thirty-three previously untreated patients with stages III and IV NSCLC have been included. Five patients are not evaluable for response and tolerance. Nine partial responses have been observed (32 %) with median response duration of 8.5 months. Five treatments were stopped due to toxicity (3 nephrotoxicity and 1 cachectic status). The limiting toxicity is clearly leukopenia (≥ 3 in 39 % of cures).

Navelbine® (vinorelbine NVB) is a new vinca alkaloid, the efficacy of which in single agent therapy has already been proved in the treatment of NSCLC by phase II trial on 78 patients, with a response rate of 33.3 % [1]. The first publication on the efficacy of cisplatin (CDDP) on the same cancers was reported in 1976 and was limited to partial responses in 17 patients (6 %) [2]; more recently better results have been obtained with this drug and a cumulative study of 17 trials involving 568 patients gave a response rate of 21 % for CDDP in single agent therapy [3]. It seems logical now to test the effects of a combination of CDDP and NVB in NSCLC.

Material and methods

In this study, 33 patients, 30 men and 3 women, have been included. They all had histologically proven NSCLC with no possibility of surgical treatment, and without previous chemotherapy or radiotherapy. Patient characteristics are summarized in *Table I*. In five cases no evaluation of response was possible, due to early disease-related deaths in three and to protocol violations (dose mistakes or treatment refusal) in two.

Table I. Patient characteristics

Characteristics	Number
Total number of patients	33
Number of patients evaluable for toxicity	28
Number of patients evaluable for response	28
Sex-ratio (M/F)	30/3
Histology : squamous cell	17
adenocarcinoma	14
large cell	2
Stage : IIIa	3
IIIb	9
IV	21

NVB was administered in a dose of 25 mg/m^2, diluted in 125 to 250 ml of normal saline, infused over at least a 20 minute period into a loarfe vein in a central venous access site. This infusion was given once a week except where there was hematologic toxicity grade $\geqslant$ 3. In this case, treatment was postponed until recovery. CDDP was administered every three weeks at a dose of 80 mg/m^2, diluted in 500 ml of normal saline with the usal hyperhydration and antiemetics.

The treatment was continued until progression occurred or until the appearance of severe clinical toxicity (grades 3 or 4 according to World Health Organization, WHO, criteria [4] used for evaluation of toxicity in this study). Except for patients with progressive disease, the first evaluation of efficacy was assessed during the 9 th week on measurable criteria established initially on thoracic X-ray, endoscopy and tomodensitometry. All the responses were then validated by a panel including at least the clinician from each center.

Efficacy

In the 27 evaluable patients, 9 achieved an objective response, corresponding to a 33 % response rate. According to histology the response rate was 4/17 in squamous lung cancer and 5/14 in adenocarcinoma, while none of two undifferentiated large cell lung cancer responded. Metastatic seemed to be the usual prognostic factor because 6/12 stage III cancers responded vs only 3/21 stage IV. Median response duration is more interesting to study than median survival because many patients received other treatments after progression. For the 9 responders, the median response duration was 8.5 months.

Tolerance

Tolerance was evaluated in 27 patients. Results of all the parameters studied are given in *Tables II* (clinical tolerance), *III* (biological tolerance) and *IV* (hematologic tolerance). Cutaneo-venous toxicity is not reported here. Although fairly frequent (venous induration, superficial phlebitis) it was generally localized to the venous puncture point and was reversible in two or three days.

NVB-CDDP tolerance may be indirectly assessed by calculating compliance to this combination. Only two patients received 100 % NVB and 100 % CDDP doses at the designated dates but 17 patients received more than 75 % of their treatment at the expected times; all the patients received more than 50 % of the planned treatment. The limiting toxicity is clearly leukopenia, with a leukocyte toxicity of grade $\geqslant 3$ of 39 %. The mean number of treatment cycles administered on the overall patient population was 12.5. Five treatments were stopped due to toxicity : 3 nephrotoxicities, 1 ototoxicity and one cachectic status (CDDP alone was stopped in the first four cases).

Table II. Navelbine®-cisplatin clinical tolerance (percent of patients)

	Grade				
	0	1	2	3	4
Nausea, vomiting	21	18	25	36	0
Constipation	57	36	7	0	0
Peripheral neuropathy	54	36	10	0	0
Alopecia	43	36	21	0	0

Table III. Navelbine®-cisplatin biological tolerance (percent of patients)

	Grade				
	0	1	2	3	4
Creatinine	79	18	3	0	0
Blood bilirubin	93	7	0	0	0
Alkaline phosphatase	68	25	7	0	0
Transaminases	79	3	15	3	0

Table IV. Navelbine®-cisplatin hematologic tolerance (percent of evaluable cycles)

	Grade				
	0	1	2	3	4
Hemoglobin	7	32	39	21	0
Leukocytes	4	18	39	39	0
Platelets	93	7	0	0	0

Discussion

In single agent therapy, NVB obtained a 33.3 % objective response rate [1]; here, with CDDP, NVB also gave a response rate of 33 %. Does the addition of the platinum salt fail to improve treatment efficacy ? This was not the case in previous studies of combination of CDDP and vinca alkaloids. With vindesine there was a 23 % objective response in single agent therapy which increased to 43 % with CDDP in the best study [5], and 32 % in a meta analysis of 636 patients [3]. Vinblastine gave similar results to vindesine, with greater hematologic toxicity [6]. The benefit of combined therapy was even stronger with CDDP-etoposide, where the single agent response rate was 10 % in NSCLC tumors and 30 % when administered with CDDP [3]. Do NVB and CDDP have no synergism ? Comparing our study with Depierre's, it is appearent that in the present one the percentage of patients with stage IV disease was (21/33) higher than in Depierre's study (41/78). A randomized trial would be necessary to really compare single agent and combination therapy, as has be done for vindesine-CDDP versus vindesine alone in three trials, all of which concluded in favor of the combination for objective response rate (33,25 and 27 % vs 7.22 and 14 %). Survival, which was not reported in one trial, was significantly longer with combined therapy in one of the two others [3]. It is already on record that for NVB the median response duration was 34 weeks in single agent therapy [1] and 8.5 months, i.e. 36 weeks, in the present study of combined treatment. It is possible that NVB alone gives a considerable degree of patient response with no further gain with the addition of CDDP. In conclusion, we wish to emphasize that the combination was well tolerated : NVB does not seem to increase the toxic effects of CDDP, such as vomiting and renal insufficiency. Constipation and peripheral neurologic effects seem less frequent than with other vinca alkaloids. Leukopenia is sometimes more disturbing, delaying some cycles, but no iatrogenic deaths have been observed.

References

1. Depierre A, Lemarié E, Dabouis G, et al. Efficacy of Navelbine® (NVB) in non-small cell lung cancer (NSCLC). *Semin Oncol* 1989; 16-2 (suppl. 4) : 26-29.
2. Rossof AH, Bearden JD, Coltman CA. Phase II evaluation of cis-diamminedichloroplatinum (II) in lung cancer. *Cancer Treat Rep* 1979; 60 : 1679-1680.
3. Bunn PA Jr. The expanding role of cisplatin in the treatment of non small cell lung cancer. *Semin Oncol* 1989 : 16-4 (suppl. 6) : 10-21.
4. The methodologic guidelines for reports of clinical trials. *Cancer Treat Rep* 1985; 69 : 1-3.
5. Gralla RJ, Casper ES, Kelsen DP, et al. Cisplatin and Vindesin combination chemotherapy for advanced carcinoma of the lung : a randomized trial investigating two dosage schedules. *Ann Intern Med* 1981; 95 : 414-420.
6. Kris MG, Gralla RJ, Kalman LA, et al. Randomized trial comparing vindesine plus cisplatin with vinblastin plus cisplatin in patients with non-small cell lung cancer, with an analysis of methods of response assessment. *Cancer Treat Rep* 1985 : 69; 387-395.

16

Phase I-II study of combination vinorelbine (Navelbine®) -cisplatin in advanced non small cell lung carcinoma

P. BERTHAUD[1], T. LE CHEVALIER[1], M. BESENVAL[2], R. ARRIAGADA[1], P. RUFFIÉ[1]

[1] *Institut Gustave-Roussy, 39, rue Camille-Desmoulins, 94800 Villejuif, France*
[2] *Pierre-Fabre Oncologie, 192, rue Lecourbe, 75015 Paris, France*

Summary

The promising results observed with NVB-CDDP in preclinical studies led us to perform the present phase I/II study. Thirty-two patients with advanced NSCLC and no prior chemotherapy were included from May 1988 to February 1989. There were 27 males and 5 females. Median age was 55 years (37-66). Median Karnofsky Index was 80 % (70-100). There were 18 adenocarcinomas, 9 large cell and 5 squamous cell carcinomas; 2 were stage IIIA, 11 stage IIIB, 12 stage IV and 7 with secondary metastases. Patients received CDDP 120 mg/m² IV day 1, 29, then every 6 weeks and NVB iv once a week. We tested 3 consecutive dosages for NVB : 20 mg/m² (9 patients), 25 mg/m² (6 patients) and 30 mg/m² (17 patients), the latter being the dose usually used in single agent phase II trials.

Introduction

Non small cell lung cancer (NSCLC) is the major cause of death from cancer in males in western countries [1]. Prognosis for inoperable patients is dismal and worsens with extensive disease [2]. The high proportion of patients who are initially inoperable because of disseminated disease at presentation explains the numerous attempts at developing systemic treatments over the past few years.

In fact few drugs have demonstrated any major efficacy in the multiple Phase II studies undertaken. Vindesine, a vinca alkaloid, and cisplatin were among the 5 drugs which had an objective response rate of better than 15 % in the retrospective analysis by Kris et al. [3]. More recently, a new synthetic alkaloid derived from the Madagascan periwinkle, vinorelbine, has joined the group of active cytotoxic agents for the treatment of NSCLC by establishing its activity during a Phase II trial of 78 patients, with a reported response rate of 33 % [4].

In view of response rates with combined cisplatin and a vinca alkaloid, and in particular the vindesine-cisplatin combination widely studied since 1981 [5] on the one hand, and on the other hand, the benefit established with this combination in terms of the duration of survival compared to the best supportive care available [6], we considered it worthwhile to test tolerance and efficacy of combined vinorelbine and cisplatin by conducting a Phase II study. Cisplatin was given in high dosage according to a protocol which previously demonstrated the value of high doses compared to lower doses [5].

Patients and methods

Thirty-two patients (27 men and 5 women) with inoperable NSCLC who had not received previous chemotherapy were included in the study from May 1988 to February 1989. Mean age was 55 years (range 37 to 60). The mean performance status according to the Karnofsky index was 80 %. All patients presented with advanced NSCLC. The histologic types were adenocarcinoma in 18 cases, large cell carcinoma in 9 cases and squamous cell carcinoma in 5 cases. The clinical staging of patients, according to the WHO classification, was as follows : 2 stage III A, deemed inoperable after exploratory surgery; 11 stage III B and 12 stage IV; 7 patients had metastatic disease after surgery and/or radiotherapy of the primary tumor. Neurological evaluation was normal in all patients, as were hepatic and renal functions. Patients received a chemotherapeutic regimen including cisplatin 120 mg/m^2 on days 1 and 29 and every 6 weeks thereafter; vinorelbine was given once weekly according to hematological toxicity. Three successive incremental dosage levels of vinorelbine were tested : 9 patients received a weekly dose of 20 mg/m^2, 6 patients 25 mg/m^2 and 17 patients 30 mg/m^2.

The onset of neutropenia in the first 24 patients caused the vinorelbine injection to be withheld until polynuclear neutrophils recovered to $2000/mm^3$. In the 8 other cases vinorelbine was given at the maximum planned dosage as long as the blood neutrophil count was at least $1500/mm^3$; the vinorelbine dose was decreased by 50 % in the event of neutropenia between 1000 and $1500/mm^3$; it was postponed for a week if neutropenia was lower than $1000/mm^3$. The objective of this dosage adaptation was to increase the intensity of the overall dose administered.

Results

Tolerance was good in most patients; only one grade 3 clinical toxicity according to WHO criteria [7] was observed, namely chronic neuropathy; in another case the onset of a reversible grade 1 renal failure was the reason why cisplatin dosage was reduced by a third, and there was no subsequent worsening of renal function.

Hematological toxicity was almost exclusively limited to effects on the granulocytes. The evaluation of toxicity for each vinorelbine dose level, for a total of 298 cycles, demonstrated that no grade 3 or 4 leukopenia occurred at the 20 mg/m² and 25 mg/m² levels. At the 30 mg/m² level leukopenia occurred in 21 % and 7 % of cases in the groups treated without and with vinorelbine dosage adjustment, respectively. Granulopenia occurred more frequently : 7 % grade 3 at 20 mg/m², 2 % grade 3 at 25 mg/m², 12 % grade 3 and 4 at 30 mg/m² without adjustment of dosages and 27 % grade 3 and 4 when vinorelbine doses were adjusted according to the degree of neutropenia so as to maximize the intensity of drug administration.

The respective dose intensities of vinorelbine and cisplatin, evaluated at the 10th week of treatment before the third planned injection of cisplatin, were 68 and 67 % at the 20 mg/m² vinorelbine level, 73 and 67 % at the 25 mg/m² level, and 64 and 67 % for the first 9 patients at the 30 mg/m² level. For the 8 other patients treated at the 30 mg/m² level with dose adjustments according to neutropenia, dose intensities were 84 and 87 % for vinorelbine and cisplatin respectively.

The evaluation of efficacy among the 28 patients with at least one measurable lesion did not reveal any objective responses in the 9 patients treated at the 20 mg/m² level. Two of the 3 patients evaluable for response at the 25 mg/m² level had a response better than 50 % : one of them was able to benefit from the satisfactory surgical removal of residual tumor. At the 30 mg/m² level, 5 objective responses were observed among the 16 evaluable patients; one of these patients also benefited from second line surgery. No complete response was observed.

Discussion

This phase I-II study has allowed us to demonstrate the good tolerance of high dosage cisplatin combined with vinorelbine when the latter is administered at the 30 mg/m² level according to the weekly schedule which has established its efficacy in monotherapy. This result is even more convincing when we note that the 25 mg/m² level is the threshold dose below which no objective response was observed in this study. Moreover cisplatin and vinorelbine dose intensities can be maximized by adjusting vinorelbine dosage according to granulopenia. Under these conditions hematological toxicity remains acceptable as no grade 3 and 4 neutropenia episodes were complicated by sepsis. The 7 objective responses (37 %) among the 19 evaluable patients who had received high dose cisplatin and vinorelbine at 25 mg or 30 mg/m^2 in a combined regimen justify the conduct of Phase III randomized trials comparing the efficacy of this combined regimen to that of the best current chemotherapeutic combinations. In view of the modest results usually obtained in advanced NSCLC it may prove to be useful to compare the duration of survival achieved in such studies.

References

1. Silverberg E, Lubera J. Cancer statistics, 1986. *CA* 1986; 36 : 9-25.
2. Lanzotti VJ, Thomas DR, Boyle LE, *et al.* Survival with inoperable lung cancer. An integration of prognostic variables based on simple clinical criteria. *Cancer* 1977; 39 : 303-313.
3. Kris M, Cohen E, Gralla R. New agents is non small cell lung cancer. *Proceedings of the fourth world conference on lung cancer* 1985; 4 : 119.
4. Depierre A, Lemarie E, Dabouis G *et al.* Phase II study of Navelbine (NVB) in non small cell lung cancer. *Proc Am Soc Clin Oncol,* 1988; 7 : abst. n° 778.
5. Gralla RJ, Casper ES, Kelsen DP, *et al.* Cisplatin and Vindesine combination chemotherapy for advanced carcinoma of the lung : a randomized trial investigating two dosage schedules. *Ann Intern Med* 1981; 95 : 414-420.
6. Rapp E, Pater J, Willian A, *et al.* A comparison of best supportive care to two regimens of combination chemotherapy in the management of advanced non small cell lung cancer (NSCLC). A report of a Canadian multicentre trial. *Proc Am Soc Clin Oncol* 1987; 6 : abst. n° 662.
7. WHO. Handbook for reporting results of cancer treatment. Genève, *WHO Offset publ* 1979; n° 48.

17

Phase II study of combination of Navelbine® and mitomycin C in non small cell lung cancer patients

B. MILLERON[1], C. BRAMBILLA[2], F. BLANCHON[3], F. PATTE[4], E. QUOIX[5], A. TAYTARD[6], H. NAMAN[7]

[1] Hôpital Tenon, 4, rue de la Chine, 75970 Paris Cedex 20, France
[2] CHU La Tronche, BP 217, 38043 Grenoble Cedex, France
[3] CHG, 6-8, rue Saint-Fiacre, 77104 Meaux Cedex, France
[4] CHU, 350, avenue Jacques-Cœur, 86021 Poitiers Cedex, France
[5] CHU, 1, place de l'Hôpital, 67000 Strasbourg, France
[6] CHU, 146, rue Léo-Saignat, 33076 Bordeaux Cedex, France
[7] Clinique Le Méridien, 93, avenue du Dr-Picaud, 06150 Cannes, France

Introduction

In the light of the chemotherapeutic value of mitomycin C (MTC) in non small cell lung cancer (NSCLC), especially when combined with vinca alkaloids, we decided to test this agent in combination with Navelbine® (NVB).

Patients and methods

Twenty-five patients (21 males and 4 females, mean age 59.7 ± 7.8 years) were entered into the study. All presented with previously untreated and histologically proven NSCLC (10 squamous cell, 7 adenocarcinomas and 8 large cell carcinomas), with at least one measurable or evaluable tumor. Expected survival of at least 3 months and

Table I. TNM classification (n = 25)

	Number	Stage	
T3 N2 M0	1	III A	(1)
T2 N3 M0	1		
T3 N3 M0	2		
T4 N0 M0	2	III B	(9)
T4 N1 M0	1		
T4 N2 M0	2		
T4 N3 M0	1		
T1 N3 M1	2		
T2 N1 M1	1		
T2 N2 M1	5		
T2 N3 M1	2	IV	(15)
T3 N2 M1	1		
T3 N3 M1	2		
T4 N2 M1	2		

a performance status (WHO scale) of ≤ 2 were required (0 : n = 4, 1 : n = 9, 2 : n = 11); 1 patient with a performance status of 3 was subsequently excluded. All patients gave their informed consent.

Upon inclusion, routine physical, laboratory and radiography examinations were performed on all patients, together with bronchofibroscopy, thoracic, brain and abdominal tomodensitometry (TDM) and abdominal ultrasound. These examinations were repeated after 9 and 18 cycles and then every 3 months. Ten patients were classified as stage III and 15 as stage IV *(Table I)*.

NVB was administered at a dose of 25 mg/m²/week by a 15 minutes i.v. infusion in 125 ml physiologic saline, flushed with 125 ml saline. MTC was given at a dose of 6 mg/m² i.v. every 3 weeks.

After 9 weeks, the therapeutic effect was evaluated according to standard WHO criteria by repeating the physical examination, chest film, bronchofibroscopy, thoracic TDM and any other tests that initially showed anomalies. Treatment was discontinued in any patients exhibiting a progression of the disease after 6 weeks. All observed responses were reviewed by a panel of clinicians on the basis of a global assessment of individual clinical and radiological case reports.

Results

Response was evaluated in 21 patients, 1 patient with a performance status of 3 was ineligible and 3 could not be evaluated (2 cases of premature deaths not related to

Table II. Treatment (n = 21)

1. Duration (n = 21)
   — 75-100 % within period planned (n = 15)
   — 50-75 % within period planned (n = 6)

2. Dose administered in 10 weeks (n = 16)
   — 100 % of theoretical dose (n = 4)
   — 75-100 % of theoretical dose (n = 5)
   — 50-75 % of theoretical dose (n = 7)

3. Number of cycles
   — 12.3 ± 8.2 cycles per patient
   — Median 10
   — Range 4-30

toxicity and 1 case in which the development of pneumothorax precluded repeated radiography and the consequent measurement of evaluable tumors).

The actual doses received by the 21 patients are presented in *Table II*. These patients showed 5 partial responses (23.8 %), 4 minor responses (19 %), 3 stabilizations (14.3 %) and 9 progressions (42.9 %).

Safety and toxicity were evaluated in 24 eligible patients according to the WHO criteria :

— *Gastrointestinal* : nausea, vomiting : grade 0 : n = 10, grade 1 : n = 4, grade 2 : n = 3, grade 3 : n = 4; constipation : grade 0 : n = 14 (58.3 %), grade 1 : n = 4, grade 2 : n = 5, grade 3 : n = 1.

Table III. Safety (2). Hematologic tolerance (n = 24)

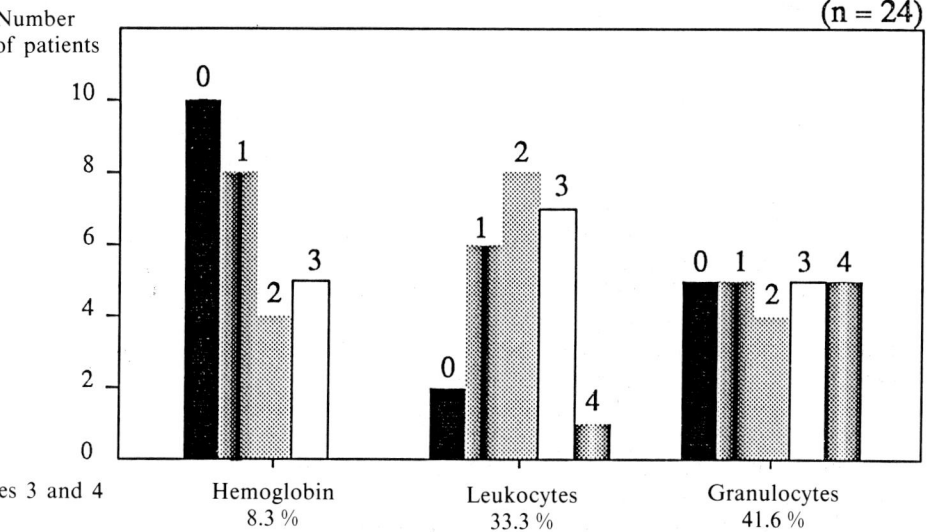

Table IV. Safety (3). Hematologic tolerance for all cycles

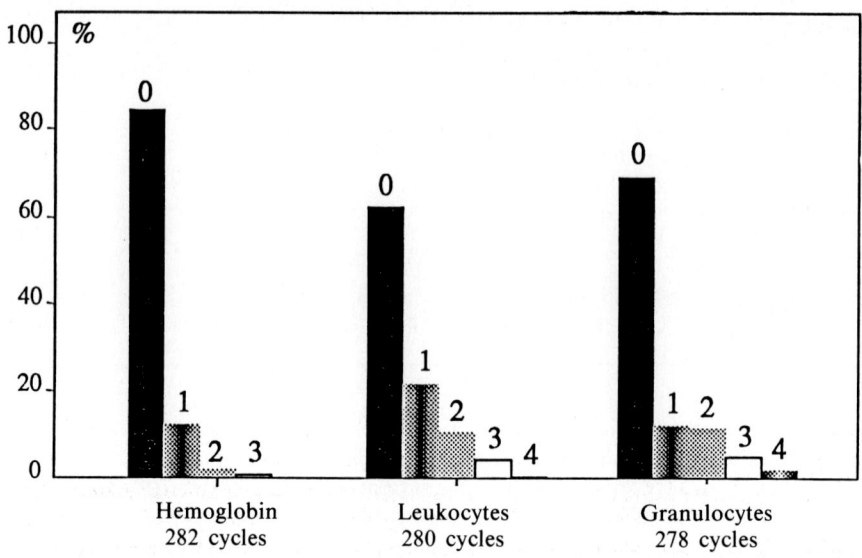

- *Paresthesia* : grade 0 : n = 20 (79.2 %), grade 1 : n = 3, grade 2 : n = 1.
- *Venous* : grade 0 : n = 21 (87.5 %), grade 1 : n = 2, grade 2 : n = 1.
- *Alopecia* : grade 0 : n = 17 (70.9 %), grade 1 : n = 4, grade 2 : n = 3.
- *Pulmonary* : absent.
- *Hematologic* : individual *(Table III)* and overall *(Table IV)* toxicity was very low.

Discussion

Many studies have investigated the use of MTC in the treatment of lung cancer in recent years. Current therapeutic regiments use MTC, alone or in combination with cisplatin (CDDP), vinblastine (VBL), vindesine (VDN) or etoposide (VP16).

Response rates with MTC-VLB, MTC-VDN, or MTC-VP16 bi-therapy range from 4.7 % to 24 % [2, 8-10]. Response rates with MTC-CDDP/VLB, VDN or VP16 show considerable variation, ranging from 10 % to 73 % [1, 3-7] and cause significant hematologic toxicity (leukopenia : 40 % [7]).

Overall survival is relatively short in these 2- and 3-drug combinations, from 18 weeks [8] to 52 weeks for responders [6].

Comparison with these results reveals the response rates obtained with the NVB-MTC combination to be comparable or superior to other MTC or vinca alkaloid combinations, in addition to the absence of serious toxicity. The high response rates seen with CDDP-MTC and vinca alkaloid combinations would indicate that the logical step is now to test the CDDP-NVB-MTC combinations.

References

1. Beck TM, Zuckerman N, Ashbaugh DG, Hart NE. Treatment of advanced non-small cell lung carcinoma with Mitomycin-C, Vinblastine and Cis-Platinum. *Proceedings Amer Soc Clin Oncol,* 1987; 6 : A734.
2. Botto HG, Marantz A, Pasccon G. Chemotherapy with mitomycin C and etoposide for advanced non small cell lung cancer. A phase II study. *Proceedings Amer Soc Clin Oncol,* 1989; 8 : A900.
3. Dhingra H, Lee J, Umsawasdi T, *et al.* Phase 2 trial of mitomycin-C, etoposide, and high dose cisplatin chemotherapy in stage IV non-small cell lung carcinoma. *Proceedings Amer Soc Clin Oncol,* 1989; 8 : A961.
4. Folman RS, Rosman M. The role of chemotherapy in non-small cell lung cancer : the community perspective. *Semin Oncol* 1986; 15 (3 sup 4) : 16-21.
5. Gralla RJ, Kris MG, Potanovich LM, *et al.* Enhancing the safety and efficacy of the MVP regiment in 100 patients with inoperable non-small cell lung cancer. *Proceedings Amer Soc Clin Oncol,* 1989; 8 : A 885.
6. Koschel G, Kaukel E, Hain E. Chemotherapie des nicht-kleinzelligen bronchialkarzinoms mit Mitomycin C, Vindesin und Cisplatin *Onkologie* 1987; 10 : 90-95.
7. Latreille J, Roy DC, Letendre F, *et al.* Mitomycin-C, Vindesine and Cis-Platinum in locally advanced and metastic non-small cell lung cancer. *Proceedings Amer Soc Clin Oncol,* 1987; 6 : A685.
8. Ruckdeschel JC, Day R, Weissman CH, *et al.* Chemotherapy for Metastatic Non-small cell bronchogenic carcinoma : Cyclophosphamide, Doxorubicin, and Etoposide versus Mitomycin and Vinblastine. *Cancer Treat Rep,* 1984; 68 : 1325-1329.
9. Shinkai T, Saijo N, Tominaga K, *et al.* Comparison of Vindesine plus Cisplatin or Vindesine plus Mitomycin in the treatment of Advanced Non-small cell lung cancer. *Cancer Treat Rep,* 1985; 69 : 945-951.
10. Weick JK, Rainey JM, Livingston RB, *et al.* Treatment of non-small cell bronchogenic carcinoma with Vinblastine and Mitomycin : A Southwest Oncology Group study. *Cancer Treat Rep,* 1985; 69 : 583-585.

18

Alternatives to cisplatin : Phase II study of combined Navelbine® and etoposide

E. LEMARIÉ[1], A. TAYTARD[2], J.-F. MUIR[3], J.-F. CORDIER[4], G. DABOUIS[5], L. JEANNIN[6], A. DEPIERRE[7]

[1] Service de Pneumologie, CHU Bretonneau, 37044 Tours Cedex, France
[2] CHU, 146, rue Léo-Saignat, 33076 Bordeaux Cedex, France
[3] CHU Rouen, 76000 Rouen, France
[4] CHU, 28, avenue Doyen-Lepine, 69394 Lyon Cedex, France
[5] Hôpital Laennec, BP1005, 44035 Nantes Cedex, France
[6] CHR La Trouhaude, rue Docteur-Calmette, 21000 Dijon, France
[7] CHU, 2, place Saint-Jacques, 25000 Besançon, France

Summary

A phase II study of combined Navelbine® (NVB) and etoposide was conducted in 23 patients with inoperable non small cell lung cancer (NSCLC) (7 adenocarcinomas, 12 squamous cell and 4 undifferentiated carcinomas) with the following stage distribution : stage I (1), stage II (1), stage IIIa (1), stage IIIb (6) and stage IV (14). NVB was administered at a dose of 25 mg/m^2/week and etoposide at a dose of 80 mg/m^2 on days 1, 2 and 3 every third week. The response could not be evaluated in 5 cases. Of the 18 patients evaluated, 3 showed partial responses (PR) (16.6 %) lasting 2, 5 and 11 months. Compliance with treatment was good. Clinical and biological tolerance was evaluated over a total of 139 3-week cycles in 21 patients : grade 1-2 nausea and vomiting were observed in 80.9 % of cycles, grade 1-2 constipation in 42.9 % and grade 1-2 neurologic toxicity in 16 %. 47.5 % of cases developed grade 1-2 anemia, 23 % developed grade 1-2 leukopenia and 9.4 % grade 3-4 leukopenia. There was no evidence of platelet, hepatic or renal toxicity. Although the NVB-etoposide combination can be administered relatively easily, it would not appear to improve the response rate in relation to the administration of NVB alone.

Introduction

The response rates obtained using chemotherapeutic combinations in the treatment of inoperable NSCLC (squamous cell, adeno- and undifferentiated carcinomas) are of the order of 20 to 30 %, with responders showing prolonged survival. On the basis of the response rate achieved using NVB alone (33.3 %) in a pilot study [1], it was deemed valid to attempt to improve this result by combining NVB with a drug of proven efficacy against this type of tumor. One such combination is NVB/etoposide. The results obtained in NSCLC patients with etoposide alone vary according to the individual study considered. In an initial study conducted by Eagan [2], an 18 % response rate was recorded at a dose of 140 mg/m^2 administered on days 1, 3 and 5 every fourth week. However, cumulative results from several other studies only produced a figure of 9 % [3]. One of the most frequent combinations is cisplatin/ etoposide, which probably exerts its effect by means of a synergistic interaction between the two drugs. A pilot study using this combination [4] produced a response rate of 38 %. In a more recent randomized study (as yet unpublished) using EORTC protocol 07861 to compare the cisplatin/etoposide and carboplatin/etoposide combinations, response rates of 27 % and 14 % respectively were obtained, with median survival times of 30 and 27 weeks.

We report below the results obtained with the NVB/etoposide combination in a randomized phase II study designed to evaluate the activity of this combination of two of the most effective drugs used to treat NSCLC.

Patients and methods

The following eligibility criteria were applied : patients aged under 75 years with a WHO performance status of 2 or less; inoperable; no prior chemotherapy or radiotherapy; presenting at least one measurable or evaluable lesion. The exclusion criteria included cerebral metastasis; the presence of a second cancer; contraindication to the administration of either of the two drugs. Normal liver function, granulocyte count in excess of 2 000/mm^3 and platelet count exceeding 100 000/mm^3 were also required before starting treatment.

The study was conducted at 8 centers in France, each center entering between 1 and 9 patients, totalling 23 (20 males and 3 females). Their mean age was 61 years (range 45-72). The histologic type distribution included 7 adenocarcinomas, 12 squamous cell and 4 undifferentiated carcinomas. Tumor extension according to the TNM classification included 1 stage I, 1 stage II, 1 stage IIIa (all 3 functionally inoperable), 6 stage IIIb and 14 stage IV cases. Of the patients with stage IV carcinomas, 2 exhibited solitary and nonresectable recurrences. The remaining 12 stage IV patients had a mean of 2 metastatic sites, involving the following tissues : bone (2), lung (5), liver (4), chest wall (3), supraclavicular and axillary nodes (2) and adrenal glands (1).

NVB was administered at a dose of 25 mg/m² on days 1, 8 and 15 and etoposide at a dose of 80 mg/m² days 1, 2 and 3 every third week. The protocol included the provision that, in the event of severe hematologic toxicity appearing in the first 3 patients, thus preventing the administration of at least 1 cycle of combined treatment and an injection of NVB alone over a 3-week period, the dose of etoposide should be reduced stepwise at 25 % intervals. Adjustment of the frequency of administration was not permitted, except for temporary delays due to hematologic toxicity. A minimum duration of 9 weeks was required before the therapeutic effects could be evaluated.

Results

The reponse could not be evaluated in 5 (22 %) of the 23 patients entered in the study. Of these 5, 2 died before completion of the study (acute pulmonary oedema unrelated to treatment and cerebrovascular accident); 1 patient was obliged to discontinue treatment during the fifth cycle owing to acute thrombosis of the legs requiring urgent surgery; and 2 declined to continue treatment following the administration of 3 and 5 cycles respectively in accordance with the study protocol.

The 18 patients in whom the response was evaluated included 3 cases of PR (16.6 % of evaluable patients and 13 % of the entire population) consisting of an undifferentiated stage IIIb carcinoma responding for 11 months, a stage IV adenocarcinoma with nodal and axillary invasion responding for 2 months, and a stage IV adenocarcinoma (isolated pulmonary recurrence) responding for 5 months. The remaining 15 evaluable patients included 3 minor responses, 2 stable diseases and 10 cases of progression.

Overall tolerance to the treatment was good. Clinical tolerance was evaluated in 21 patients over 139 cycles : 57.1 % of cases reported grade 1 nausea and 57.1 % did not develop constipation; grade 2 neurologic toxicity was observed in only 11 % of patients; grade 1-2 alopecia appeared in 56 % of patients *(Table I)*. Additionally, 2 cases of stomatitis were noted, 2 cases of asthenia and 1 case of trismus of uncertain origin. Biological tolerance was also evaluated in 21 patients over 139 cycles. 67.6 % of patients exhibited no leukocyte toxicity and 52.5 % exhibited no erythrocyte toxicity *(Table II)*. There was no evidence of platelet, hepatic or renal toxicity. The cumulative

Table I. Clinical tolerance evaluated over 139 cycles in 21 patients

	Grade 0	Grade 1	Grade 2	Grade 3	Grade 4
Nausea, vomiting	19.1 %	57.1 %	23.8 %	0	0
Constipation	57.1 %	28.6 %	14.3 %	0	0
Neurologic problems	84 %	5 %	11 %	0	0
Alopecia	25 %	23.8 %	32.1 %	19 %	0

Table II. Biological tolerance evaluated over 139 cycles in 21 patients

	Leukocytes	Hemoglobin
Grade 0	67.6 %	52.5 %
Grade 1	12.2 %	43.9 %
Grade 2	10.8 %	3.6 %
Grade 3	8.6 %	0
Grade 4	0.8 %	0

Table III. Cumulative dose given to 14 patients in the first 9 weeks of treatment

Navelbine® dose	100 %	70-100 %	50-70 %
Etoposide dose			
100 %	1	3	
70-100 %		8	1
50-75 %			1

dose of each drug administered during the first 9 weeks was calculated in 14 cases, showing that 1 patient received the scheduled dose and 11 patients received 70-100 % of this dose. Only 2 patients received as little as 50-70 % of the scheduled dose *(Table III)*. It should be noted that, owing to the leukopenia induced by the NVB/etoposide combination administered at the start of each cycle, most cycles contained 2 injections of NVB instead of 3.

This pilot study does not provide sufficient justification for continued investigation of the NVB/etoposide combination, since only 3 objective responses were obtained from 23 patients. The patient population included in this study did not appear to differ from those receiving combinations of NVB with other cytotoxic agents known to be active against NSCLC. It would therefore seem that the low response rate can be attributed to the combination itself. Although this series was short, it does not imply antagonism between NVB and etoposide, but rather that etoposide exerts no complementary effect. It is also possible that the low response rate obtained was due to the fact that, owing to the hematologic toxicity of the combination administered at the start of each cycle, the total dose of NVB given was lower than that used in the previous pilot study in which NVB was evaluated alone. Although there appears to be no antagonism or synergism between NVB and etoposide, the synergistic action observed between cisplatin and etoposide, and possibly between cisplatin and NVB, could provide grounds for testing these drugs in a triple combination (platin/etoposide/NVB).

References

1. Depierre A, Lemarié E, Dabouis G, et al. Efficacy of Navelbine® (NVB) in non-small cell lung cancer (NSCLC). *Semin Oncol*, 1989; 16 :26-29.
2. Eagan RT, Ingle JN, Creagan ET, et al. VP16-213 chemotherapy for advanced squamous cell carcinoma and adenocarcinoma of the lung. *Cancer Treat Rep*, 1978; 62:843-844.
3. Issel BF, Crooke ST. Etoposide (VP16-213). *Cancer Treat Rep*, 1979, 6:107-124.
4. Longeval E, Klastersky J. Combination chemotherapy with cisplatin and etoposide in bronchogenic squamous cell carcinoma and adenocarcinoma. *Cancer*, 1982; 50:2751-2756.

19

Alternative to cisplatin : 5FU-Navelbine® combination

J. TREDANIEL[1], V. DIERAS[2], C. FERME[3], M. MARTY[2], A. HIRSCH[1]

[1] Service de Pneumologie (Pr Hirsch), Hôpital Saint-Louis, 1, avenue Claude-Vellefaux, 75475 Paris, France
[2] Service d'Oncologie médicale, Hôpital Saint-Louis, 1, avenue Claude-Vellefaux, 75475 Paris, France
[3] Centre médico-chirurgical de Bligny, 91460 Bris-sous-Forges, France

Summary

The scheme developed and currently employed by the authors in a phase II study of the treatment of inoperable forms of non small cell lung cancer (NSCLC) consists of a chemotherapeutic combination (FUN) of 5-Fluorouracil (5FU) and Navelbine® (NVB). 5FU is administered at a dose of 750 mg/m²/day from day 1 to day 5 and NVB at a dose of 30 mg/m² on days 1 and 5 avery third week. The fundamental objective of this study is to obtain results that are as positive as those obtained with cisplatin but without the adverse gastrointestinal and renal effects noted with the latter. A sequential method of evaluation (triangular test) is used to assess therapeutic efficacy. Evaluation of tolerance in the first 13 patients entered reveals no severe hematologic or gastrointestinal toxicity.

Introduction

The current lung cancer epidemic, for which incidence and mortality are virtually synonymous, continues to rise in France, being responsible for the deaths of

20 110 individuals in 1985 (15 % of all cancer-related deaths and approximately 4 % of the overall mortality rate) [1]. While the only hope of prolonged survival is given by surgery [2], this only applies to a small percentage of cases, probably less than 20 %. The development of a therapeutic strategy for the majority of patients who are initially inoperable due to extensive local tumor, metastases or poor respiratory function constitutes the main problem.

Withholding therapy in the event of non small cell lung cancer (NSCLC) used to be the only option available to clinicians, justified by the fact that chemotherapy showed only moderate efficacy and had no effect on survival [3]. Such an attitude had a devastating effect on patients, who, with a diagnosis of untreatable terminal disease, faced an inevitable deterioration in functional and general well-being [4].

Table I. Non small cell lung cancer (stages III and IV) — Median survival (weeks). Supportive care (SC) + Chemotherapy (CT)/Supportive care (SC)

Authors	Year	Number of patients	SC + CT	SC	P	Ref.
Cormier	1982	37	30.5	8.5	0.0005	[5]
Williams	1988	188	23	16	NS	[6]
Cellerino	1988	89	34	20	NS	[7]
Rapp	1988	233	32.6/24.7*	17	0.024	[8]
Ganz	1989	63	20.4	13.6	NS	[9]

* According to the chemotherapy protocol used.

More recently, 5 trials have been published *(Table I)* [5-9] comparing no treatment («best supportive care») with chemotherapy, the only therapeutic modality that lends itself to such an approach. They all showed increased survival in patient receiving combination chemotherapy : in 2 cases [5, 8], this gain was statistically significant.

Several of the combination chemotherapy protocols used were based on cisplatin. This product no longer represents a therapeutic novelty with regard to NSCLC; while standard non-cisplatin chemotherapy regimens produce a 20 % response rate, that figure is doubled when cisplatin is incorporated [10]. Unfortunately, since its use is restricted by severe renal and gastrointestinal toxicity, therapeutic options have usually been considered in terms of the toxicity of treatment, representing a choice between prolonged survival that may prove difficult to tolerate and abstention from treatment. Notwithstanding our current detailed understanding of the link between prognostic factors and response to treatment [11-13] establishing guidelines on which to base this choice, there is still a clear need for therapeutic combinations exhibiting equivalent activity to those currently available, but with improved tolerance. The patient's quality of life should no longer have to be diminished by excessive toxicity, and all the more so in the light of the finding that active treatment actually improves the quality of life, even in nonresponders [14].

Why test the chemotherapeutic combination 5-fluoro-uracil-Navelbine® in the treatment of non small cell lung cancer ?

We considered it important to test the 5 fluoro-uracil (5FU) and Navelbine® (NVB) combination in palliative chemotherapy of NSCLC for the following reasons :
— we believe that it is generally accepted that chemotherapy produces a slight but significant increase in survival with this type of tumor;
— such prolonged survival should not be counterbalanced by a decline in the quality of life;
— phase II studies have revealed a 33 % response rate and tolerable toxicity, distinguishing Navelbine® from other recently developed drugs and ranking it as a major anti-tumor agent;
— 5FU, in combination with cisplatin, has been established as one of the most important drugs available against this pathology [16];
— although 5FU has not yet been tested in combination with Navelbine® (FUN), theoretic considerations imply that it should produce response rates identical to those of combinations already in use but with much lower toxicity, perhaps allowing the possibility of ambulatory treatment.

Patients and methods

The following eligibility criteria were applied under this protocol : patients aged under 75 years with an estimated survival of at least 8 weeks and histologically (or cytologically) confirmed inoperable NSCLC. A measurable lesion was indentified at the start of treatment and was selected as the evaluation target. In view of the difficulty frequently presented by this requirement, certain patients were entered without measurable lesions. A signed consent form was required in all cases.
　The exclusion criteria included : foreseeable noncompliance with treatment, prior chemotherapy, concomitant radiotherapy of target lesion or lesions (not excluding patients for whom palliative irradiation was indicated for non-target lesions), severe impairment of any major organ and a WHO performance status of 4.
　The initial examination included complete physical screening (testing for signs of existing peripheral neuropathy), standard laboratory tests and analysis of principal tumor markers (ACE, CA_{19-9}, SCC, NSE). The initial assessment was based on front and profile lung radiography, lung fibroscopy and biopsy, and CT scan of the thorax and upper abdomen (used to assess the condition of the liver and adrenals). Bone scintiscan and CT brain scan were performed when clinically indicated.
　The therapeutic regimen consisted of the following combination :
— 5-fluoro-uracil : 750 mg/m²/day — 5-day continuous infusion (D1-D5);
— Navelbine® : 30 mg/m²/day — 30 minute infusion on D1 and D5.

These drugs were given via a catheter surgically implanted into a central vein. It was permissible for an ambulatory medical service to administer all treatment at the patient's home. Cycles were repeated every 21 days.

Dose reductions were made according to toxicity :
— Hematologic toxicity :
WBC > 2.5 g/1 plat > 100 g/1, 5FU 100 % and NVB 100 %,
WBC > 2   g/1 plat > 75 g/1, 5FU 70 % and NVB 70 %.
Lower values required treatment to be postponed for 7 days :
— mucous toxicity : ≥ grade 3 mucitis required 30 % reduction in 5FU dose.
— neurologic toxicity : ≥ grade 3 peripheral neurotoxicity or constipation required 30 % reduction in Navelbine® dose.

Blood count was monitored every 10 days. A clinical examination, standard X-ray assessment of the target lesion and hepatic function tests were performed during every cycle. Initially elevated tumor markers were monitored every other cycle. Tolerance was evaluated according to the WHO scale (hematologic, mucous, gastrointestinal and neurologic toxicities).

Evaluation

The main objective was to evaluate the activity of the 5FU-Navelbine® combination against inoperable NSCLC on the basis of the objective response of the primary target (identified at the beginning of the study) after two cycles of chemotherapy (D42).

Complete remission was defined as the disappearance of all clinical, radiological and biological anomalies. A reduction of ≥ 50 % in the target tumor mass was defined as partial remission while a reduction of 25 % < 50 % without progression noted in other tumors was defined as stable disease. Progression was defined as the growth of the target tumor or the appearance of a tumor in a new location.

Responders exhibited complete or partial remission of the primary tumor and nonresponders showed progressive disease. Stability or any evaluation other than progression, particularly in patients with no measurable lesion, was considered an index of satisfactory therapeutic activity.

It is often unrealistic to expect responses comparable with those generally seen with most other types of cancer in patients such as these, who present extremely serious form of the disease. We consider progression-free survival and, most importantly, overall survival to be the best evaluation criteria for this protocol.

All patients were evaluated during every other cycle. Upon completion of two cycles, treatment was continued for up to 6 cycles or until progression in cases exhibiting stable disease or response. Tumoral progression was recorded as a failure of treatment.

Upon completion of six cycles :
— patients with histologically confirmed complete responses were transferred to maintenance treatment of 1 FUN cycle every 6 weeks for 8 months;

— patients exhibiting regular and progressive partial response continued to receive the treatment until an improved response was obtained, at which point they were transferred to maintenance treatment;
— where the partial response failed to improve after two cycles, maintenance treatment was commenced;
— in patients with stable disease, the treatment was continued every 4 weeks until progression.

Statistic analysis

The triangular test was selected for analysis of the results, using a sequential grouping procedure adapted from phase II studies. Taking into account the success rates recorded with existing protocols, it was decided that a final efficacy level of 20 % or less would be disregarded (justifying abandonment of the protocol) while 40 % or more would provide grounds for continuing to phase III studies. First and second type error risks were set at 5 %. This methodology required a partial analysis to be routinely performed following the inclusion of each 9 new patients.

Preliminary results

A feasibility study was conducted initially on 13 patients (mean age : 61.5 years, range : 45.5-75.2) of the following histologic types : 7 squamous cell, 3 adenocarcinomas and 3 undifferentiated carcinomas. The disease was localized within the thorax (stage III) in 5 patients and there were 8 cases of metastasis (stage IV). No patient had received prior radio- or chemotherapy. The WHO performance status scale was as follows : 0 : 3 patients; 1 : 2 patients; 2 : 5 patients; 3 : 2 patients; 4 : 1 patient.

In general, this protocol was characterized by excellent gastrointestinal, hematologic and neurologic tolerance. Toxicity was evaluated over a total of 43 cycles : 4 cycles (9 %) caused leukopenia of < 2 000/mm^3 and 9 % also caused the development of anemia < 10 g. In this preliminary analysis, hematologic toxicity seems to be sporadic and non-cumulative. Although 3 cycles caused low grade mucitis, none induced thrombocytopenia < 100 000, nausea or vomiting, evidence of neuropathy or abnormal hepatic, cardiac, renal or cutaneous function. 1 case of partial alopecia was noted during the fourth cycle.

Conclusion

The 5FU-Navelbine® combination appears to be well tolerated by patients with advanced lung cancer and shows no cumulative toxicity. Ambulatory administration is feasible. As a result of this excellent tolerance, and in accordance with the new FDA regulations governing phase II clinical studies, it has been decided to enter patients with a WHO performance status of 3. Fourteen patients are currently entered and undergoing treatment. At this preliminary stage, response rates are within permissible limits.

References

1. Hill C, Benhamou E, Doyon F, Flamant R. Statistiques de santé. *Evolution de la mortalité par cancer en France entre 1980 et 1985.* Editions INSERM, 1989.
2. Naruke T, Goya T, Tsuchiya R, Suemasu K. Prognosis and survival in resected lung carcinoma based on the new international staging system. *J Thorac Cardiovasc Surg,* 1988; 96 : 440-447.
3. Mulshine JL, Glatstein E, Ruckdeschel JC. Treatment of non small cell lung cancer. *J Clin Oncol,* 1986; 4 : 1704-1715.
4. Depierre A. La chimiothérapie apporte-t-elle un bénéfice réel aux patients porteurs d'un cancer bronchique épidermoïde non opérable ? *Rev Mal Resp,* 1986; 4 : 169-171.
5. Cormier Y, Bergeron D, La Forge J, et al. Benefits of polychemotherapy in advanced non small cell bronchogenic carcinoma. *Cancer* 1982; 50 : 845-849.
6. Williams CJ, Woods R, Levi J, Page J. Chemotherapy for non small cell lung cancer : a randomized trial of cisplatin/vindesine v no chemotherapy. *Sem Oncol* 1988; 15 : 58-61.
7. Cellerino R, Tummarello D, Porfiri E, et al. Non small cell lung cancer (NSCLC). A prospective randomized trial with alternating chemotherapy CEP/MEC versus no treatment. *Eur J Cancer Clin Oncol* 1988; 24 : 1839-1843.
8. Rapp E, Pater JL, Willian A, et al. Chemotherapy can prolong survival in patients with advanced non small cell lung cancer. Report of a Canadian multicenter randomized trial. *J Clin Oncol,* 1988; 6 : 633-64.
9. Ganz PA, Figlin RA, Haskell CM, et al. For the Ucla Solid Tumor Study Group. Supportive care versus supportive care and combination chemotherapy in metastatic non small cell lung cancer. Does chemotherapy make a difference ? *Cancer* 1989; 63 : 1271-1278.
10. Chauvergne J, Chomy P. Perspectives de la chimiothérapie des cancers bronchiques. *Rev Mal Resp* 1989; 6 : 409-416.

11. Lanzotti VJ, Thomas DR, Boyle LE, et al. Survival with inoperable lung cancer. An integration of prognostic variables based on simple clinical criteria. *Cancer*, 1977; 39 : 303-313.
12. Aisner J, Hansen HH. Current status of chemotherapy for non small cell lung cancer. *Cancer Treat Rep*, 1981; 65 : 979-986.
13. O'Connell JP, Kris MG, Gralla RJ, et al. Frequency and prognostic importance of pretreatment clinical characteristics in patients with advanced non small cell lung cancer. *J. Clin Oncol*, 1986; 4 : 1604-1614.
14. Fernandez C, Rosell R, Abad-Esteve R, et al. Quality of life during chemotherapy in non small cell lung cancer patients. *Acta Oncologica* 1989; 28 : 29-33.
15. Depierre A, Lemarie E, Dabouis G, et al. Phase II Study of Navelbine® (NVB) in non-small cell lung cancer. *Proc Am Soc Clin Oncol* 1988; 7 : 201 (Abst 778).
16. Gralla RJ, Kris MG. Chemotherapy in non small cell lung cancer : results of recent trials. *Sem Oncol*, 1988; 15 : 2-5.

20

Study of combined Navelbine®-cisplatin-VP16 in the treatment of non small cell lung cancer

P. JACOULET, A. DEPIERRE, G. GARNIER, J.-C. DALPHIN

Service de Pneumologie, CHR de Besançon, 25000 Besançon, France

Summary

The objective of the present study was to evaluate the toxicity and efficacy of the combination of Navelbine®-cisplatin and VP16 (NVB-CDDP-VP16) in nonresectable small cell lung cancer (NSCLC) using the following dose regimen : CDDP : 25-30 mg/m^2 × 3 days; VP16 : 50-80 mg/m^2 × 3 days every 3 weeks; NVB : 25 mg/m^2 × 1 day/week. Thirty-three patients were included in the study the following eligibility criteria : previously untreated histologically proven evaluable or measurable stage III or IV NSCLC. No patients were excluded on the basis of age, performance status or the presence of brain metastases (irradiated in 6/7 cases). Eleven (42 %) objective responses (OR) were observed in the 26 patients evaluated, with a median duration of 7 months (evaluated in 9/11 cases) and median survival (11 responders) of 11 months.

Hematologic toxicity was the primary limiting factor, with grade 3-4 leukopenia observed in 55 % of patients. Owing to the absence of patient selection, infectious complications developped with aplasia. The nonhematologic toxicity observed mainly consisted of gastrointestinal (21 %), renal (12 %) and local (12 %) effects. In spite of this toxicity, the response rate achieved with this regimen justifies further study.

Introduction

Although a number of drug combination protocols are effective in small cell lung cancer, no therapeutic modality has given comparable results in NSCLS, which accounts for about 75 % of all lung cancers.

While various drug combination regimens appear to have improved on the results obtained in monotherapy, complete responses (CR) are nevertheless rarely seen. The current median survival of stage IV patients is 22-26 weeks, depending on the series studied, with 17-31 % OR [1]. OR rates seen in NSCLC with monotherapy are 33 % - NVB [2], 17-26 % - cisplatin [3] and 18 % - VP16 [4]. In view of the 20-40 % OR seen with cisplatin and VP16 in first-line treatment, the addition of NVB has aroused considerable interest. We present below the results seen with combined NVB-CDDP-VP16.

Materials and methods

All patients initially presented with evaluable or measurable histologically proven stage III or IV NSCLC and had received no prior treatment.

Pretherapeutic assessment included a chest film, bronchial endoscopy and biopsy, thoracic/abdominal and brain CT scan and hepatic ultrasound. Bone scans and myelograms were not performed unless clinically indicated. No exclusion criteria were established in respect of age, performance status (PS) or metastatic dissemination. The presence of brain metastases did not preclude entry, provided that they did not serve as evaluable chemosensitivity targets.

The chemotherapy regimen used consisted of : NVB : 25 mg/m^2/week; CDDP : initial dose of 30 mg/m^2/day iv × 3 days every 3 weeks; VP16 : initial dose of 80 mg/m^2/day iv × 3 days every 3 weeks. This regimen was administered only if the leukocyte count remained over 3 000/mm^3, the platelet count remained over 150 000/mm^3 and serum creatinine remained below 120 µmol/l. If these biological parameters were not found to satisfactory, 1 or 2 of the weekly NVB cycles was eliminated in order to maintain the triple combination every 3 weeks. CDDP was suspended if serum creatinine aroused over 200 µmol/l and was reduced at 120-200 µmol/l.

Rehydration with 1 500 ml physiologic saline solution was administered over 5 h during the 3 days when CDDP was given. An injection of 120 mg methylprednisolone was given 1 h before and 4 h after the CDDP dose, together with 200 mg alizapride.

Six/seven patients with brain metastases had undergone irradiation at the start of treatment.

Clinical examination, chest film and full blood count were performed every 3 weeks. Therapeutic activity was evaluated after 2 months and then every 3 months in stable disease or response cases on the basis of the following : bronchial endoscopy with biopsy, thoracic CT scan and abdominal ultrasound. Brain CT scans were only performed in patients initially presenting with brain metastases or in the event of central nervous symptoms. Toxicity was graded according to WHO criteria [5].

A complete response (CR) was defined as the complete disappearance of tumors, confirmed by the above paraclinical examinations. A partial response (PR) corresponded to > 50 % reduction in the perpendicular diameters of the target lesion. Stabilization (S) signified either no change or < 25 % neoplastic regression.

Progression (P) was indicated by an increase in measurable or evaluable tumors and/or the appearance of new tumor sites. Treatment was continued in CR, P and S patients until progression, unless unacceptable cumulative toxicity was noted > 50 % decrease in evaluable tumor size was defined as a partial response. Response duration was calculated from the first day of the first cycle to the date of relapse. Survival corresponded to the period from the first day of the first cycle until death.

Table I. Patient characteristics (n = 33)

Sex :
    Males : 29 (87.8 %)
    Females : 4

Age :
    ≤ 70 years : 27 (81,8 %)
    > 70 years : 6
    Median = 59 (37-77)

PS :
    ≤ 2 : 20 (60.6 %)
    > 2 : 13

Histological type :
    Squamous cell carcinoma : 14
    Adenocarcinoma : 16
    Large cell carcinoma : 3

Stage :
    III : 9 (III a : 4, III b : 5)
    IV : 24 (72.7 %)

Metastatic sites :
    Liver : 9
    Bone : 8
    Brain : 7
    Lung : 5
    Lymph nodes : 4
    Adrenals : 3
    Skin : 3
    Bone marrow : 2

Results

Thirty-three patients were entered in the study between September 1987 and September 1989. Their characteristics are shown in *Table I*. 72.7 % presented with stage IV NSCLC at 3 predominant metastatic sites : liver (n = 9), bone (n = 8) and brain (n = 7). Three histological types were found : adenocarcinoma (n = 16), squamous cell (n = 14) and large cell carcinoma (n = 3). 81.8 % were aged under 70 and 60.6 % had a PS (ECOG) of 2 or less.

Efficacy

Seven patients (21 %) could not be evaluated (3 deaths from septicemia with aplasia during the first month. 1 death from an intercurrent disease condition and 3 refusals to continue treatment). The 26 patients evaluated exhibited : 11 (42 %) objective responses (CI : 23-61 %), 10 stabilizations and 5 progressions. The overall response rate was 33 % (CI : 17-49 %). The response duration, evaluated in 9/11 patients (1 secondary lobectomy and 1 withdrawal after 4 months) was 2, 3^+, 4, 7, 7^+, 11, 13^+, 17^+ months (median 7 months). Survival in the 11 responders was 2, 3^+, 4, 7, 9, 11, 11^+, 13^+, 13^+, 15^+, 17^+ months (median 11 months). Median response rates and survival are shown in *Table II*, with the responses categorized by sex, age, PS and histological type in *Table III*.

Table II. Median response duration and survival classified according to chemotherapeutic results

Result	Number of patients	Response duration (months)	Median survival (months)
RC	1	13 +	13 +
PR	10	median 7	10
		(range : 2-17 +)	(range : 2-17 +)
			1 withdrawal : 13 +
			1 lobectomy : 11 +
S	10		4.5
P	5		2
Total	26		5

Table III. Objective responses classified according to age, PS, histological type and stage (n = 11)

		No of OR/ Total No	(%)
Sex :	Males	11/29	(38 %)
	Females	0/4	
Age :	≤ 70 years	11/27	(41 %)
	> 70 years	0/6	
PS :	≤ 2	8/20	(40 %)
	> 2	3/13	(23 %)
Histological type :	Squamous cell carcinoma	4/14	(29 %)
	Adenocarcinoma	6/16	(37 %)
	Large cell carcinoma	1/3	(33 %)
Stade :	III	4/9	(44 %)
	IV	7/24	(29 %)

Toxicity

Hematologic toxicity was the primary limiting factor with this regimen as summarized in *Table IV*. Anemia and thrombocytopenia were readily compensated and in no case gave rise to clinical repercussions. However, in 12,5 % of cycles, grade 4 leukopenia was responsible for 5 infectious complications involving irreversible septic shock.

Table IV. Hematologic toxicity (n = 33)

Leukopenia :
  G3 : 14.6 % of cycles
      Mean duration : 2.5 days
      (Range : 1-8 days)
  G4 : 12.5 % of cycles
      Mean duration : 2.4 days
      (Range : 1-5 days)

Anemia :
  G1 : 5 cases

Thrombopenia :
  G3 : 3 cases

Cumulative toxicity was evaluated in 33 patients. Seven (21 %) reported nausea and/or vomiting (grade 1 : n = 2; grade 2 : n = 4; grade 3 : n = 1). Grade 1 renal toxicity (slight reversible elevation in serum creatinine, but less than 2.5 times normal peak value) was observed in 4 patients (12 %). Local venous toxicity was noted in 4 cases (12 %) : grade 1 : n = 1, grade 2 : n = 2, grade 3 : n = 1. There were 2 reported cases of peripheral neuropathy (grade 1 : n = 1, grade 2 : n = 1), 2 cases of grade 2 constipation and 2 cases of grade 3 asthenia. Grade 2 alopecia was seen in 36 % of patients.

Discussion

A high response rate (42 %) was obtained with NVB-CDDP-VP16. This result is highly promising when compared with those obtained with 3 other cisplatin-based drug combinations [1, 6, 8, 9, 11, 12]. The median response duration was 28 weeks, with 44 week median survival in responders and overall median survival of 20 weeks. These results do not surpass previous findings.

The fact that the benefit in response rates was not expressed in terms of survival can partly be explained by the absence of preliminary patient selection. Fewer than 1/3 of responses were observed in patients with a performance status over 2 and no responses were noted in patients aged over 70. Brain metastases did not affect the therapeutic response seen in 7/24 stage IV cases (29 %). No conclusions can be drawn on the basis of histological distribution. The response rate in patients aged under 70 years with a PS of 2 or less was 50 % (8/16).

The highest degree of hematologic toxicity was observed with the initial doses used (NVB : 25 mg/m^2 × 1 day/week; VP16 : 80 mg/m^2 × 3 days every 3 weeks, CDDP : 30 mg/m^2 × 3 days every 3 weeks). It proved necessary to adjust this regimen as the study progressed : dose reductions were required (VP16 to 60 mg/m^2 and CDDP to 25 mg/m^2) in order to reduce myelotoxicity and hence maintain regular treatment. Hematologic toxicity was dose-dependent and related to interactions between the leukopenia induced by the triple combination (D1-D21) and the weekly injections of NVB (D8-D15). The administration of NVB on D8 coincided with a fall in the WBC count and so precipitated the development of aplasia. Consequently, the NVB dose due on D15 could not be given unless the count had recovered sufficiently. Secondary infectious complications of chemically-induced myelosuppression were only noted in cases of associated morbidity, PS > 2 and advanced disease.

Conclusion

The NVB-CDDP-VP16 combination is only suitable for carefully selected patients, and then only in moderate doses (especially of VP16) in order to avoid antagonism between the drop in blood count caused by the triple combination and the weekly dose of NVB. Under such circumstances, the response rates obtained provide some justification for further study.

References

1. Ruckdeschel JC, Finkelstein DM, Ettinger DS, et al. A randomized trial of the four most active regimens for metastatic non small cell lung cancer. *J. Clin Oncol,* 1986; 4 : 14-22.
2. Depierre A, Lemarie E, Dabouis G, et al. Efficacy of Navelbine® (NVB) in non small-cell lung cancer. *Semin Oncol* 1989; 16 : 26-29.
3. Klastersky J. Cisplatin and carboplatin in combination with etoposide as a treatment for non-small cell lung cancer : the experience of the EORTC Lung Cancer Working Party. *Cancer Treat Rev,* 1988; 15 : 33-40.
4. Itri LM, Gralla RJ. A review of etoposide in patients with non-small-cell lung cancer (NSCLC). *Cancer Treat Rev* 1982; 9 : 115-118.
5. The methodologic guidelines for reports of clinical trials. *Cancer Treat Rev,* 1985; 69 : 1-3.
6. Ruckdeschel JC, Finkelstein DM, Mason BA, Creech RH. Chemotherapy for metastatic non small cell bronchogenic carcinoma : EST 2575, Generation V. A randomized comparison of four cisplatin-containing regimens. *J Clin Oncol* 1985; 3 : 72-79.
7. Klastersky J, Sculier JP, Bureau G. Cisplatin versus Cisplatin + Etoposide in the treatment of advanced non small cell lung cancer. *J Clin Oncol* 1989; 7 : 1087-1092.
8. Dhingra HM, Valdivieso M, Carr DT, et al. Randomized trial of three combinations of Cisplatin with Vindesine and/or VP16-213 in the treatment of advanced non small cell lung cancer. *J Clin Oncol* 1985; 3 : 176-183.
9. Hainsworth JD, Johnson DH, Hande KR, Greco FA. Chemotherapy of advanced non small cell lung cancer : A randomized trial of three Cis-platin-based chemotherapy regimens. *Am J Clin Oncol* 1989; 12 : 345-349.
10. Veronesi A, Magri MD, Tirelli U, et al. Chemotherapy of advanced non-small-cell lung cancer with Cyclophosphamide, Adriamycin, Methotrexate, and Procarbazine versus Cisplatin and Etoposide. *Am J Clin Oncol* 1988; 11 : 566-571.
11. Sridhar KS, Varki J, Donnelly E. Toxicity of FED chemotherapy in non-small-cell lung cancer. *Am J Clin Oncol* 1987; 10 : 499-506.
12. Kesketh PJ, Cooley TP, Finkel HE, et al. Treatment of advanced non-small-cell lung cancer with Cisplatin, 5-Fluoro-uracil, and Mitomycin C. *Cancer* 1988; 62 : 1466-1470.

21

Combination Navelbine®-cisplatin-etoposide in bronchial adenocarcinomas

J.-L. BREAU, J.-F. MORERE, C. BOAZIZ, L. ISRAEL

Service d'Oncologie médicale, CHU Avicenne, 93000 Bobigny, France

Bronchial adenocarcinomas represent 20 % of non small cell lung cancer (NSCLC). This disease has clinical features and prognosis that distinguish it from others, such as epidermoid and large cell cancers [1, 2]. Its chemotherapeutic treatment has been studied far less than for other forms of lung cancer. Navelbine® (NVB) in monotherapy achieved a 20 % objective response rate (OR). In animals, synergism was observed in P388 leukemia with the combination NVB - cisplatin (CDDP) and NVB - etoposide (VP16-213) [3].

Therefore, it was considered interesting to evaluate the efficacy and the tolerance in a triple combination with NVB-CDDP and VP16 as a first line treatment in patients with inoperable bronchial adenocarcinomas.

Material and methods

Patients

Twenty-two patients were included in a study from March 1988 until June 1989. There were 17 men and 5 women, whose average age was 56 years (range 41-72). The object of the study was to evaluate the efficacy of a triple combination with NVB, CDDP and VP16 in bronchial adenocarcinoma. All of the patients had histologically confirmed primary bronchial adenocarcinoma. There were 11 patients with intrathoracic locoregional localization, 6 stage IIIA's, and 5 stage IIIB's. Eleven patients had metastatic disease : 4 lung, 5 bone, 2 liver, 3 skin and 1 adrenal.

Patients with brain metastasis were ineligible. The average WHO/ECOG performance status was 1 (range 0-2). Weight loss during the last six months before inclusion in the study was less than 10 % in 15 patients and greater than 10 % in 7 patients. All the patients had complete blood counts and kidney function within normal limits, allowing treatment to be started. None of the patients had received previous treatment with chemotherapy. The target sites chosen for evaluation had not been irradiated. These characteristics are summarized in *Table I*.

The initial work-up included : lung endoscopy in localized disease forms, tomodensitometric examination of the brain, thorax and abdomen.

Table I. Patient characteristics

General characteristics
 Number of eligible patients : 22
 Number of evaluable patients : 20
 Sex : men 17, women 5
 Average age 56 years (41-72)
 Median Performance Status 1 (0-2)
 Weight loss during the 6 months prior to inclusion :
 > 10 % : 7 patients; < 10 % : 15 patients.

Tumor stages
 III A : 6
 III B : 5
 IV : 11 initially metastatic

Metastatic sites
 Lung : 4
 Bone : 5
 Liver : 2
 Skin : 3
 Kidney : 1

Treatment

Treatment consisted of a daily i.v. dose of CDDP 15 mg/m^2 and VP16 50 mg/m^2 for 5 days every 21 days. NVB was given on days 1, 8 and 15 according to hematologic toxicity. Weekly perfusions of NVB were not given unless platelet count was greater than or equal to 100,000/mm^3 and polymorphonuclear neutrophils were greater than or equal to 2,000/mm^3. NVB was given in a dose of 20 mg/m^2 in the first 3 patients and at 25 mg/m^2 in the next 19 patients. This treatment was continued until progression or severe toxicity.

Results

Responses

Evaluation of response was made according to WHO criteria after nine weeks of treatment (3 complete cycles). It included the assessment of clinically measurable lesions (supraclavicular adenopathies or cutaneous lesions), chest X-ray (thoracic cliches), lung endoscopy and tomodensitometric examination of the thorax and/or abdomen as required by the clinical situation.

Two patients were not evaluable due to early death from cardiovascular accidents. Twenty patients were evaluable for response (Table II).

Table II. Responses : 20 evaluable patients

Partial responses :	9	45 %
Stabilizations :	8	40 %
Progressions :	3	15 %

No complete response was observed: 9 out of 20 patients had Partial Response (PR 45 %), 8 had stable disease (40 %), and 3 had progression (15 %).

The duration of response, and its relationship with stage of disease is reported in Table III. One treatment was interrupted for neurotoxicity in the ninth week, and

Table III. Duration of response according to stage

Stages	Partial responses	Duration of response (weeks)
III A	2	9* 34
III B	2	15** 31
IV	5	12 19+ 24 24 34+

* Treatment interrupted for neurotoxicity
** Lost sight of patient

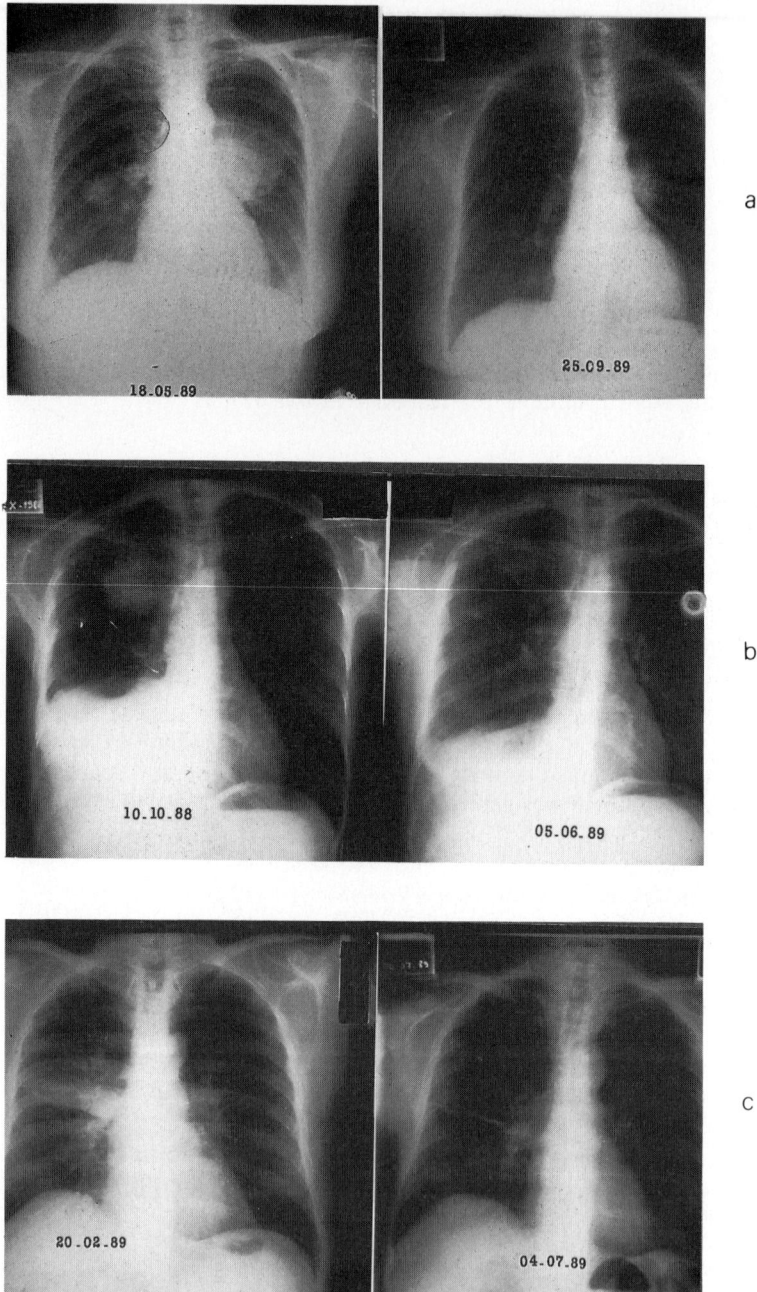

Figure 1. Partial responses after NVB-CDDP-VP16

contact was lost with one patient after fifteen weeks. Both of them were responders. *Figures 1, 2 and 3* illustrate partial responses on chest X-ray.

Survival

Median survival for all 20 evaluable patients is 28.5 weeks (range 4-76) and 34 weeks (range 16^+ - 76) for the responders.

Toxicity

Toxicity was evaluated according to WHO criteria.

Hematologic Toxicity

Hematologic toxicity was analysed in function with the number of cycles of the triple combination with NVB, CDDP and VP16, and NVB alone.

Grades II, III and IV leukopenia were observed in 18.5 %, 17.5 % and 3.8 % of the cycles respectively, and granulocytopenia, grades II, III and IV, in 9.3 %, 18.2 % and 17.6 % of the chemotherapy cycles.

Over 85 cycles, the injection of NVB at D15 could not be given in 77 % of the cases. Treatment with the triple association had to be postponed from D22 to D28 in 45.8 % and from D22 to D36 in 8 % of the patients. No case of thrombocytopenia was observed.

Other toxicities

The other toxicities are described in *Table IV*. They were minimal, with only one case of ileus, grade IV, which forced the interruption of treatment in the ninth week, and one case of distal paresthesia, grade III being observed.

Table IV. Non-hematologic toxicities

	WHO Grades (No of patients)			
	I	II	III	IV
Alopecia	5	2	3	—
Nausea, vomiting	3	5	2	—
Stomatitis	2	2	—	—
Local phlebitis	1	1	—	—
Constipation	1	—	—	1
Paresthesia	—	—	1	—
Asthesia	—	—	1	—

Discussion

The objective response rate of 45 % PR obtained in this study, 25 % of the cases having metastatic disease, confirms the efficacy of the combination NVB-CDDP-VP16 in bronchial adenocarcinomas. This rate was superior to that observed for other cisplatin-based double combinations : CDDP-vindesine (VDS), CDDP-vinblastine and CDDP-VP16 which range between 10 % and 40 %, and is similar to the rates observed in triple combinations with CDDP-VDS base and mitomycin C, VP16 or bleomycin (objective response rates ranging between 0 % and 60 %) in 18 studies that were the object of a recent review [3], as well as in our own experience [4]. Toxicity for this combination is acceptable, especially neurotoxicity.

The administration schedule with the doses used here can be recommended for other studies, if we eliminate the administration of NVB at D15, which was not given in 77 % of cases and was responsible for a delay in treatment from D15 to D22 in 54 % of the cases.

These results justify the introduction of NVB in other protocols for the treatment of this form of lung cancer, and the evaluation of this triple combination in the treatment of large cell and epidermoid cancers. The combination CDDP-VP16 has also proven active [5], as well as NVB [6] in monotherapy for this indication.

References

1. Sorensen JB, Clerici M, Hansen HH. Single-agent chemotherapy for advanced adenocarninoma of the lung. A review. *Cancer Chemother Pharmaco* 1988; 21 : 84-102.
2. Sorensen JB, Basberg JH, Hansen HH. Response to cytostatic treatment in inoperable adenocarninoma of the lung : critical implications. *Br J Cancer* 1990; 60 : 389-393.
3. Sorensen JB, Hansen HH. Combination chemotherapy for advanced adenocarcinoma of the lung. A review. *Cancer Chemother Pharmacol* 1988; 21 : 103-116.
4. Israel L, Breau JL, Morere JF. Lung cancer. *In* : JJ Lokich Ed. *Cancer chemotherapy by infusion*. Chicago, Precept Press; 1987 : 338-352.
5. Longeval E, Klastersky J. Combination chemotherapy with Cisplatin and etoposide in bronchogenic squamous cell carcinoma and adenocarcinoma. A study by the EORTC Lung Cancer Working Party (Belgium). *Cancer* 1982; 50 : 2751-2756.
6. Depierre A, Lemarie E, Dabouis G, *et al.* Efficacy of Navelbine® (NVB) in non small cell lung cancer (NSCLC). *Semin Oncol* 1989; 16 (Suppl 2) : 26-29.

22

Navelbine® (vinorelbine) tolerance in non small cell lung cancer

M. BESENVAL[1], F. LERAY[1], F.M. DELGADO[2], S. MERLE[2], A. KRIKORIAN[2], A. HERRERA[1]

[1] Pierre-Fabre Oncologie, 192, rue Lecourbe, 75015 Paris, France.
[2] Pierre-Fabre Médicament, 192, rue Lecourbe, 75015 Paris, France.

Introduction

Tolerance of Navelbine® has been closely studied during phase II trials of patients with non small cell lung cancer (NSCLC) [1].

The evaluation of this tolerance provided data on the biological and clinical effects, and more specifically on hematological and neurological toxicities. The results of a phase I trial by Mathe (department of hemato-oncology) showed evidence that Navelbine® (NVB) has a dose-limiting hematologic toxicity, primarily involving granulocytes [2]. Furthermore, the fact that this agent is a compound of the spindle poison family imposes a strict requirement for surveillance for neurologic toxicity. This neurologic toxicity was reported infrequently and in moderate degree in the patients included in the phase I trial. All of the patients had been heavily pretreated by cytostatics, including other spindle poisons.

The results of a phase II study of NVB given weekly in a dose of 30 mg/m^2 confirmed the efficacy (33 % objective response rate) of the drug against NSCLC, with a dose-limiting, non-cumulative hematoxicity.

The need to increase the efficacy of chemotherapy for this disease, which has a reputation for low chemosensitivity, has lead to research into the potential therapeutic effects of NVB along with other cytostatics used in the treatment of NSCLC.

With this in mind, several pilot studies have been done with NVB in combination with either mitomycin C (Mito C), etoposide (VP16) or cisplatin (CDDP) [3-6].

The evaluation of tolerance for these combinations can be defined in two situations : in the first, NVB was combined with a drug known to have a potentially high dose-limiting myelotoxicity; and in the second, NVB it was combined with a drug with low myelotoxicity but with another dose-limiting toxicity in common with NVB.

Tolerance of NVB in monotherapy

A phase II study by Depierre (Besançon), Dabouis (Nantes), and Lemarie (Tours) used NVB in monotherapy in weekly doses of 30 mg/m^2. Seventy-eight patients less than 76 years of age with inoperable NSCLC, and who had not received previous chemotherapy, were included in the study.

The hematologic toxicity of the drug was expressed mainly in the leukocyte count; grades III and IV leukopenia and granulocytopenia were reported in 12.5 % and 21.4 % of treatment cycles respectively *(Table I)*. No platelet toxicity was observed. Erythrocyte precursor toxicity was moderate, with grade III anemia being reported in only 1.6 % of the cycles.

Table I. Hematologic tolerance

	Grades WHO (% of cycles)				
	G0	G1	G2	G3	G4
Leucocytes	46.5	22.1	18.9	10.3	2.2
Granulocytes	51.7	12.7	14.2	12.6	8.8
Platelets	100.0	0.0	0.0	0.0	0.0
Hemoglobin	58.7	32.2	7.5	1.6	0.0

Clinical side effects of NVB were infrequent *(figure 1)*. Among the most frequently observed adverse effects, nausea and vomiting, alopecia and local reactions in the injection site were generally not severe, and affected less than 12 % of the patients with more than grade III toxicity. There was no reported grade IV toxicity.

Particular attention was given to the neurotoxic effects of the drug and the principal effects are described in a histogram *(figure 2)*. Paresthesia was rarely observed, affecting less than 6 % of the patients. It was of moderate severity and only one patient reported an intolerable, grade III paresthesia.

Constipation was frequently noted (41 % of patients), and in the majority of cases was not serious and of short duration. One patient, however, had a paralytic ileus which led to discontinuation of treatment. Deep tendon reflexes were commonly affected, with areflexia in 25 % of the patients.

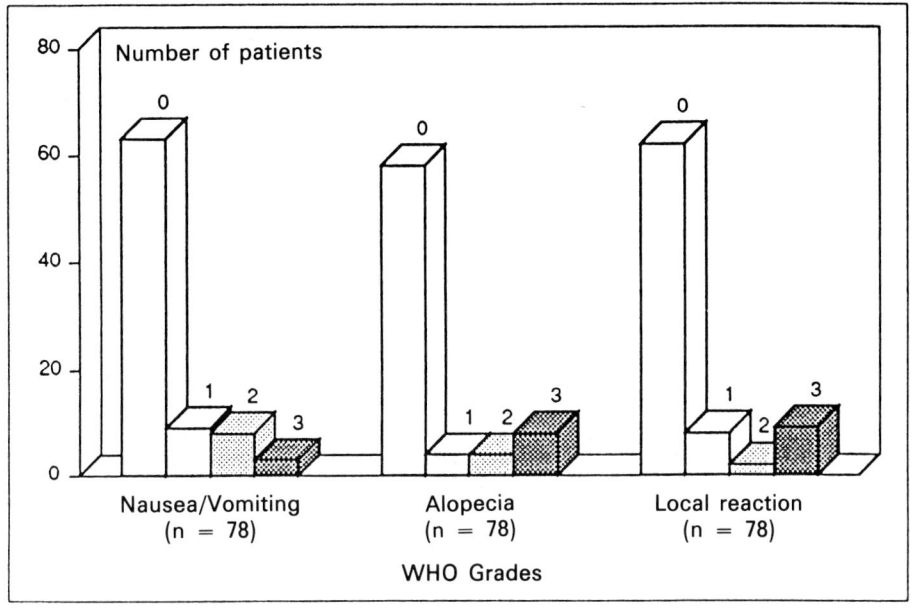

Figure 1. Clinical tolerance

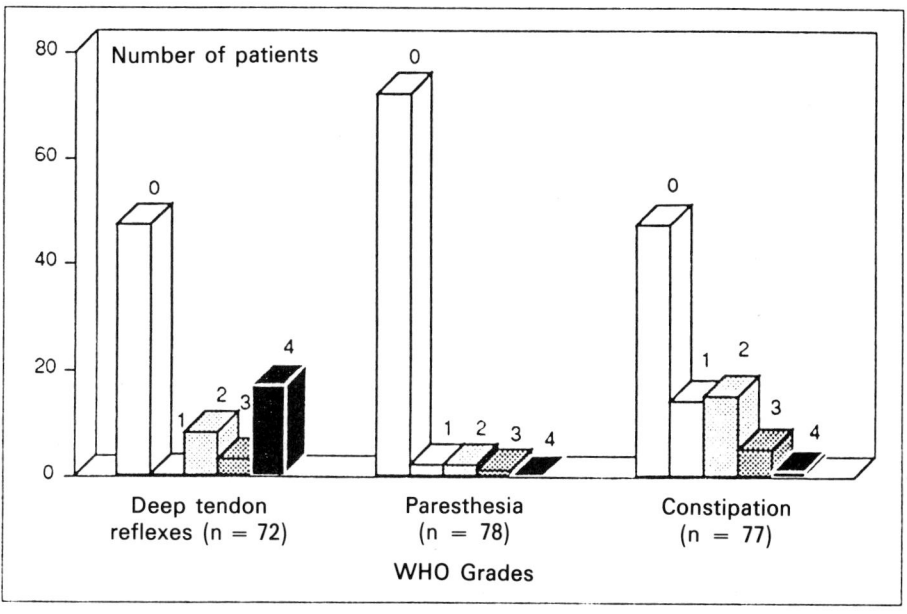

Figure 2. Neurologic tolerance

Table II. Neurotoxicity compared with other vinca alkaloids

	Vincristine	Vindesine
Number of patients	329	318
Doses	2 mg/m²/10-14 D	3-4 mg/m² /7-14 D
Decrease to deep tendon reflexes	100 %	64 %
Paresthesia	57 %	45 %
Constipation	33 %	23 %
Myalgia	6 %	23 %
Muscular weakness	23 %	22 %
Paralytic ileus	3 %	4 %

Comparison of the neurotoxicity of NVB with that of other vinca alkaloids (VA) from previously published studies [7] *(Table II)* shows that :
— areflexia is a common neurotoxic effect of all VAs;
— compared to NVB, the incidence of paresthesia is significantly higher with vincristine (57 % of patients) and with vindesine (45 % of patients);
— although there was a higher frequency of constipation with NVB, it was relatively less severe : 3 % to 4 % of paralytic ileus were reported respectively with vincristine and vindesine, against 1.3 % with NVB.

Tolerance to NVB in combination chemotherapy

After examining the results of phase II monotherapy studies, il was concluded that NVB is generally well tolerated and is genuinely active in NSCLC (29 % objective responses in stages III and IV).

The objectives of the studies of NVB in combination with other agents were to increase the benefits of chemotherapy treatment without increasing the toxicity. To achieve this, weekly administration of NVB was maintained but the dose was decreased by approximately 15 % (25 mg/m²).

Two principal types of combination were studied : combinations with other drugs with high myelotoxic potential (Mito C and VP16); and combinations with other drugs with low myelotoxic potential, but with toxicity in common with NVB. Such was the case of CDDP, which has known neurotoxicity.

Myelotoxic combinations

NVB plus Mito C was the first combination tested. In this study, Mito C was given in a dose of 6 mg/m^2 every 3 weeks, in combination with NVB (25 mg/m^2/week).

A study including lung cancer patients showed that Mito C, at a total dose of 10 mg/cycle, was responsible for leukopenia in 17 % and thrombocytopenia in 6 % of the patients. The hematotoxicity also led to the delay of treatment in nearly 12 % of the cycles. Furthermore, this myelotoxicity was cumulative [8]. Thus the combination of Mito C and NVB was predicted to increase hematologic toxicity, particularly in leukocytes.

The comparison of histograms (figure 3) gives a visual outline of the leukogranulopenias observed with NVB in monotherapy and with polychemotherapy using the combination of NVB plus Mito C (figure 3), indicating that the incidence of granulocytopenias with bitherapy was not greater than with monotherapy.

This combination induced severe leukopenias or granulocytopenias (grade III and IV) in only 5 % and 7 % of cycles respectively.

The second combination, NVB-VP16, could have been expected to produce a lower degree of hematologic tolerance than monotherapy. Issel reported that VP16 at a dose of 60 mg/m^2, 5 days consecutively, induced severe leukopenia ($<2 000$/mm^3) in 25 % of the patients and thrombocytopenia in 4 % [9].

In this pilot study, VP16 was combined with NVB and given at low doses: 80 mg/m^2, 3 days consecutively, every 3 weeks. As with NVB-Mito C, hematologic tolerance with the NVB-VP16 combination was comparable to that of monotherapy. Leukopenia and granulocytopenia, grades III and IV were observed in 10 % and 14 % of cycles respectively (figure 4).

Cisplatin combinations

The low myelotoxicity of CDDP allowed two different studies to be conducted: in the first CDDP was given in standard doses of 80 mg/m^2, every three weeks, and in the second a higher dose of CDDP was used: 120 mg/m^2 days 1 and 29, then every 6 weeks.

The major objective of these two pilot studies was to evaluate the potential increase of neurotoxicity for the combination compared to monotherapy, and to determine an eventual dose effect in relation to the dosages of CDDP.

CDDP in monotherapy, given in a dose of 80 mg/m^2 every 3 weeks, induced sensory peripheral neuropathy in almost 10 % of the patients. This was cumulative since it was generally observed after a total dose of 300 mg. The clinical picture is dominated by chronic, disabling, and often painful paresthesia [10].

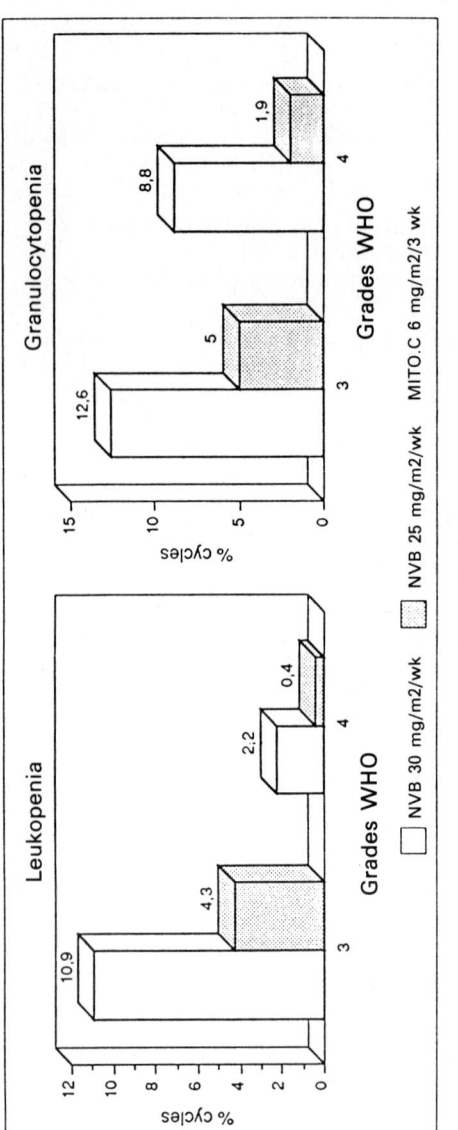

Figure 3. Hematotoxicity NVB-bitherapy NSCLC

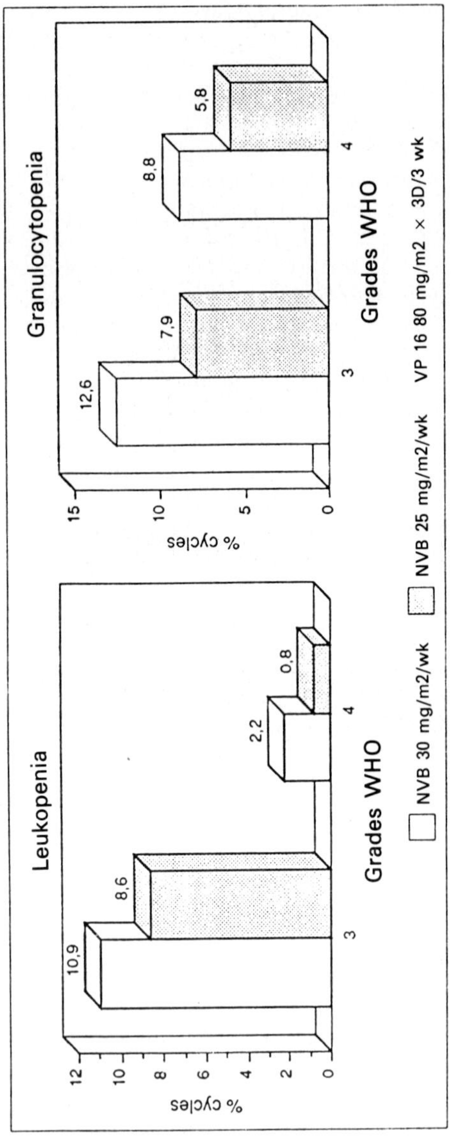

Figure 4. Hematotoxicity NVB-bitherapy NSCLC

Thus it seems of fundamental importance to determine if the incidence of paresthesia increased with treatment with the NVB-CDDP combination. This incidence is reported in the histograms shown in *figure 5*, in which it can be seen that the combination appears to be responsible for an increase of paresthesia compared to NVB monotherapy. However, only paresthesia of low degree (grade I) increased significantly, affecting nearly 28 % of patients given doses of 80 mg/m² of CDDP every 3 weeks, and 18 % of patients receiving larger doses of CDDP at 6 week interval after the first two doses on days 1 and 29.

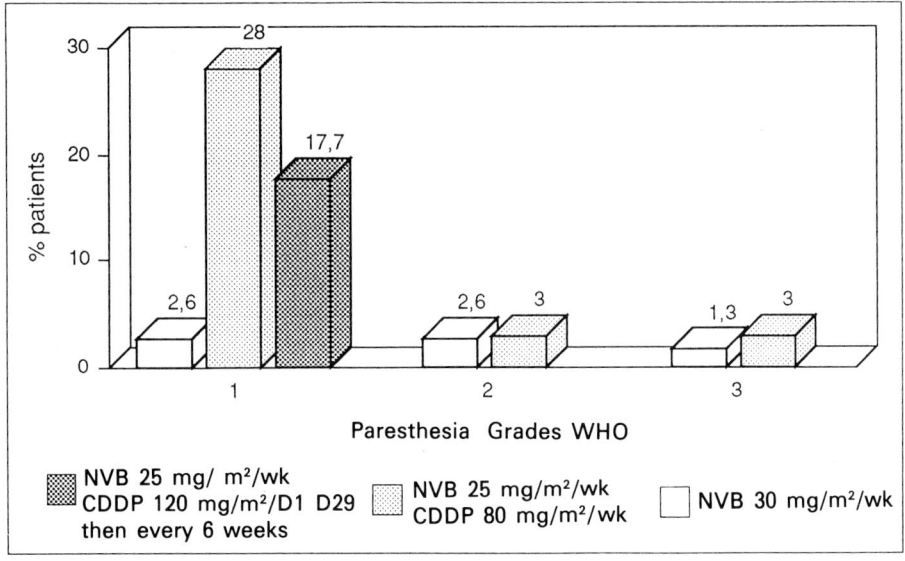

Figure 5. Neurotoxicity

Dose intensity

Satisfactory tolerance of the combinations, from both a hematologic and a neurologic standpoint, confirms the possibility of safely combining NVB with other drugs, even if they are myelo- or neurotoxic. Nevertheless, such a combination may not be satisfactory if the dose intensity administered in each bitherapy combination is not comparable to that of monotherapy. It is therefore essential to show that the good tolerance to bitherapies was not just the result of a decrease in the overall doses the patients actually received, biased by an increase in cycle intervals.

The histograms shown in *figure 6* represent the dose intensities of NVB in monotherapy, and in the various combinations used : NVB - Mito C, NVB - VP16,

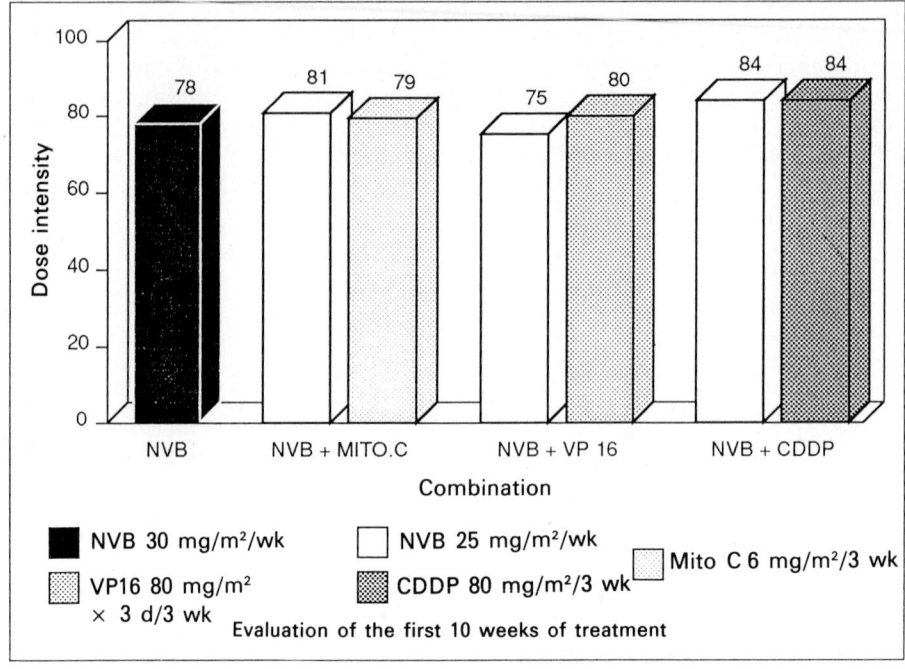

Figure 6. Dose intensity. NVB - Bitherapy - NSCLC

and NVB - CDDP. The results described represent the average values of dose intensities calculated from the total patient population after the first ten weeks of treatment.

More than 75 % of the theoretical dose was given for the double combinations as a whole. In the phase II study NVB given in monotherapy was also given at 78 % of the theoretical dose. This result justifies (retrospectively) the decrease in the NVB dose in the combination schemas. The study of the combination with CDDP, which is known for having low myelotoxicity, led to our research into optimizing the dose/effect by increasing the levels of NVB from 20 mg/m^2 to 25 and 30 mg/m^2. The moderate hematotoxicity which characterized the 30 mg/m^2 level prompted indirectly the proposal of a schedule adapting the weekly dose of NVB to the polymorphonuclear (PN) neutrophil cell count. Decreases of 25 % to 50 % of the NVB doses for PN values between 1,500 and 1,000/m^3 allowed an increase in the total cumulative dose of NVB.

The results of the different therapeutic schedules show little variation in dose intensities, whether CDDP is given at a dose of 80 mg/m^2 every 3 weeks, or at the dose of 120 mg/m^2 on days 1 and 29 and then every 6 weeks, in combination with NVB at a dose of 25 mg/m^2/week *(figure 7)*. On the other hand, the administration of a dose of NVB at 30 mg/m^2 with CDDP at 120 mg/m^2, when PN rates were at least 2,000 mm^3, led to a sharp drop in the dose intensity of both drugs.

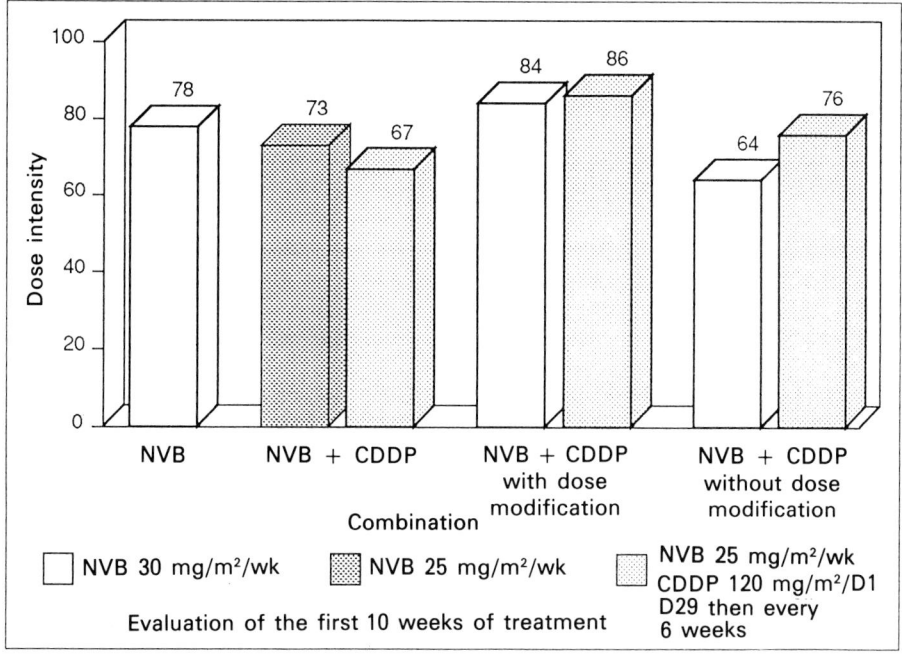

Figure 7. Dose intensity. NVB - Bitherapy - NSCLC

Finally, the schedule for modifying the weekly NVB doses in relation to PN rates between 1,500 and 1,000/mm³ allowed the optimization of dose intensities for both NVB and CDDP.

Conclusion

The efficacy of Navelbine® in the treatment of inoperable NSCLC was established in a phase II study, in monotherapy at a dose of 30 mg/m² administered weekly.

The good clinical tolerance and the dose-limiting hematotoxicity led us to undertake bitherapy combination studies, in which the weekly schedule of NVB was conserved and the dose decreased by 15% (25 mg/m²).

At a dose of 25 mg/m² per week, can be given in combination with Mito C (6 mg/m²/3 weeks), VP16 (80 mg/m² × 3 days/3 weeks), and CDDP (80 mg/m²/3 weeks) without a significant increase in myelotoxicity or neurotoxicity.

At a dose of 30 mg/m² per week, NVB can be given in combination with CDDP (120 mg/m², days 1 and 29/6 weeks) without a significant increase in myelotoxicity or neurotoxicity provided that a schema adapting doses to the granulocytes count is introduced.

References

1. Depierre A, Lemarié E, Dabouis G, *et al.* Efficacy of Navelbine® (NVB) in Non-Small Cell lung Cancer (NSCLC). *Semin Oncol* 1989; 16 (suppl. 4) : 26-29.
2. Mathé G, Ribaud P, Gouveia J. *Pierre Fabre International Report on Navelbine,* part IV B, Vol 2/38. Paris, Pierre Fabre, 1988.
3. Milleron B, Brambilla C, Blanchon F, *et al.* Essai Phase II d'une association de Navelbine (NVB) et Mitomycine C (MTC) chez 25 patients atteints de Cancer Bronchique non à petites cellules (CBNPC) étendu. *Symposium Navelbine,* Biarritz, Nov 1989; Abstract : pp. 42.
4. Lemarié E, Taytard A, Muir JF, *et al.* Les alternatives au Cisplatine : Etudes de Phase II Navelbine + Etoposide. *Symposium Navelbine,* Biarritz, Nov 1989; Abstract : pp. 43.
5. Lebeau B, Clavier J, Kleisbauer JP, *et al.* Etude de phase II Navelbine-Cisplatine. *Symposium Navelbine,* Biarritz, Nov. 1989; Abstract : pp. 39.
6. Le Chevalier T, Berthaud P, Ruffie P, *et al.* Etude pilote de l'association Navelbine-Cisplatine dans les cancers bronchiques non à petites cellules. *Symposium Navelbine,* Biarritz, Nov. 1989; Abstract : pp. 40.
7. Brade W. Critical Review of Pharmacology, Toxicology, Pharmacokinetics of Vincristine, Vindesine, Vinblastine. Proceedings of the International Vinca Alkaloïd. *Symposium Vindesine.* Frankfurt, Nov. 1980; pp. 95-123.
8. Samson MK, Comis L, Baker LH, *et al.* Mitomycin C in Advanced Adenocarcinoma and Large Cell Carcinoma of the Lung. *Cancer Treat Rep* 1978; 62 : 163-165.
9. Issels BF, Krooke ST. Etoposide. *Cancer Treat Rev* 1979; 6 : 107-124.
10. Hadley D, Herr HW. Peripheral neuropathy associated with Cis-Diammineplatinum (II) treatment. *Cancer* 1979; 44 : 2026-2028.

PART III

Navelbine® : Perspectives

A. Advanced breast cancer

23

Phase II pilot study of Navelbine® in advanced breast cancer

F.M. DELGADO[1], L. CANOBBIO[2], F. BOCCARDO[2], F. BREMA[3], V. FOSSER[4]

[1] Centre de Recherche Pierre-Fabre, 192, rue Lecourbe, 75015 Paris, France.
[2] Instituto Nazionale per la Ricerca sul Cancro, viale Benedetto XV, n° 10, 16132 Genova, Italia.
[3] Ospedale San Paolo, corso Italia 30, Savona, Italia.
[4] Ospedale San Bortolo, via Rodolfi, 36100 Vicenza, Italia.

Summary

The objective of this phase II pilot study, conducted at three centers in Italy, was to determine Navelbine® (NVB) efficacy and tolerance in advanced breast cancer.

The 36 patients included in the study received NVB in a 20 minutes i.v. infusion at a dose of 30 mg/m²/week. Toxicity was evaluated in all cases and efficacy in 34 only. The median age was 61 years (range 37-75) with a median performance status of 1 (0-2 scale). The patients were divided into two groups : pretreated (10 patients, 9 evaluable for response) and not pretreated (26). The first group showed two responses out of a total of nine. Since this group included so few patients, analysis was based on the 26 patients in the second group. The objective response rate was 60 % (41 %-79 %) for 25 evaluable patients : 5/25 complete responses and 10/25 partial responses. The response rate obtained for cutaneous, nodal and visceral lesions was 79 %. Two/nine responses and 3/9 stabilizations were observed with osseous lesions. The response rates observed in measurable targets (80 %) and evaluable targets (61 %) represented 52 % and 48 % respectively of the 36 sites studied.

The most severe toxic effect demonstrated by NVB was leukopenia : 35 % of patients (grade 3-4) corresponding to 4 % of 386 cycles evaluated. Anemia was frequent (69 %) but not severe (grade 1-2). No cases of thrombocytopenia were detected. Biological and clinical tolerance were good : grade 3 alopecia (7 %);

grade 1-2 nausea and vomiting (26%); grade 1-2 (11%) and 3 (4%) paresthesia; grade 1 (11%) and 2 (4%) constipation.

Although the present study was restricted to a small patient sample, it does suggest that NVB is one of the most effective drugs available in the treatment of advanced breast cancer. A number of phase I and II studies are currently being conducted in an attempt to confirm this finding in a larger number of patients.

Introduction

Breast adenocarcinoma is the most common form of malignancy seen in women [1]. While about 50% of these cancers can be cured by standard therapeutic means, the development of metastases generally indicates an incurable condition with a median survival of approximately two years [2]. Polychemotherapy is the most widely used and effective treatment in such cases, with objective response rates of 50-70%. The median response duration is of the order of 9 months.

Irrespective of the mode of administration or type of polychemotherapy employed, it does not appear that current efficacy levels are improving [3 4]. The motivation underlying the search for new molecules is to find more active therapeutic agents and schemes and increase median survival.

The activity of vinca alkaloids in advanced breast cancer has been recognized for 25 years, exhibiting response rates of between 20 and 29%. Many protocols therefore contain alkaloids derived from the periwinkle plant. Navelbine® (NVB) or vinorelbine (5' noranhydrovinblastine), a semisynthetic vinca alkaloid derivative, has shown significant cytotoxic activity against P388 and L1210 leukemias, B16 melanoma, VCR-resistant P388 leukemias and many other experimental tumors. This strongly suggests that NVB possesses a wide spectrum of activity [5].

Following preliminary phase I studies showing the maximum tolerated dose to be 30 mg/m²/week (limited by the development of leukopenia but with minimal levels of neurotoxicity), a phase II pilot study was conducted in order to investigate the efficacy of NVB in advanced breast cancer.

Materials and methods

The study was carried out at three Italian centers [6]. All patients entered were suffering from objectively measurable advanced breast cancer. Eligibility criteria included: age ≤ 75 years, performance status ≤ 2 (WHO scale) and expected survival of a least 3 months. Patients previously receiving vinca alkaloids, receiving more than one type of chemotherapy for the advanced cancer, or with only previously irradiated lesions were excluded. Upon inclusion, NVB treatment was delayed for 4 weeks from the date of the last treatment. Other eligibility criteria included:

polynuclear neutrophils $\geq 2\,000/\mu l$ and platelets $\geq 100\,000/\mu l$; bilirubin, SGOT, SGPT and creatinine $< 1.25 \times N$ (normal limit); the absence of clinically detectable brain metastases or peripheral neuropathy. Evaluation before treatment was based on : history of the disease and physical examination, measurement and evaluation of target lesions, blood count and formula, laboratory tests, ECG, chest film, hepatic ultrasound and other radiological scanning or ultrasound examinations as indicated. Physical examination, blood count and formula and laboratory tests were repeated weekly. Chest film, bone scintiscan and hepatic ultrasound were repeated after the first 8 administrations and every 4 cycles in order to evaluate the response.

NVB, diluted in 250 ml physiological saline, was given at a dose of 30 mg/m^2/week as a 20 min i.v. infusion. Treatment was discontinued in the event of progression, unacceptable toxicity or noncompliance on the part of the patient. In the event of neutropenia $\leq 2\,000/\mu l$ or thrombopenia $\leq 100\,000/\mu l$, the NVB dose was postponed. If hematologic toxicity imposed an interruption of more than 3 weeks, the dose could be decreased to 25 mg/m^2/week. Therapeutic efficacy was evaluated on the basis of WHO/EORTC/NCI criteria.

Results

Thirty-six patients were entered between 3 August 1986 and 10 November 1987. Of these, 10 had previously received chemotherapy for metastatic carcinoma. In order to be able to evaluate the efficacy of the test substance in a homogeneous population, the panel of investigators decided to stratify the population into 2 groups : pretreated and not pretreated. Owing to the small number of patients in the first group, analysis was performed on the 26 patients not previously treated for advanced cancer with chemotherapy. Their characteristics are shown in *Table I*.

The primary tumors had been operated in all of these cases. Twenty patients had also received adjuvant chemotherapy either alone or combined with hormone therapy, and 10 of these 26 patients had also undergone radiotherapy *(Table II)*.

Tolerance was evaluated in all 26 patients and efficacy in 25. One patient died within a week of the second NVB injection and could not therefore be evaluated. The most severe toxic effects caused by NVB were hematologic in nature, mainly affecting polynuclear neutrophils; grade 3-4 neutropenia *(Tables III and IV)* was observed in 57 % of patients in 11 % of cycles. Although anemia was also frequent, noted in 69 % of patients in 31 % of cycles, it was of low intensity (grade 1-2). Thrombocytopenia was not observed. Despite the high incidence of leukopenia (WHO grade 3-4 : 31.6 %, corresponding to 6.9 % of the total number of cycles), it was possible to maintain weekly administrations in 69 % of cycles and only 6 % of cycles were postponed for more than 15 days (dose intensity : 80 %).

Biological tolerance was satisfactory, with moderate (grade 1-2) rises in transaminases occasionally noted in 2 % of cycles *(Table V)*.

Overall clinical tolerance was also good. Alopecia was observed in 50 % of patients but only reached grade 3 in 2/26. It appeared over a period of time rather than immediately *(Table VI)*. Nausea and vomiting were infrequent (noted by 15 % of

Table I. Patient characteristics

• Number of patients entered	26
• Number of patients in whom toxicity was evaluable	26
• Number of patients in whom response was evaluable	25
• Age (years)	
Mean	59.6 ± 9
Median	61
Range	42-75
• Performance status	
Median	1
Range	0-2
• Interval between breast cancer diagnosis and first NVB dose (months)	
Median	36
Range	3-132
• Target sites	
Lymph nodes	10 patients
Bone	9 «
Lung	8 «
Skin	7 «
Liver	3 «
• Number of metastatic sites	
1 site	17 patients
2 sites	4 «
3 sites	4 «

• Distribution between measurable and evaluable sites

	Total number of sites	M	E
Lymph nodes	11[1]	10	1
Bone	9	1	8
Lung	8	2	6
Skin	7	5	2
Liver	3	2	1

(1) Two different sites in one patient

patients in 2 % of cycles) and always low in intensity (< grade 2), although it should be stressed that antiemetics were often prescribed *(Table VI)*. Neurotoxicity was very carefully evaluated : 4 cases were observed (2 grade 1, 1 grade 2, 1 grade 3), usually manifesting as paresthesia. Neurotoxicity was reversible in all cases. Constipation was reported by 5 patients (3 grade 2, 2 grade 3).

Of the 26 patients evaluated, treatment was discontinued in 3 cases owing to excessive toxicity : neurotoxicity in one case and unacceptable local tolerance in two cases (responders).

Table II. Previous treatment

	Number of patients
Adjuvant chemotherapy	
CMF[1]	10
CMF + Adriamycin	1
CMF + palliative hormones therapy	2
Adjuvant hormone therapy	3
Palliative hormone therapy only[2]	4
No previous medical treatment	6

(1) CMF : cyclophosphamid + methotrexate + 5-fluorouracil
(2) Hormone therapy : tamoxifen or tamoxifen + medroxyprogesterone

Table III. Hematologic tolerance : leukopenia

Number of evaluable patients	WHO grades[1] 0	1	2	3	4	Number of evaluable cycles	WHO grades 0	1	2	3	4
26	2	3	12	8	1	386	148	113	111	13	1
%	7.7	11.5	46.2	30.8	3.8	%	38.3	29.3	28.8	3.3	0.3

(1) Maximum toxicity/patient

Table IV. Hematologic toxicity : granulopenia

Number of evaluable patients	WHO Grades[1] 0	1	2	3	4	Number of evaluable cycles	WHO grades 0	1	2	3	4
26	3	2	6	12	3	264	127	59	50	24	4
%	11.5	7.7	23.1	46.2	11.5	%	48.1	22.3	18.9	9.1	1.6

(1) Maximum toxicity/patient

The objective response rate was 60 % (confidence interval 41-79 %) for the 25 patients evaluated *(Tables VII and VIII)*. A 79 % response was obtained for skin, nodal and visceral sites. Although it proved difficult to evaluate osseous metastases, 2 responses and 3 stabilizations were observed out of a total of 9. Equivalent objective responses were observed in measurable targets (80 %) and evaluable targets (61 %), representing 50 % and 48 % respectively of the total 38 sites shown in *Table I*.

The median response duration was 23 weeks (range : 9-58 weeks). Seven of the 15 responders interrupted treatment in the absence of objective signs of progression or toxicity.

Table V. Biological tolerance

	Number of evaluable patients	WHO grades[1] 0	1	2	3	4	Number of evaluable cycles	WHO grades[1] 0	1	2	3	4
Creatinine	26	26					294	294				
Urea	26	26					268	268				
SGOT	26	21	5[2]				301	293	8			
SGPT	26	17	5	4[3]			301	265	31	5[2]		
Bilirubin	26	26					265	265				
Alkaline phosphatase	22	18	4				278	250	28			

(1) Maximum toxicity/patient.
(2) 1 patient with elevated SGOT upon inclusion (G1).
(3) 1 patient with elevated SGPT upon inclusion (G1).

Table VI. Clinical tolerance

	Number of patients	WHO grades[1] 0	1	2	3	4	Number of cycles	WHO grades[1] 0	1	2	3	4
Alopecia	26	13	7	4	2		407					
Pruritis	26	26					407	100				
Allergies	26	26					407	100				
Skin rash	26	25	1				407	>99	<1			
Nausea/vomiting	26	19	3	4			407	91	7	2		
Stomatitis	26	25	1				407	99	1			
Diarrhea	26	25	1				407	99	1			
Paresthesia	26	22	2	1	1		407	86	11	2	1	
Constipation	26	21	3		2		407	83	11	4	2	

(1) Maximum toxicity/patient.

Table VII. Response

	Complete remission	Partial remission	Stabilization	Progression
n	5	10	5	5
%	24	36	20	20
	60 %			

Table VIII. Response according to target site

Site	n	CR	PR	Stab.	Prog.
Nodes	11	5	4	2	—
Liver	3	—	1	1	1
Lungs	8	1	5	2	—
Skin	7	2	5	—	—
Bone	9	—	2	3	4

Discussion conclusion

It has been clearly established that many cytolytic drugs exert an antitumor action in breast cancer. Among these, cyclophosphamide, mitomycin C, adriamycin, methotrexate and 5-fluorouracil generally exhibit response rates in excess of 30 % [8]. At present, adriamycin and its analogues are considered to be the most active. The efficacy of combinations of these drugs is more evident in terms of improved quality and longer duration of the objective responses observed than by an actual increase in the response rate and, consequently, most studies have focused interest on this group of drugs [9]. Nevertheless, other substances have also been shown to be effective for this indication, the vinca alkaloids for example, with response rates in metastatic cancer of between 20 % and 29 % [10].

Many protocols have included a vinca-rosea alkaloid and obtained 40-77 % response rates [11, 12]. The application of these drugs is, however, limited by a number of side effects; vincristine is particularly neurotoxic, for instance. Following the detection of the low neurotoxicity of NVB and the proven efficacy of other vinca alkaloids in advanced breast cancer, this pilot study has confirmed the activity of this drug in this indication. An overall objective rresponse rate of 60 % was achieved, with a confidence interval of 40-79 % in a population of 25 patients. This response rate represents a significantly improvement over drugs generally regarded as more active in addition to a number of combinations in current use. Evaluation of tolerance established leukopenia as the dose-limiting toxicity; biological and clinical tolerance was satisfactory. Gastrointestinal tolerance was good, with only 15 % of patients reporting nausea and/or vomiting during 2 % of cycles. Overall neurological toxicity was good, with 4 % grade 3, 4 % grade 2 and 8 % grade 1 neurotoxicity observed in 14 % of cycles.

If the very encouraging results obtained in this study, especially in relation to efficacy and tolerance, are confirmed in mono- and polychemotherapy studies in larger patient populations, it may prove possible to improve the overall quality and duration of the therapeutic response seen in advanced breast cancer.

References

1. Silverberg E, Lubera J. *Cancer Statistics* 1987; CA 37 : 2-19.
2. Clark GM, Sledge GW, Osborne KC. Survival form first recurrence. Relative importance of prognosis factors in 1 015 breast cancer patients. *J Clin Oncol* 1986; 4 : 62-70.
3. Tormey D, Gelman R, Falkson G. Prospective evaluation of rotating chemotherapy in advanced breast cancer. An Eastern Cooperative Oncology Group trial. *Am J Clin Oncol* 1983; 6 : 1-7.
4. Powles TJ, Smith IE, Ford HT, *et al.* Failure of chemotherapy to prolong survival in a group of patients with metastatic breast cancer, *Lancet* 1980 : *8168* : 580-583.
5. Cros S, Wright M, Morimoto M, *et al.* Experimental Antitumor Activity of Navelbine. *Sem in Oncol* 1989; 16 (2) supp 4 : 15-20.
6. Canobbio L, Pastorino G, Gasparini G, *et al.* Phase II study of Navelbine in advanced Breast Cancer Patients. *Proc Second International Congress on Neoadjuvant Chemotherapy* Fev 19th 1988 : 15.
7. Miller AB, Hoogstraten MD, *et al.* Reporting results of cancer treatment. *Cancer* 1981; 47 : 207-214.
8. De Vita V, Hellman S, Rosenberg S. Cancer Principles and practice in Oncology. Philadelphia, JB Lippincott Company 1989; 1197.
9. Lomprizi C, Carbone P. Breast Cancer in Cancer Chemotherapy. Amsterdam, Annual 7 HM Pinedo and BA Chalone, Elsevier 1985.
10. Holland JF, Scharlau C, Gailani S. Vincristine treatment of advanced cancer : a cooperative study of 392 cases. *Cancer Res* 33 : 1258-1264.
11. Smith I, Powles TJ. Vindesine in the treatment of breast cancer. *Cancer Chemother Pharmacol* 1973; 2 : 261-262.
12. De Lena M, Brambilla C, Morabito A, Bonadonna G. Adriamycinil chemotherapy with cyclophosphamide, Methotrexate and 5-Fluorouracil for advanced Breast Cancer. *Cancer* 1975; 35 (4) : 1108-1115.

24

Preliminary results of a phase II study of Navelbine® in the first line treatment of advanced breast cancer

P. FUMOLEAU[1], T. DELOZIER[2], P. KERBRAT[3], F. BURKI[4],
A. MONNIER[5], R. KEILING[6], Ph. CHOLLET[7], E. GARCIA-GIRALT[8],
M. NAMER[9], C. BRUNE[10], F.M. DELGADO[10]

[1] *Centre René-Gauducheau, quai Moncousu, 44035 Nantes Cedex, France*
[2] *Centre François-Baclesse, route de Lion-sur-Mer, BP 5026, 14021 Caen Cedex, France*
[3] *Centre Eugène-Marquis, Pontchaillou, 35011 Rennes Cedex, France*
[4] *Institut Jean-Godinot, 1, rue du Général-Kœning, BP 171, 51056 Reims Cedex, France*
[5] *CHR Bouloche, rue du Dr-Flamand, 25209 Montbéliard, France*
[6] *Centre Paul-Strauss, 3, rue de la Porte-de-l'Hôpital, 67085 Strasbourg Cedex, France*
[7] *Centre Jean-Perrin, 30, place Henri-Dunant, BP 392, 63001 Clermont-Ferrand Cedex, France*
[8] *Institut Curie, 26, rue d'Ulm, 75231 Paris Cedex 05, France*
[9] *Centre Antoine-Lacassagne, 36, voie Romaine, 06054 Nice Cedex, France*
[10] *Pierre-Fabre Médicament/CRPF, 192, rue Lecourbe, 75015 Paris, France*

Introduction

The phase II study of Navelbine® (NVB) in the treatment of advanced breast cancer conducted in Italy by L. Canobbio et al.[1] in 25 non-pretreated patients produced an objective response rate which exceeded 50 %. This finding has allowed to include NVB among the most active antitumor drugs available for the treatment of breast cancer. The objective of the present multicenter study is to confirm this result in a larger population (establishing the response rate according to the location of metastatic sites) and to determine the tolerance of weekly administrations of NVB.

Materials and methods

Patients *(Table I)*

Since October 1989, 75 patients with histologically confirmed metastatic breast cancer have been entered in this study. Their median age is 57 years (range : 32-74). Thirty-four received prior adjuvant chemotherapy, completed at least 1 year before inclusion. No patient has received first line chemotherapy for the disease, although 25 patients have received palliative hormone therapy. Fifty-eight are menopausal. Their mean performance status (WHO scale) is 1 (range : 0-2) and the mean interval from initial diagnosis and the start of NVB treatment is 65 months (range : 1-216). Twenty-one patients initially presented with 1 measurable site, 15 with 2 and 15 with 3 or more. The measurable metastatic sites seen in the 51 patients currently evaluable are shown in *Table II*.

Table I. General characteristics of patients entered.

Number of patients	75
Median age	57 years (range : 32-74)
Hormonal status	
- menopausal	58
- pre-menopausal	11
- not determined	6
Mean performance status (WHO scale)	1 (range : 0-2)
Prior chemotherapy	
- metastatic phase	0
- adjuvant phase ($\geq$ 1 year)	34
Prior hormone therapy	
- metastatic phase	25
- adjuvant phase	19

Treatment

The drug regimen consists of a weekly dose of NVB (30 mg/m² i.v.) given in the form of a 20 minute infusion in 250 ml physiological saline. In the event of unsatisfactory hematologic parameters (polymorphonuclear neutrophils < 1 500/mm³ and/or platelets < 100 000/mm³) recorded on day 8, the cycle is delayed for 1 week. If cytopenia is still noted after 3 weeks, the treatment is regarded as myelotoxic and is discontinued.

Table II. Distribution of measurable sites in 51 patients evaluated.

Measurable sites	n = 70
Lymph nodes	18
Liver	16
Lung	12
Cutaneous	11
Primary tumor	10
Bone	2
Other	1

Evaluation

Tolerance is evaluated on the WHO scale. Efficacy is only evaluated in patients who have received at least 4 weekly NVB cycles. Objective responses are defined according to standard WHO criteria [2]. The response duration (calculated from the first day of treatment) has exceeded 4 weeks for all patients assessed to date.

Results

Tolerance

Safety has been evaluated in 56 patients over a total of 380 cycles.

Hematologic toxicity

The distribution of toxic effects reported is summarized in *Table III*. Hematologic toxicity is the main factor limiting the weekly NVB dose, expressed as anemia (Hb < 5.89 mmol/l in 9 % of cases), leukopenia (< 2 000/mm^3 in 11 %) and neutropenia (< 1 000/mm^3 in 19 %; < 500 in 5 %). No cases of thrombocytopenia (< 50 000/mm^3) have been noted. For the 51 patients in whom response was evaluated receiving at least 4 cycles (total 373 cycles), hematologic toxicity caused the next cycle to start :
— on D8 (no delay) in 67 % of cases (250 cycles);
— on D15 (1 week delay) in 23 % of cases (86 cycles);
— on D21 (2 week delay) in 9 % of cases (34 cycles);
— on D28 (3 week delay) in < 1 % of cases (3 cycles).
The mean dose intensity was therefore 72.5 % ± 18 of the theoretical dose.

Table III. Hematologic toxicity.

Treatment cycles (%)						
Grade		0	1	2	3	4
Hemoglobin	n = 368	57	33	8	1	0
Leukocytes	n = 373	39	24	26	9	2
Neutrophils	n = 368	47	16	17	14	5
Platelets	n = 371	98	1	1	0	0

56 patients (%)					
Grade	0	1	2	3	4
Hemoglobin	29	55	12	4	0
Leukocytes	2	20	32	39	7
Neutrophils	16	7	12	39	25
Platelets	95	2	3	0	0

Other toxicities (Table IV)

All other toxic effects are mild : grade 3 nausea-vomiting (1 %), grade 3 infection (1 %), grade 1 (7 %) and grade 2 (2 %) peripheral neuropathy, grades 1, 2 (11 %) and 3 (4 %) constipation over 380 evaluable cycles. Venous toxicity was evaluated over 293 cycles (without using a chamber implant) and was classified separately.

- Grade 0 : absent   232 cycles (79 %)
- Grade 1 : pain along the course of the vein ≤ 2 days   57 cycles (19 %)
- Grade 2 : pain along the course of the vein 2-5 days, and/or erythema, and/or vesicles   2 cycles (1 %)
- Grade 3 : pain along the course of the vein > 5 days, and/or erythema, and/or vesicles   2 cycles (1 %)
- Grade 4 : intolerance necessitating discontinuation of treatment   0 cycle (0 %)

Table IV. Other toxicities (380 treatment cycles, 56 evaluable patient.

Grade	0	1	2	3	4
Nausea/vomiting	62	29	8	1	0
Diarrhea	93	3	3	0	0
Constipation	85	9	2	4	0
Alopecia	69	25	5	0	0
Peripheral neuropathy	91	7	2	0	0
Stomatitis	91	3	3	2	0
Infection	97	1	1	1	0

Therapeutic results

Response was evaluated in 51 patients : 51 % overall response rate with 6 complete (12 %) and 20 partial responses (> 50 %) (CI : 37-65 % with 95 % probability). These responses are classified by evaluable metastatic sites in *Table V,* and by dose intensity in *Table VI.*

Table V. Responses classified according to tumor site.

Overall response	n 51	CR 6	PR 20	% CR + PR 51 %	Stab. 18	Prog. 7
Measurable sites	70					
Lymph nodes	18	5	5	56 %	7	1
Liver	16	2	3	31 %	10	1
Lung	12	2	2	33 %	8	0
Skin	11	1	8	81 %	3	1
Primary tumor	10	1	5	60 %	3	1
Bone	2	1				
Others	2				2	

CR : complete response; PR : partial response; Stab : stabilisation; Prog : progression.

Table VI. Response classified according to dose intensity.

Percentage of theoretical dose actually administered	Number of patients	Objective response rate
> 75 %	20	55 %
50-75 %	24	54 %
50 %	7	43 %

Conclusion

The preliminary results of this study have confirmed those obtained in a previous Italian pilot study. NVB shows a 51 % response rate, with neutropenia exhibiting limiting toxicity at a dose intensity of 72.5 % and good clinical tolerance. The findings justify continuation of the study.

References

1. Seminars in Oncology, Vol 16, N° 2, Sup 4, Avril 1989, 33-36.
2. Cancer, Janvier, 1981.

25

Phase II study of vinorelbine in first and second line treatment of advanced breast cancer

J.-M. EXTRA[1], S. LEANDRI[1], V. DIERAS[1], C. FERME[2], L. MIGNOT[3], F. MORVAN[4], M. ESPIÉ[1], M. MARTY[1]

[1] *Service d'Oncologie médicale, Hôpital Saint-Louis, 1, avenue Claude-Vellefaux, 75010 Paris, France.*
[2] *Centre médico-chirurgical de Bligny, 91640 Bris-sur-Forges, France.*
[3] *Service d'Oncologie médicale, CMC Foch, 40, rue Worth, 92151 Suresnes Cedex, France.*
[4] *Service d'Oncologie médicale, Centre Dubos, avenue de l'Île-de-France, 95301 Cergy-Pontoise, France.*

Summary

Vinorelbine or Navelbine® (NVB) is a semisynthetic vinca alkaloid with a strong affinity for tubulin. Although it has demonstrated a high level of antitumor activity in experimental studies, its toxicity, especially hematologic, is far from negligible. The response rate with NVB in previously untreated advanced breast cancer exceeds 50 %. The present study included heavily pretreated breast cancer patients. The 33 patients who met the eligibility criteria received NBV by infusion at a dose of 30 mg/m²/week. Eighty-five % had previously received adjuvant chemotherapy and all had undergone 1 or 2 courses of chemotherapy.

Neutropenia (grade > 2) was the limiting toxicity in more than 50 % of cases and resulted in a prolongation of the intervals between cycles. The doses received ranged from 66 % to 76 % of the theoretical dose. Grade 1-2 neuropathy was observed in 20-35 % of patients and alopecia in 20-25 %. NVB proved slightly emetic (< 18 % of cycles). No renal, hepatic, cardiac, respiratory or cutaneous toxicity was reported. Ten responses were obtained (2 CR, 8 PR) giving a response rate of 30.3 %. Using such a 2-stage methodology, the fundamental hypothesis is rejected if the response rate is less than 20 % with > 95 % probability. The results of this study, together with the low extra-hematologic toxicity of NVB, therefore provide further evidence that this anti-tumor agent is effective in the treatment of advanced breast cancer.

Introduction

Navelbine® or vinorelbine (nor-5 anhydrovinblastine) (NVB) is a new molecule which is distinguished from other vinca alkaloids by substitution of the catharanthine moiety [9]. It acts on microtubule structure and inhibits tubulin polymerization [1]. Although NVB is almost as active as vincristine on mitotic spindle microtubules, much higher concentrations are needed to achieve an effect on axon microtubules and induce tubulin spiraling [1, 6]. This could account for the low grade neurotoxicity reported with NVB.

Experimental studies on murine tumors, human cancer cell lines and tumor xenografts in athymic mice have demonstrated that the antitumor activity of NVB is at least equal to that of vinblastine or vincristine [3].

In a phase I study in patients with hematologic or solid malignancies, the dose-limiting toxicity was reversible and non-cumulative neutropenia. Alopecia and vomiting were observed in fewer than 20 % of patients. Neurologic toxicity was relatively low and comparable with that of vincristine. The recommended dose of NVB was 30 mg/m²/week, given as a 15 minute i.v. infusion in 125 ml physiologic saline [5, 8].

NVB exerts significant antitumor activity in non small cell lung cancer [4] and advanced breast cancer previously untreated by chemotherapy [2].

We have conducted a further phase II study of NVB in patients with advanced breast cancer previously treated with 1 or 2 chemotherapy regimens for metastatic progression of the disease. Our initial objectives were to demonstrate that NVB achieves response rates in excess of 20 % under a 2-stage protocol [7] and to establish the major side effects experienced by chemotherapeutically pretreated patients.

Materials and methods

The following eligibility criteria were retained : patients aged under 75 years, histologically proven breast cancer; 1 or 2 prior chemotherapy protocols for metastatic advance; progressive disease or tumors refractory to all other therapeutic modalities at the time of inclusion; expected survival of a least 12 weeks; at least 1 measurable lesion; performance status of 2 or less (WHO scale); absence of major visceral organ impairment unrelated to the tumor mass (granulocytes $> 2.10^9/1$, platelets $> 100.10^9/1$, bilirubin, transaminases, alkaline phosphatase and creatinine < 1.25 N); absence of clinical signs of peripheral neuropathy (except problems related to tumor compression); informed patient consent.

Patients were excluded from the study if they had received more than two prior chemotherapy or vinca alkaloid regimens for the treatment of metastatic advance and in cases of brain or meningeal involvement and/or target tumor subjected to local treatment (resection or radiotherapy).

NVB was supplied in vials containing 10 or 50 mg ditartrate solution of NVB. On the basis of the safety established during phase I and II studies in solid tumor patients, the drug was administered at a dose of 30 mg/m^2/week in 125 ml physiologic saline, given by a 15 minute i.v. infusion. No antiemetic premedication was given with the first injection.

Safety was evaluated according to WHO criteria. If toxicity, especially neutropenia, exceeded grade 2, the dose was reduced and/or the interval between cycles prolonged. Treatment was continued until progression or limiting toxicity was noted. Calculation of the actual dose received (dose intensity) was based on any dose reduction and prolongation of the intervals between cycles.

Upon inclusion, a routine physical examination was performed and measurable target lesions were evaluated, in addition to neurologic state and performance status. Blood cell and platelet counts, renal and hepatic function tests, analysis of tumor markers, chest film, abdominal ultrasound and bone radionuclide scintiscan were routinely performed. Other more specific tests were also performed where clinically indicated.

During treatment, a physical examination, full blood count and electrolyte, renal and hepatic tests were performed before each cycle to detect any adverse effects. All evaluable parameters were assessed every 4 cycles. Efficacy was evaluated on the condition of measurable tumor targets after 8 cycles : disappearance of the target was taken as a complete response (CR) and a decrease of 50 % for a two-dimensional tumor or 30 % for a one-dimensional tumor in the initial size of the target (other lesions remaining stable) was taken as a partial response (PR). These responses were confirmed every 4 weeks. Death or premature discontinuation of treatment was recorded as failure of treatment.

Results

Thirty-three patients, with a median age of 48 years (range 28-66), were included in the evaluation of safety. The median period between diagnosis and the first metastasis was 502 days (range 0-1670) and the median period between diagnosis and inclusion in the study, 756 days (103-2277). The main tumor targets and organs primarily involved are shown in *Table I*. Ten patients initially presented with metastases at the initial diagnosis.

The various pretreatments received included radiotherapy (n = 28) and adjuvant chemotherapy (CMF n = 5, anthracyclins n = 11). The median number of chemotherapeutic protocols was 6 (range 2-8); the types of agents and median doses given are shown in *Table II*. The optimum response to pretreatment, CR, was seen in 7 patients (21 %), with PR in 10 patients (30 %), minor response or stabilization in 5 (16 %) and progression in 11 patients (33 %).

Table I. Sites involved and target lesions.

Site	Number	Target lesion
Lung	6	5
Pleura	5	0
Liver	13	11
Lymph nodes	11	3
Skin	11	11
Bone	25	3
Bone marrow	6	0
Breast	6	0

Table II. Prior chemotherapy.

AAC	Number	Median dose (mg/m²) (range)	
DOX + EDOX	27	420	(40-720)
DHAD	14	72	(20-100)
CPM	33	6 400	(800-14 400)
5FU	29	7 200	(1 200-33 000)
MTX	24	3 600	(85-13 400)
VCR	18	5.5	(2-15)

Upon entry, all patients had a performance status (WHO scale) of 2 or less. Grade 1-2 alopecia was present in 30 % of patients, grade 3 in 3 %, grade 1-2 neuropathy in 9 % and grade 3 in 3 %.

The dose intensity ranged from 66 % to 76 % of the theoretical dose (66 % in cycles 1 to 4, n = 33 patients; 72 % in cycles 5 to 8, n = 31; 72 % in cycles 8 to 12, n = 28; 76 % in cycles 12 to 16, n = 18; 72 % from cycle 16, n = 13).

The only acute and frequent adverse effect was myelosuppression, that is, neutropenia. The median nadir of the leukocyte count was between $2.2 \times 10^9/l$ and $4 \times 10^9/l$ and was unaffected by repeated administrations of NVB. Neutropenia was always rapidly reversible, but did reach grade 4 on occasion, necessitating a prolongation of interval between cycles or, less often, a dose reduction. The overall dose intensity therefore amounted to only 66-76 % of the theoretical value. Although neutropenia in excess of grade 2 was observed in over 50 % of patients, infection only developed in 2 cases. NVB induced significant thrombocytopenia in only 1 patient, who also exhibited bone marrow involvement. Grade 1 or more anemia was reported in 25 % of patients.

Bilirubin and transaminase levels, expressed as multiples of their standard maximum values, were not significantly affected, even in patients with liver metastases causing biochemical anomalies in tests of liver function. These cases showed no

Table III. Hematologic, hepatic and renal toxicity.

	C1	C2	C3	C4	C5	C6	C7	C8	C12	C16	post
Number of patients	33	33	33	33	31	31	31	28	18	14	13
Day min. max.	1	7 7 14	18 13 29	28 21 63	38 28 77	46 34 86	55 42 99	68 49 107	102 77 147	145 105 196	
Dose (%) med. min. max.	100 66 115	100 56 115	100 50 115	100 50 115	100 56 115	100 56 100	100 56 115	100 50 115	60 50 115	100 50 115	100 56 115
DI (%)	-----66-----				-----72-----				—76—	—72—	
WBC med. min. max.	4.0 0.9 11	2.1 0.4 8.0	2.8 0.7 12	3.2 0.8 5.7	2.7 1.0 5.9	2.9 1.0 7.2	3.6 0.8 8.2	2.6 1.1 8.5	2.3 0.8 3.8	2.2 0.9 3.8	2.3 1.1 3.6
Plat med. min. max.	211 54 455	240 63 426	248 44 517	249 19 580	261 3 728	263 89 440	232 60 384	280 48 420	230 75 426	242 90 430	240 160 347
SGOT SGPT med. (*N) min. max.	1 1 4	1 1 4	1 1 3	1 1 4	1 1 2	1 1 2	1 1 3	1 1 8	1 1 3	1 1 1	1 1 2
Alk ph med. (*N) min. max.	1 1 3	1 1 *5	1 1 *7	1 1 *9	1 1 3	1 1 1	1 1 3	1 1 2	1 1 4	1 1 1	1 1 2
Bili med. (*N) min. max.	1 1 1	1 1 1	1 1 1	1 1 1	1 1 1	1 1 1	1 1 1	1 1 1	1 1 1	1 1 1	1 1 1
Creat med. min. max.	76 61 111	74 61 91	74 60 91	78 59 111	76 62 99	74 62 89	74 67 91	72 53 107	74 53 93	78 55 91	77 64 91

Table IV. Other toxicities.

	C1	C2	C3	C4	C5	C6	C7	C8	C12	C16	post
Number of patients	33	33	33	33	31	31	31	28	18	14	13
Day	1	7	18	28	38	46	55	68	102	145	
min.		7	13	21	28	34	42	49	77	105	
max.		14	29	63	77	86	99	107	147	196	
Dose (%)											
med.	100	100	100	100	100	100	100	100	60	100	100
min.	66	56	50	50	56	56	56	50	50	50	56
max.	115	115	115	115	115	100	115	115	115	115	115
DI (%)	————66————				————72————			—76—	—72—		
Muc. (%)											
Gr 0	100	100	100	97	97	93	100	100	100	100	100
Gr 1-2	0	0	0	3	3	7	0	0	0	0	0
Gr > 2	0	0	0	0	0	0	0	0	0	0	0
NV (%)											
Gr 0	82	88	91	94	97	86	97	93	100	100	85
Gr 1-2	18	12	9	6	3	14	3	7	0	0	15
Gr > 2	0	0	0	0	0	0	0	0	0	0	0
Alop (%)											
Gr 0	91	91	87	80	76	75	81	88	79	77	85
Gr 1-2	8	8	12	20	20	21	11	4	17	23	15
Gr > 2	0	0	0	0	4	4	8	8	6	0	0
Neuro (%)											
Gr 0	84	81	71	81	76	70	68	77	72	69	75
Gr 1-2	13	19	29	19	24	30	32	23	28	31	25
Gr > 2	*3	0	0	0	0	0	0	0	0	0	0
Cardiac (%)											
Gr 0	100	100	100	100	100	100	100	100	100	100	100
Gr 1-2	0	0	0	0	0	0	0	0	0	0	0
Gr > 2	0	0	0	0	0	0	0	0	0	0	0
Pulm (%)											
Gr 0	100	100	100	100	100	100	100	100	100	100	100
Gr 1-2	0	0	0	0	0	0	0	0	0	0	0
Gr 1-2	0	0	0	0	0	0	0	0	0	0	0

* 1 patient with spinal compression.

enhancement of hematologic toxicity. No renal toxicity was detected. Grade 1-2 nausea and vomiting were observed in 18 % of cycles but did not represent a dose-limiting factor and were controlled by standard doses of antiemetics. No case of gastrointestinal toxicity exceeded grade 2. In addition to the 8 % of patient with alopecia upon inclusion, grade 1-2 alopecia appeared in 20-25 % of patients during treatment. It appeared to be unrelated to the number of cycles administered. 13 % of patients initially presented with grade 1-2 neuropathy and 1 patient (3 %) with grade 3 neuropathy (spinal compression). Grade 1-2 neuropathy (reduced tendon reflexes) was observed in 20-35 % of patients after the third cycle but was not accompanied by dysesthesia or severe constipation. No respiratory or cutaneous toxicity was detected. These results are summarized in *Tables III and IV*.

Of the 33 patients in whom efficacy was evaluated, 10 exhibited a response to treatment (8 PR, 2CR), giving an overall response rate of 30.3 % (confidence interval : 13.75-49 %). A 2-stage analysis was performed. The first stage, completed after observing 5 responses in the first 14 patients evaluated, confirmed the inititial hypothesis with a 13 % alpha risk (false-positive). The second stage, following the evaluation of 11 additional patients (25 patients : 9 responses), confirmed that the probability of a genuine response rate to NVB of more than 20 % exceeds 95 % (4.7 % alpha risk).

There did not appear to be any link between the response to NVB and the responses obtained to the drugs administered previously (2 patients who formerly proved refractory to chemotherapy exhibited partial responses), the target tumor site, or the dose intensity after 8 cycles. The responses were observed between days 56 and 112. The median response duration was 14 weeks (range : 8-52).

Discussion

Ten responses (2 CR, 8 PR) were obtained among the 33 patients evaluated, giving an overall response rate of 30.3 % (CI : 13.75-49 %). NVB is active when administered alone, with a response rate of more than 20 % in advanced breast cancer patients who had received 1 or 2 prior courses of combined chemotherapy containing anthracyclines and/or mitoxantrone. Only a few compounds (ametycin, ellipticinium) have produced comparable results in such a patient population. No vinca alkaloid, even when used as a first line treatment, has demonstrated comparable results in this particular indication. It should also be noted that, unlike in standard phase II studies, the 2-stage statistical method of analysis used in this study provided a much earlier interpretation (25 patients in this study).

The limiting toxicity seen with NVB was neutropenia, which exceeded grade 2 in more than 50 % of cycles. Although it was short-lived, this neutropenia resulted in a prolongation of the intervals between cycles and, less often, a dose reduction. The dose intensity was 66-76 % of the therapeutic dose. Thrombocytopenia and anemia were rarely reported and were not dose-limiting.

Grade 1-2 neuropathy (reduced tendon reflexes) was seen in 20-35 % of patients, increasing in frequency, though not cumulative, as treatment progressed. Grade 1-2 alopecia was noted in 20-25 % of patients; the problem was eased slightly with the use of a cooling cap. 18 % of cycles were accompanied by grade 1-2 nausea and vomiting. No renal, hepatic, cardiac, respiratory or cutaneous toxicity was reported.

The activity of NVB in advanced breast cancer will be better defined by the following studies (currently in progress):

— NVB administered in monotherapy as a first line treatment: more than 100 patients entered;

— NVB administered in combined forms to patients with no prior chemotherapy against advanced carcinoma: combination of NVB 30 mg/m^2 on days 1 and 5 plus 5FU 750 mg/m^2 on days 1-5 every 3 weeks; factorial group analysis is performed every 9 patients with $HO = 50\%$, $H_a = 70\%$, alpha = 5 % and beta = 5 % as baseline parameters.

References

1. Binet S, Fellous A, Lataste H, *et al.* In situ analysis of the action of Navelbine on various types of microtubules using immunofluorescence. *Semin Oncol,* 1989; 16 : 5-8.
2. Canobbio L, Boccardo F, Pastorino G, *et al.* Phase II study of navelbine in advanced breast cancer. *Semin Oncol,* 1989; 16 : 33-36.
3. Cros S, Wright M, Morimoto M, *et al.* Experimental antitumor activity of Navelbine. *Semin Oncol,* 1989; 16 : 15-20.
4. Depierre A, Lemarie E, Dabonis G, *et al.* Efficacy of navelbine in non-small cell lung cancer. *Semin Oncol,* 1989; 16 : 26-29.
5. Favre R, Garnier G, Depierre A, *et al.* A phase I study of Navelbine (Nor-5'-anhydro-vinblastine). *Proc. of the 14th International Congress of Chemotherapy,* Kyoto 1985; Anticancer section 1 : 641-642.
6. Fellous A, Ohayon R, Vacassin T, *et al.* Biochemical effects of Navelbine on tubulin and associated proteins. *Semin Oncol,* 1989; 16 : 9-14.
7. Lee YJ, Staquet M, Simon R, *et al.* Two-stage plans for patient accrual in phase II cancer clinical trials. *Canc Treat Rep,* 1979; 63 : 219-223.
8. Mathé G, Reizenstein P. Phase I pharmacologic study of a new vinca-alkaloid : Navelbine. *Canc Lett* 1985; 27 : 285-293.
9. Potier P. The synthesis of Navelbine, prototype of a new serie of vinblastine derivates. *Semin Oncol* 1989; 16 : 2-4.

26

Navelbine® - 5-fluorouracil combination in first line treatment of advanced breast cancer

V. DIERAS, C. VARETTE, C. LOUVET, M. ESPIÉ, P. COLIN, M. MARTY

Service d'Oncologie médicale, Hôpital Saint-Louis, 1, avenue Claude-Vellefaux, 75785 Paris Cedex 10, France

Summary

Eighteen patients with advanced breast cancer are receiving first line treatment with a 5-fluorouracil-Navelbine® (5FU-NVB) combination under a sequential group protocol. The response rate is used to establish efficacy. All are currently included in the response and safety analysis; 13 have exhibited objective responses with acceptable tolerance.

Introduction

Metastatic progression of invasive breast cancer can be confirmed upon diagnosis or following initial treatment in over 40% of cases. With the use of combination chemotherapy in the treatment of metastatic carcinoma, it has been established that, with an objective response, median survival is more than 24 months; this figure falls to under 18 months with stable disease and to just a few months if the first line treatment fails.

Table I. Principal active cytotoxic antitumor agents in the first line treatment of breast cancer.

Agent (INN)	Abbreviation	Standard dose (mg/m^2)	Response rate (%) 1st line
Doxorubicin	DOX; ADR	30-75	40-50 %
Epirubicin	EDOX	50-90	40-50 %
Mitoxantrone	DHAD	10-14	20-35 %
Cyclophosphamide	CPM	400-600	34 %
Methotrexate	MTX	60	34 %
Altretamin	HMM	150/d × 7	27 %
Melphalan	MELP	2-6/d × 5	23 %
Ametycin	MITC	10	20-25 %
Elliptiniume	NMHE	80/d × 3	20-30 %
Vincristine	VCR	1.4	21 %
Chlorambucil	CLB	2-6/d × 5	20 %

Drugs active in advanced breast cancer primarily include anthracyclines with 40-50 % first line response rate (RR), cyclophosphamide (35 % RR), methotrexate (35 % RR) and melphalan, ametycin and elliptinium, all with 20-25 % RR *(Table I)*.

Vinorelbine (Navelbine®) is a semi-synthetic vinca alkaloid with response rates of approximately 60 % in first line treatment and 30 % in second line treatment. It does however cause toxic, especially hematologic, effects [3, 4, 7]. 5FU also ranks as one of the most active agents, with response rates of 25-35 %. When 5-day continuous infusions are used, 5FU can be given in higher doses but with low toxicity [6].

In the light of these facts, we decided to investigate the 5FU and NVB as a combination (FUN).

Materials and methods

Eligibility criteria

— Histologically proven breast cancer;
— stage I metastasis;
— patient aged under 70 years;
— expected survival of more than 8 weeks;
— at least 1 measurable metastatic tumor (with the exception of isolated brain tumors); the primary target tumor selected upon entry will be used to evaluate the response.

Exclusion criteria

— Prior chemotherapy treatment for the first metastatic progression (excluding adjuvant chemotherapy preceding metastatic progression);
— concomitant radiotherapy of evaluable target tumor/s;
— concomitant hormone therapy;
— severe impairment of any visceral organ.

5FU is given at a dose of 750 mg/m^2/day in a 5-day continuous infusion. NVB is given at a dose of 30 mg/m^2/day on days 1 and 5 in a short i.v. infusion (20 minutes in 250 ml 5% glucose solution), this treatment cycle being repeated at D21. All patients are to receive at least two cycles. Response is evaluated upon completion of these two cycles. Where a partial response or stable tumor is seen, treatment is continued for up to six cycles or until progression occurs. Tumor progression is regarded as a failure of treatment.

The protocol permits a dose reduction in the event of significant toxicity (70% reduction in 5FU dose for mucitis > grade 3; 70% reduction in NVB dose for hematologic or neurologic toxicity > grade 3).

The main objective of this study is to evaluate efficacy every two treatment cycles on the basis of the objective response shown by the primary target selected upon entry.

Secondary objectives criteria

In addition, three secondary objectives have also been defined :
— overall objective response after six cycles;
— evaluation of response duration, that is, the interval preceding treatment failure, progression of the disease, premature discontinuation of the protocol owing to unacceptable toxicity or patient refusal of treatment or treatment-or disease-related death;
— evaluation of the safety of the drug combination used.

Statistical analysis is based on a sequential group protocol [2] since the single-stage method requires a large patient population and frequently results in unplanned analysis of too few cases, reducing statistical significance or increasing the first-class risk (false positive results). The sequential group method of analysis retained for this study is Whitehead's triangular test adapted for use in phase II studies.

Following the success rates previously reported with existing protocols, an efficacy of 50% or less (po) will be disregarded and will justify abandoning the protocol. The definition of a "maximum" level allows the beta risk to be defined. First and second-class risks are set at 5%. Analysis will be performed after each additional 9 patients (k = 9). Rejection of the zero hypothesis allows confirmation that the response rate exceeds 50%.

The following computations will be made upon completion of the evaluation of every 9 consecutive patients :
— Z statistic = S-Npo, the difference between the number of observed responses (S) and the number of expected responses (Npo) under the zero hypothesis following evaluation of N patients.

— variance V = Npo (1-po), under Ho.
The value obtained will be plotted on the sequential plan :
— if it falls within the triangle, then the study will continue with the inclusion of 9 more patients;
— if it appears below the Ho acceptance line, the study will be discontinued and the zero hypothesis will not be rejected (success rate equal to or less than 50 %);
— if it appears above the Ho rejection line, the study will be discontinued and the zero hypothesis rejected (success rate over 50 %).

The expected mean number of subjects required to obtain a conclusion is 34 under Ho (p = 0.50), 37 under Ha (p = 0.70) and 45 for p = 0.60 (for which the sequential group plan requires a higher number of subjects).

Presentation of patients

Efficacy and safety are currently being evaluated in 18 patients with a median age of 54 years (range : 41-68). Ten have received prior adjuvant anthracycline-based chemotherapy. The mean interval between initial diagnosis and metastatic progression is 32.5 months (range : 0-78 months). Upon initial diagnosis, hormonal receptor tests proved negative in 7 patients, positive in 5 and were not performed in 6 cases. The primary target tumors show the following site distribution : lung n = 6, liver n = 8, lymph nodes n = 2, skin n = 2 and bone marrow n = 1. Five patients have only 1 metastatic site while the remaining 13 patients have multiple metastases *(Table II)*.

Table II. Combinations of metastatic sites.

Lungs-Pleura	1
Lungs-Bone	1
Lungs-Liver	4
Lymph nodes	2
Lymph nodes-Bone marrow	1
Liver	3
Liver-Bone	2
Liver-Breast	1
Liver-Breast-CNS	1
Skin-Breast-Bone	2

Results

Thirteen patients have demonstrated an objective response : 3 complete remissions (liver n = 1, lymph nodes n = 2), 10 partial responses (lung n = 3, liver n = 4, skin n = 2, bone marrow n = 1), giving an overall objective response rate of 72.2 %. Although the primary target defined upon inclusion is used to evaluate response, there should not be any disparity between the response of this tumor and those at other metastatic sites. Five patients have been classified as nonresponders (2 stable diseases, 3 progressions). The duration of response cannot yet be evaluated.

Toxicity

The main forms of toxicity observed are hematologic and mucous (presented in *Table III* in accordance with WHO criteria). Hematologic toxicity primarily consists of leukopenia (13/18 grades 3-4 with a nadir at D10 and transient neutropenia not exceeding 1 week). Thrombocytopenia is rare with only 1 case of grade 4 toxicity noted (patient with previous bone marrow involvement). Mucous toxicity is highly significant, with 8/18 patients showing grade 3-4 toxicity. As a result of the above effects, dose reductions have been made with NVB (3 cases) and 5FU (8 cases). Alopecia has been noted in 12/18 patients. Neurotoxicity is rare, with only 2 cases reported (1 grade 1 and 1 grade 3).

Table III. Principal toxicities (WHO scale).

Grade	0	1	2	3	4
Hematologic					
Leukocytes	2	1	2	8	5
Platelets	14	1	2	0	1
Mucitis	6	2	2	6	2

Discussion

With the 18 patients entered in this study, the current response rate is 72.2 % ($\pm$ 38.6). Factorial analysis reveals that the response rate calculated from the 2 analyses falls within initial limits. Since no threshold values have been exceeded (Ho or Ha), inclusions in the protocol should continue *(figure 1)*.

While this initial evaluation is highly encouraging, it is but a preliminary result and the follow-up is as yet insufficient for the response duration to be determined.

Moreover, in terms of Disease Free Survival (DFS) it would seem beneficial to propose the use of some form of maintenance treatment, the optimal modalities of which remain to be defined.

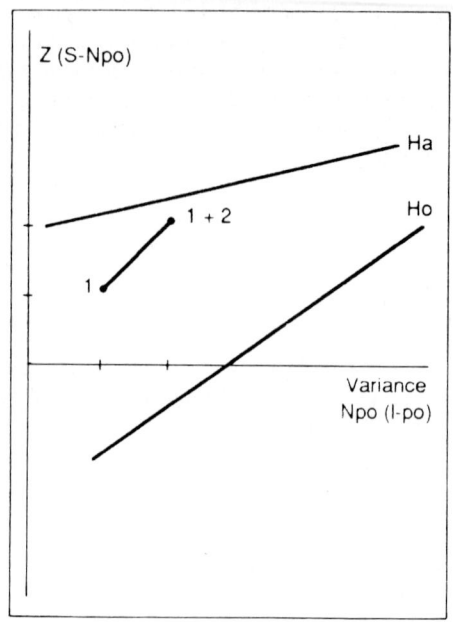

Figure 1. Triangular test.
Z = statistic; V = variance; 1 = 1st stage (n = 9); 1 + 2 : 2nd stage (n = 18).

We should perhaps at this point stress the value of factorial group analysis in cancer studies since they enable the efficacy of treatment to be assessed in a reduced patient population.

This study appears to demonstrate the acceptable safety of this combination, with most treatments administered on an out-patient basis. Dose reductions were required in only 3/18 patients (NVB) and 8/18 (5FU). Hematologic toxicity (grade 3 : n = 8, grade 4 : n = 5) was severe in only two cases, involving febrile episodes and hospitalization for parenteral antibiotic administration. Mucous toxicity was mainly observed in patients with liver metastases who initially presented with anomalous hepatic function. In cases of efficacy, these toxic effects have subsequently regressed, enabling the full doses established by the protocol to be resumed. No toxicity-related deaths have occurred.

Provided that the final result does not entail complete rejection with a response rate of less than 50 %, this study therefore confirms that :

1) NVB is active in breast cancer, which is very unusual for a vinca alkaloid. Response rates exceed 20 % in second line combination chemotherapy and reach 50-60 % in first line therapy, with acceptable safety. Navelbine® appears to be one of the most active molecules in breast cancer, particularly among intercalating agents.

2) This combination constitutes just one approach; other possibilities should also be studied in the future. The use of a sequential group plan enables such research

to be conducted in smaller patient populations before deciding whether to proceed with comparative studies.

3) This combination provides a potential alternative to first line cyclophosphamide-intercalant-based chemotherapy which may prove difficult to administer in the case of patients having received prior adjuvant anthracycline-based chemotherapy (10/18 patients in the current series).

References

1. Aisner J, Weinberg V, Perlof M, et al. Chemo-hormonotherapy for advanced breast cancer : a randomized comparison of 6 combinations each with or without MER hormonotherapy. A CALG study. *Am Soc Oncol* 1981; 22 : 443.
2. Benichou J, Bellissant E, Chastang C. Analyses séquentielles d'essais thérapeutiques en Hématologie et en Cancérologie. *Eurocancer,* Avril 1989.
3. Besenval M, Delgado M, Demarez JP, Krikorian A. Safety and tolerance of Navelbine in phase I-II clinical studies. *Lugano,* October 1988.
4. Brunner KW, Sontag RW, Martz G, et al. A controlled study in the use of combined drug therapy for metastatic breast cancer. *Cancer* 1975; 36 : 1208-1219.
5. Canobio L, Pastorino G, Brema F, Santi L. Efficacy of Navelbine (NVB) in advanced breast cancer. *Lugano* october 1988.
6. Lokich J. Optimal schedule for 5 Fluoro-Uracile chemotherapy : intermittent bolus or continuous infusion ? *Ann J oncol* 1985; 8 : 445-448.
7. Marty M, Extra JM, Espié M, et al. Advances in vinca-alkaloids : Navelbine. *Nouv Rev Fr Hematol* 1989; 31 : 77-84.
8. Nemoto T, Vana J, Bedwani RN, et al. Management and survival of female breast cancer : results of a national survey by the American College of Surgeons. *Cancer* 1980; 45 : 2917-2924.

B. Advanced ovarian carcinoma

27

Phase II study of Navelbine® as second or third line treatment in advanced ovarian carcinoma

J.-F. HÉRON[1], M.J. GEORGE[2], P. KERBRAT[3], J. CHAUVERGNE[4],
A. GOUPIL[5], D. LEBRUN[6], J.-P. GUASTALA[7], M. NAMER[8], R. BUGAT[9],
Y. AYME[10], C. LHOMME[2], C. TOUSSAINT[2], S. MERLE[11], M. BESENVAL[11],
J.-P. BURILLON[11]

[1] Centre François-Baclesse, route de Lion-sur-Mer, BP 5026, 14021 Caen, Cedex, France
[2] Institut Gustave-Roussy, rue Camille-Desmoulins, 94805 Villejuif, France
[3] Centre Eugène-Marquis, Pontchaillou, 35011 Rennes Cedex, France
[4] Fondation Bergonié, 180, rue de Saint-Genès, 33076 Bordeaux, France
[5] Centre René-Huguenin, 35, rue Dailly, 92211 Saint-Cloud, France
[6] Institut Jean-Godinot, 1, rue du Général-Koening, BP 171, 51056 Reims Cedex, France
[7] Centre Léon-Berard, 28, rue Laennec, 69373 Lyon Cedex, France
[8] Centre Antoine-Lacassagne, 36, voie Romaine, 06054 Nice Cedex, France
[9] Centre Claudius-Regaud, 20-24, rue du Pont-Saint-Pierre, 31052 Toulouse Cedex, France
[10] Institut Paoli-Calmette, 232, boulevard de Saint-Marguerite, 13273 Marseille Cedex 9, France
[11] Pierre-Fabre Médicament/CRPF, 192, rue Lecourbe, 75015 Paris, France

Introduction

Navelbine® is a new semisynthetic vinca alkaloid, with a strong experimental antitumor activity against L 1210 and P 388 murine leukemias, as well as against human tumor xenografts in nude mice [1].

A phase I clinical study demonstrated a maximal tolerated dose of 27.5 mg/m² to 35.4 mg/m², with a weekly intravenous bolus schedule; thus the recommended dose for further phase II studies was 30 mg/m², every week [2].

We present the results of a multicenter phase II study of Navelbine® in advanced ovarian cancers, in relapse or progressive disease, after the previous administration of one or two chemotherapy regimen(s) including cisplatin. Preliminary results were published in 1988, at the Lugano meeting of ESMO [3].

Patients and methods

Inclusion criteria

Patients with epithelial ovarian adenocarcinoma, relapsing after an effective pretreatment of polychemotherapy, or progressing under polychemotherapy (including a platinum compound), were eligible. Patients with secondary tumor malignancies (except in situ cervix carcinoma or basal cell skin carcinoma) were excluded.

The following criteria were also required:

Age had to be under 75 years, performance status less than WHO's grade 3; no prior treatment with vinca alkaloids was allowed and no more than two previous chemotherapy regimens. Neurological clinical examination had to be normal; the blood count had to show granulocytes above 2,000/mm^3 and platelets above 100,000/mm^3. Adequate renal, cardiac and liver function had to be demonstrated.

At least one measurable lesion, as assessed by clinical and/or radiological and/or ultrasound examination, was required. Tumor markers were not used to assess outcome. An interval of at least 4 weeks after prior treatment was necessary before beginning the treatment with Navelbine®.

Treatment protocol

Treatment consisted of Navelbine®, 30 mg/m^2, over 20 minutes, injected into a running IV infusion line. Treatment was given weekly, for at least 8 weeks, unless evident progression or unacceptable toxicity was observed.

Evaluation of the treatment was made after 8 cycles, with the same examinations used in the pretherapeutic workup. However, if at the weekly consultation, clear progression was observed, the patient could be withdrawn from the trial, and considered as a treatment failure.

The drug administration was postponed for 1 week, if full haematological recovery had not occurred. A dose reduction to 25 mg/m^2 was made, if the treatment had been postponed for more than 2 weeks. The treatment was discontinued, if full haematological recovery was not obtained after 3 weeks. Responses and toxicities were defined according to the WHO criteria.

Patients

The treatment was begun in 58 patients; however only 56 clinical records could be assessed. Fifty patients were eligible, the 6 other patients being excluded due to too short an interval between previous treatment and Navelbine®, too numerous previous chemotherapeutic regimens, a previous treatment with a vinca alkaloid or the absence of a clear measurable lesion.

One patient refused further treatment after one injection; thus only 49 patients are evaluable for toxicity. Seven patients are unevaluable for response : 2 early post-surgical deaths, one due to patient's refusal after 3 cycles, 2 patients due to toxic side-effects (allergy, haematological toxicity), and 2 patients were lost to follow-up : thus, only 42 patients are evaluable for response.

The clinical characteristics of the patients are as follows : the median age was 54 years (range 23-72 years), and the WHO performance status was grade I for 16 patients, grade II for 23 patients, grade III for 11 patients. FIGO initial staging was stage I for 2 patients, stage II for 6 patients, stage III for 31 patients, stage IV for 11 patients.

Thirty-four patients had no disease-free interval between initial treatment and the Navelbine® trial; for the 14 other patients, the interval ranged from 1 to 30 months.

All the patients had undergone at least one surgical procedure, 26 patients 2 procedures, 5 patients 3 procedures and 4 patients 4 procedures. Thirty patients had previously received one chemotherapy regimen, while the 20 others had received two regimens. All but one patient had previously been treated with cisplatin, 42 with cyclophosphamide, 33 with adriamycin and 22 with hexamethylmelamine. Furthermore, 12 patients had been irradiated : 8 to the pelvis and the abdomen, 1 to the abdomen alone, and 3 to the pelvis alone.

Results

Treatment tolerance

Median number of cycles per patient was 8, ranging from 1 to 49. Twelve patients received less than 4 cycles, 26 patients between 4 and 8 cycles, and 12 patients more than 8 cycles.

Delays in the administration due to the haemotologic toxicity were very often necessary. 37 % of the cycles were delayed, due to granulocytopenia less than 1 500. The intervals between two cycles were respectively one week for 63 %, 2 weeks for 22 %, 3 weeks for 14 % and 4 weeks for 1 % of the cycles. The reduction of the dose, as recommended by protocol, was performed in 16 % of the cycles (to 25 mg/m² for 13 %, and 20 mg/m² for 3 % of the cycles).

A study of the progress of treatment showed that it was very difficult to follow the proposed treatment protocol schedule : only 16 % of the patients received their first 4 cycles during the first 4 weeks, whereas not a single one could receive the 8 injections during the time limit of 8 weeks *(Figure 1)*.

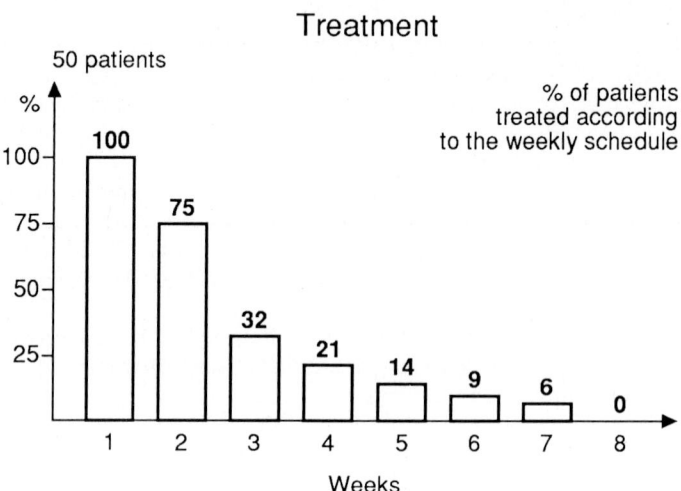

Figure 1. % of patients treated according to the weekly schedule

Clinical toxicity

Clinical toxicity was not severe

Nausea and vomiting of grade I or II intensity occurred in 25 patients, with only 5 patients being debilitated by grade III vomiting. Alopecia was observed for 16 patients, although it is not always easy to evaluate it, due to previous treatments. Grade I or II paresthesiae occurred in 13 patients. Previous treatment with cisplatin (almost every patient received more than 600 mg/m^2) might interfere, making the evaluation of the role of Navelbine® in the onset of neurological toxicity incertain. Constipation (grade I or II) was observed in 21 patients, and more severe sub-occlusions (grade III-IV) were observed in 8 patients : since at this nearly preterminal period of their disease most patients suffer from occlusion or constipation, it is not clear whether or not Navelbine® played a significant role in this toxic side effect. On the other hand, diarrhea was observed in 10 patients, and for one patient, it was severe (grade III). Phlebitis was very common (25 % of the patients).

Haematological toxicity

It is summarized in *Table I*.

Anemia was common; however only 12 % of the weekly blood counts showed a haemoglobin level low enough to justify blood transfusions.

Almost no toxicity was seen on the platelet line. On the other hand, granulocytopenia was very common, explaining the delay of 34 % of the cycles.

Table I. Haematological toxicity (percentage of cycles with toxicity; WHO grading for haematological toxicity).

Blood lineage	0	1	2	3	4
Haemoglobin	24	39	25	11	1
Leucocytes	41	23	22	12	2
Granulocytes	57	9	13	14	7
Platelets	97	0	1	1	1

Clinical responses

We observed one complete clinical response, 6 partial responses, 3 stabilizations and 32 patients progressed under treatment.

Table II. Presentation of responses.

Age	First staging	Previous treatments	Sites of relapse	Free interval	Duration response
Complete response					
37 years	II	CPM ADM CDDP	Pelvis Rectum	12 months	72 wks
Partial responses					
58 years	II	CDDP CPM Radioth.	Abdomen Pelvis	None	11 wks
43 years	III	ADM CPM HMM CDDP	Abdomen Pelvis Ing. node	None	15 wks
43 years	IV	ADM CPM HMM VP16 IFM	Abomen Pelvis	None	42 wks
23 years	III	ADM CDDP CPM HMM	Pelvis	None	22 wks
62 years	III	ADM CPM CDDP	Pelvis	30 months	31 wks
51 years	IV	ADM VM26 CPM CDDP	Axill. node	6 months	17 wks

Discussion

We treated a group of patients with advanced ovarian cancers, relapsing or progressive after an intensive chemotherapy regimen, including a platinum compound [4]. Such a population of patients is known to be very refractory to new treatment, and up to now, only high doses of platinum compounds have been shown to be active, but with a high incidence of severe toxicities [5, 6]. Most other drugs only give very transient insignificant responses (below 5 %).

The toxicity of Navelbine® treatment, in those heavily pretreated patients (surgery, chemotherapy with platinum, radiotherapy) was moderate and quite acceptable. Non hematological toxicity was limited to paresthesiae, without motor compromise, or to a constipation which could just as well be a consequence of the disease itself. Nevertheless these neurological complications appeared to be reversible when the treatment was discontinued [7].

Hematological toxicity was more severe, notably in patients previously irradiated. However, we observed no septic or bleeding complications.

Since we observed such a high efficiency in a population of refractory patients, we are now planning a pilot study of first fine Navelbine®, in combination with the two major drugs platinum and cyclophosphamide, for the patients remaining with a heavy tumor burden after first laparotomy.

References

1. Cros S, Wright M, Morimoto M, *et al.* Experimental Antitumor Activity of Navelbine®. *Semin Oncol* 1989; 16, 2 (suppl 4) : 15-20.
2. Mathé G, Reizenstein P. Phase I pharmacologic study of a new vincaalkaloid : Navelbine®. *Cancer Lett* 1985; 27 : 285-293.
3. George MJ, Héron JF, Kerbrat P, *et al.* Navelbine® in advanced ovarian epithelial cancer : a study of the French Oncology Centers. *Semin Oncol* 1989; 16, 2 (suppl 4) ; 30-32.
4. Ozols RF, Young RC. Chemotherapy of ovarian cancer. *Semin Oncol* 1984; 11 : 251-265.
5. Ozols RF, Ostchega Y, Curt G. High dose carboplatin in refractory ovarian cancer patients. *J Clin Oncol* 1987; 4 : 197-201.
6. Héron JF. Traitements adjuvants des cystadénocarcinomes de l'ovaire. *Rev Prat* 1989; 39, 26 : 2325-2329.
7. Besenval M, Delgado M, Demarez JP, Krikorian A. Safety and tolerance of Navelbine® in Phase I-II Clinical Studies. *Semin Oncol* 1989; 16, 2 (suppl 4) : 37-40.

28

Study of the combination vinorelbine - hexamethylmelamine (V-H) in advanced ovarian adenocarcinoma : prelimimary results of a phase I-II study NHO-88, from the ARTAC multicentric ovarian carcinoma study group

M.C. PINEL[1], G. PINON[2], M.J. GOUDIER[3], B. COIFFIER[4], M.H. FILIPPI[5], A. GOUPIL[6], B. ROULLET[7], T. FACCHINI[8], L. MIGNOT[9], P. TRESCA[1], F. HERITIER[1], M. DELGADO[10], D. BELPOMME[15]

[1] Centre de Recherche Clinique Cancérologique (CRCC) de l'Association pour la Recherche Thérapeutique Anti-Cancéreuse (ARTAC), 38, rue de Silly, 92100 Boulogne/Seine, France
[2] Polyclinique de Courlancy, 38, rue de Courlancy, 51100 Reims, France
[3] Centre Hospitalier de Lorient, 27, rue du Dr-Lettry, 56100 Lorient, France
[4] Centre Hospitalier Lyon Sud, 165, chemin du Grand-Revoyet, 69310 Pierre-Bénite, France
[5] Hôpital Bichat, 46, rue Henri-Huchard, 75018 Paris, France
[6] Centre René-Huguenin, 35, rue Dailly, 92211 Saint-Cloud, France
[7] Centre Hospitalier, 2, avenue Alexis-Carrel, 87042 Limoges, France
[8] Centre Hospitalier de Metz-Thionville, 57038 Metz, France
[9] Hôpital Foch, 40, rue Worth, 92151 Suresnes Cedex, France
[10] Pierre-Fabre Médicament/CRPF, 192, rue Lecourbe, 75015 Paris, France

Summary

The lack of decisive progress in ovarian cancer chemotherapy in recent years led us to re-initiate its study with a hypothesis based on collateral sensitivities. In this work, the V-H combination, combining vinorelbine and hexamethylmelamine, was studied in patients with previously treated ovarian adenocarcinoma, most of whom had

become resistant to previous chemotherapy. The aim of the study was to find an active combination without complete cross-resistance with first line platinum salt-based combination such as CAP, FAP or CACb-300. A pilot feasibility study was first carried out to determine the maximal tolerated weekly doses (MTWD) of vinorelbine (20 mg/m²/week), hexamethylmelamine being administered per os on days 1 and 14 of every 28 day cycle at a standard dose of 250 mg/m²/day. Then an open phase IIA study was done according to a two-step sequential analysis method for phase II studies. We observed :
   1) a good tolerance of the V-H combination aside from frequent neutropenia;
   2) a response rate of 35 % (confidence interval : 24.5 % − 54.5 %);
   3) a median response duration of 5 months (range : 1-10);
   4) and the absence of a complete cross-resistance between the V-H regimen and the previous CAP or FAP combinations therapy.
   These encouraging results which are currently being validated (phase IIB ongoing), are the first step in the search for an efficient treatment of advanced ovarian adenocarcinoma with alternate or sequential chemotherapeutic combinations.

Introduction

With an incidence of around 4 000 cases per year in France and a mortality rate of 3 000/year, ovarian adenocarcinoma still rises difficult therapeutic problems.
   Considering the difficulty of an early diagnosis and the lack of efficient screening methods, advanced FIGO stages IIB/C, III and IV remain the most frequent, approximately 70 % of the cases [2]. Surgery and chemotherapy are clearly two active treatments, but a certain number of immediate failures occur, as do relapses after an initial complete regression [3, 4].
   Among the first line chemotherapies, the CAP combination (cyclophosphamide, adriamycin and cisplatin) is the most frequently used [5, 6]. The macroscopic response rate (complete and partial responses) however is 40-70 %, not significantly different from the rate we obtained with the FAP combination, in which cyclophosphamide is replaced by 5-fluorouracil [4, 7, 8]. Moreover, the replacement of cisplatin in the CAP combination by carboplatin (or cisdiammine 1-1 cyclobutane-dicarboxylate-platinum), administered in a dose of 300 mg/m²/cycle (CACb-300 combination) [9, 10] brought about a better gastrointestinal and renal tolerance, but its efficacy was not superior, as shown by a preliminary analysis of a phase III study comparing these two combinations [11].
   Therefore, even though ovarian adenocarcinomas are generally considered to be chemosensitive tumors, these results indicate the need to find new chemotherapeutic regimens, without cross-resistance to the classical ones [12].
   Nor-5'-anhydro-vinblastine or vinorelbine (VNB) (Navelbine®) is a new alkaloid derived from the Madagascar periwinkle plant, selected for its therapeutic index, which is potentially superior to that of vincristine (VCR) and vinblastine (VLB) [13-15]. *In vitro*, VNB inhibits the polymerization of tubulin of the mitotic microtubules as efficiently as the former two alkaloids, but induces a lower spiralization of

axonic microtubules [16]. In animals, the molecule is at least as active as VCR or VLB in L1210 leukemia line and B16 melanoma [17, 18]. In studies with this same leukemia line, (P388/MDR+) with a multi-drug resistance phenotype or only to VCR (P388/VCR), VNB was still active and thus showed only a weak degree of cross-resistance to VCR and other drugs inducing the MDR phenotype. These preclinical observations justified the clinical development of the product. In a phase I study, it was confirmed that VNB had little neurotoxicity and an acceptable hematologic tolerance. The Maximum Tolerated Weekly Dose (MTWD) was evaluated at 30 mg/m^2/week [19]. In addition, in the course of a phase II study in patients with ovarian adenocarcinoma pretreated with multiple chemotherapies, VNB was shown to be still active [20] with a response rate of approximately 15 %. Considering that the drug was given as a second, third of fourth line treatment, there seems to be a relative lack of cross resistance with the drugs given previously.

Hexamethylmelamine (HMM) is an S-triazine drug, derived from ethylene immine, proposed for the treatment of ovarian adenocarcinoma [21, 22]. The molecule is activated essentially by oxidative N-demethylation in hepatic microsomes, and also, although to a lesser degree, in tumor cells [23, 24]. During this activation, the hydroxymethylmelamine derivatives, known to be the most cytotoxic *in vitro,* might be the metabolites responsible for the observed clinical activity. Although the mechanism of action of this drug and its hydroxymethylmelamine derivatives is not clear, an alkylating action is not demonstrated *in vivo* (and there are many possible interactions with numerous macromolecules), obviously hexamethylmelamine is active in ovarian adenocarcinoma. The response rate is about 30-40 % as a first line treatment [21, 25, 26] or in patients not previously treated with alkylating agents [27, 28] and also from 5-25 % as a second line treatment [29, 33]. These results suggest the absence of complete cross-resistance with classical alkylating agents and anthracyclines and explain the use of this drug in a number of combinations, not only in first line but also in second line treatment [21].

The purpose of the present stydy was to evaluate the tolerance and efficacy of the V-H combination in patients with ovarian adenocarcinoma previously treated by chemotherapy. The protocol was designated to determine first the MTWD of VNB, with a standard constant HMM dose in a limited number of patients, and secondly, the efficacy and the tolerance of this combination in a classic open phase II study.

We present here the preliminary results of this study, from an intermediary analysis done in September 1989.

Patients and methods

Patients

Inclusion criteria were as follows :
— Age less than 70 years.
— Histologically proven ovarian adenocarcinoma with a measurable lesion in its two largest diameters.

— Previous treatment with a chemotherapy combination containing at least one platinum compound (cisplatin or carboplatin).
— No contraindication to the administration of vinorelbine or hexamethylmelanine.
— A World Organization (WHO) performance status inferior or equal to 2.
— No second cancer, except for in situ cervix or skin cancer considered as cured at the time of inclusion.
— Possibility of follow-up.
— An informed consent to the treatment.

Exclusion criteria were as follows : 1) tumor of low malignancy; 2) clinically detectable brain metastases; 3) signs of severe neuropathy, revealed by electromyography or clinical examination (WHO, grade > 1); 4) a lesion within an irradiated field; 5) previous treatment with VNB and/or HMM.

Protocol design

HMM was given per os at a dosis of 250 mg/m^2/day, from day 1 to day 14, and VNB as a bolus intravenous injection on day 1, 7, 14 and 21, with 28-day cycles (V-H combination). HMM being given at the dose indicated above, the MTWD for VNB was determined in a limited number of patients in a preliminary feasibility trial. A dose of 20 mg/m^2/week was given in the first cycle (first step dose), 25 mg/m^2/week in the second step dose, and 30 mg/m^2/week in the third step dose. *Table I* summarizes the VNB doses adaptation in this preliminary trial. Once the MTWD of VNB was determined, it was used in the first cycle for the other patients. The treatment was continued until disease progression, following the dose adaptation schedule shown in *Table II*.

Evaluation criteria

The evaluation of tolerance and antitumor response followed the WHO criteria [35]. The degree of response was evaluated considering measurable lesions, in their largest diameters, and the appearance of new lesions. Thus, in the case of an unmeasurable lesion (either clinically or by imaging), evaluation could be made only after a second look laparotomy.

Evaluation and statistical analysis

After determining the MTWD of VNB, the study consisted in a classical open phase II trial using a two-step sequential method. The initial hypothesis in the first step (phase IIA), assumed that the V-H combination could induce a response rate of at least 20 % or greater, considering the previous multitreatments of the patient population, and accepting a beta risk of 5 % [36, 37]. As the MTWD of VNB was found to be the first dose-step, 20 mg/m^2/week (described below), most of the patients included in the feasibility trial were considered as available for the phase II A study, insofar as they had measurable lesions. However, only the patients who received at least 1 cycle of the V-H regimen were considered as evaluable for response.

Table I. Feasibility study of the V-H combination : adaptation of VNB doses.

	Polynuclears/mm³	Platelets/mm³	
Before each V-H cycle	≥ 2 000	≥ 120 000	Increase to the next step-dose.
	1 000 – 2 000	50 – 120 000	1 week delay. If longer than 1 week, decrease to the previous step-dose.
	< 1 000	< 50 000	Decrease to the previous step-dose.
Before each administration of VNB	≥ 1 500	≥ 100 000	Full dose.
	1 000 – 1 500	50 – 100 000	1 week delay. If longer than 1 week, decrease to the previous step-dose.
	< 1 000	< 50 000	Decrease to the previous step-dose.

Table II. Adaptation of VNB doses in patients treated at the MWTD.

	Polynuclears/mm³	Platelets/mm³	
Before each V-H cycle	≥ 2 000	≥ 120 000	Full dose.
	1 000 – 2 000	50 – 120 000	1 week delay.
	< 1 000	< 50 000	1 week delay; dismissal from the study if it persists the second week.
Before each administration of VNB	≥ 1 500	≥ 100 000	Full dose.
	1 000 – 1 500	50 – 100 000	1 week delay
	< 1 000	< 50 000	1 week delay; dismissal from the study if it persists the second week.

Results

Patient population

From February 1988 to September 1989, 34 consecutive patients (median age = 58 years, range : 36-70) were included. Thirty patients were eligible. One case of pre-existing neuropathy (WHO grade 1), and three cases of bone marrow insufficiency secondary to previous chemotherapies, with polymorphonuclear count

Table III. Patient population

	Number of patients
Median age : 58 (36-70)	
Included	34
Not eligible	4
Eligible	30
FIGO stage	
II	1
III	22
IV	7
Number of previous treatments	
1	16
2	8
>2	5
Unknown	1

< 2.000 at the time of inclusion, were considered as non-eligible. Of the 30 eligible patients, 22 presented with FIGO stage III, seven with stage IV and one with stage IIB disease. Sixteen patients (53 %) received the treatment as a second line, eight (27 %) as a third line and five (17 %) at an even later stage. In one case the number of chemotherapeutic regimens already received could not be determined. These data are summarized in *Table III*.

Feasibility study of the V-H combination : determination of the MTWD of VNB

With a HMM dose of 250 mg/m^2/day from D 1 to D 14 of each cycle, the MTWD of VNB was determined in 10 patients by a progressive increase in doses, with 4-week dose steps. Each dose step corresponded to a cycle of the previously described protocol. *Table IV* summarizes the results. The step doses of 25 mg/m^2/week and 30 mg/m^2/week could be reached in only three and one patient respectively, because of the appearance of a neutropenia in six patients in the first step, preventing the progression to higher step-doses. Therefore, the MTWD of VNB retained for the V-H combination was 20 mg/m^2/week.

Table IV. Feasibility study of the V-H combination.

Level of VNB doses reached	1st level 20 mg/m^2/week	2nd level 25 mg/m^2/week	3rd level 30 mg/m^2/week
Number of patients	6	3	1

Tolerance of the V-H combination

Of the 30 eligible patients, 24 were evaluable for tolerance (Table III) : one patient was lost to follow-up and five were not considered evaluable because of too short a delay between their inclusion and the time of the analysis.

Hematologic tolerance

The results are shown in *Table V*. The tolerance is excellent as far as platelet and red blood cells are concerned. However the protocol's limiting toxicity concerns neutrophils essentially. WHO grade III-IV neutropenia occurred in approximately 2/3 of the patients, and appeared after a median span of five weeks (range : 2-10), after the beginning of the V-H combination, resulting in a VNB dose modification.

Table V. Hematologic tolerance of the V-H combination (24 patients).

Parameter	WHO grade	
	≤2*	>2
Hb	21 (87 %)	3 (13 %)
Leukocytes	15 (62 %)	9 (38 %)
Polynuclears	7 (29 %)	17 (71 %)
Platelets	23 (96 %)	1 (4 %)

* The WHO grades were determined for each patient after evaluation of the Nadir during the whole treatment.

General tolerance

The results are shown in *Table VI*. Nausea/vomiting, often with a moderate intensity, were the most frequent complications and were reported by all patients (role of HMM). Alopecia was minimal (grade I) and observed in only 21 % of the cases. Even though some of the patients had already been treated with cisplatin, peripheral neuropathies were rare and of very minor intensity. There was only one reported case of grade I neuropathy. At the time of inclusion, five patients presented a grade I neuropathy secondary to a previous cisplatin treatment. In three of them, the neuropathy remained unchanged, whereas in the others, it increased to a grade II. Constipation which occurred in only 16 % of the patients was always moderate, as well as diarrhea. Signs of hepatic toxicity were observed in five patients. The increases in the SGPT and SGOT transaminases were already present in one patient, and thus could not be attributed to the V-H combination. In two other patients however, there was a grade II and IV transitory increase in the transaminase respectively, resulting in treatment withdrawal. An isolated increase in alkaline phosphatase was observed in the two remaining patients, (grade II in one and grade III in the other), and could

Table VI. General tolerance of the V-H combination (24 patients).

Parameter	WHO grades				
	0	1	2	3	4
Nausea/vomiting		12 (50 %)	5 (21 %)	7 (29 %)	
Alopecia	19 (79 %)	5 (21 %)			
Peripheral neuropathy	28 (94 %)	1 (5 %)			
Constipation	20 (84 %)	4 (16 %)			
Diarrhea	20 (84 %)	1 (4 %)	2 (8 %)	1 (4 %)	
Hepatic toxicity	20 (84 %)		2 (8 %)	1 (4 %)	1 (4 %)
Infection	20 (84 %)		1 (4 %)	3 (12 %)	
Venous toxicity	20 (84 %)	1 (4 %)	3 (12 %)		
Mucous toxicity	22 (92 %)		2 (8 %)		

be related to the drugs rather than to the disease. Four other patients had infectious complications, reversible with antibiotic treatment. They were grade II in one patient (no detectable infectious site, no identified germ and non specific infection signs) and grade III in the other three patients : one case of candida septicimia, one case of ascitic fluid infection and finally one case of abscess, caused by a rectovaginal fistula. Venous toxicity was characterized by pain during the injection of vinorelbine (grade I) in one case and by a more significant phlebitis (grade II) in three other cases. There was no reported cutaneous, renal, or cardiac toxicity. This explains the relatively good general tolerance to the V.H. combination.

Compliance

For the 24 patients evaluated for tolerance, the ratio of actually received VNB doses and the theoretical doses, as established previously (20 mg/m^2/week) is 75 %. In all cases, dosis modifications were caused by neutropenia.

Response

Among the 20 patients evaluable for response, two had a complete and five a partial response (*Table VII*). The observed response rate is 35 % (7/20), ± 10.5 % (95 % confidence interval). Six of these seven patients had a FIGO stage III, and one a stage IV disease (*Table VIII*). Four patients presented with a relapse (early or late) and three had an initial failure. All patients had been previously treated with cisplatin and

Table VII. Response rate and duration with the V-H combination.

Response	Number of patients	Rate (%)
CR	2	35 % ± 10,5
PR	5	
S	9	45 %
P	4	20 %

Median duration : 5 months (range : 1-10 months).

Table VIII. Clinical data on patients responding to the V-H combination.

Case number	FIGO stage	Previous treatment(s)	Carcinologic status at inclusion	Measurable lesions	Type of response	Response duration (months)
1	IIIA	CAP (×6)	1st relapse (420 d)	Pelvis	RP	10
2	IV	CAP (×6)	1st relapse (680 d)	Pelvis Lymph nodes	RP	10
3	IIIB	CAP (×2)	Initial failure	Abdomen	RP	1
4	IIIB	FAP (×3)	Initial failure	Pelvis	RP	5
5	IIIA	FAP (×6)	2nd relapse	Lymph nodes	RP	4
6	IIIA	CAP (×4)	Initial failure	Lymph nodes	CR	5
7	IIIA	CAP (×6)	1st relapse (550 d)	Abdomen	CR	3(*)

III A largest diameter of the most voluminous residual post-surgical lesion < 2 cm;
III B largest diameter of the most voluminous residual lesion, ⩾ 2 cm;
(X n.) : number of administered cycles; (n. d) : delay between the initial diagnosis and relapse in days.
 Lymph nodes : retrogastic (case No. 2), supraclavicular (case No. 5), lumbaortic (case No. 6).
* Protocol interruption after three months, due to a grade IV hepatic toxicity (see text).

adriamycin. Five of these received the CAP combination, and two the FAP combination. The measurable lesions were pelvic or pelviabdominal in five cases, nodal in one, and pelvic and nodal in another. The median response duration was five months (range : 1-10).

Discussion

These results are the first step of a phase II study to evaluate the tolerance and efficacy of the V-H combination in previously treated ovarian adenocarcinoma, with at least one platinum salt. The approach of this study is part of a general strategy in oncologic research aiming to find alternate or sequential drug regimens without cross-resistance to one another [12, 38-40]. In this study as well as in others, particularly in breast cancer [38-40], one of the hypotheses we are presently testing is that a first line chemotherapy selects and/or induces the appearance of tumor cell clones, some of which are chemosensitive to the action of second line combinations. We have recently formulated the hypothesis that the chemoresistance is a consequence not only of a clonal selection phenomenon, similar to that described by Goldie-Coldman [41], but also of an induction phenomenon, which could be included at least partially, in a more general adaptation theory [12, 40, 42]. This hypothesis implies that the appearance of collateral sensitivities after a first line chemotherapy could follow a similar induction mechanism. However in numerous initially chemo-sensitive human tumors, the early appearance of pleiotropic resistance is the most frequent phenomenon, as shown by biological and clinical observations.

In a previous pilot study on ovarian adenocarcinoma, we showed that VLB when given in monotherapy at a high doses (12 mg/m^2 to 45 mg/m^2), with 28 day cycles, could induce a certain number of responses in tumors resistant to alkylating agents, antimetabolites, anthracyclines, and even VLB itself, used at classical doses [43]. However paralytic ileus, although medically manageable, was very frequent. We also showed in a second study, that the cisplatin-HMM combination could give a high response rate in tumors resistant to alkylating agents, classical antimetabolites and adriamycin [44]. The recent availability of a new vinca alkaloid, VNB, less neurotoxic and possibly more active than VLB, prompted us to use it with HMM, with a further objective of combining these two drugs with a platinum salt, considering the possible potentiation between these 3 drugs [45].

The results of the present study, although preliminary, are encouraging. The responses obtained in two cases of initial failure with the CAP combination and in one case of initial failure with the FAP combination, suggest the absence of a complete cross-resistance between the V-H combination and these regimens. Furthermore, as shown by the response rate (35 ± 10.5 %) and above all, its duration (median 5 months), the overall efficacy of the combination is interesting. This justify a phase II B complementary activation of this protocol (currently in progress), in order to include a large enough number of patients.

Although the V-H combination was relatively well tolerated, its hematologic toxicity is a limiting factor. Even if, in our study, the doses were decreased to 20 mg/m^2/week, the neutropenia induced by VNB results in a protocol compliance of only 75 %. We have proposed since 1979 that the vinca alkaloids be administered less frequently at higher doses as a bolus, and not according to the traditional weekly schedule. We showed that this modality of administration, at least for VLB in ovarian carcinoma, yields a relatively satisfactory response rate in previously treated patients, with a remarkable hematologic tolerance even at high doses. Obviously such a therapeutic schedule, less demanding on the patients and on their veins, would make VNB easier to manage in combination regimens. This approach should be tested in the future, using this new drug, at least in the treatment of solid tumors, especially ovarian carcinoma.

* A preliminary publication of this study was reported at the ECCO 5 Congress, September 1989 [34].

References

1. INSERM, *Causes médicales de décès, résultats définitifs.* France, 1986.
2. Belpomme D. Acquisitions récentes dans le traitement des adénocarcinomes de l'ovaire : le pronostic, la place des traitements locorégionaux, les nouveaux médicaments et nouvelles stratégies, la chimio-radiothérapie lourde suivie d'autogreffe de moelle osseuse. *In* : A. Netter (eds), *Actualités gynécologiques,* Paris, Masson, 1987; 1-23.
3. Levardon M, Sibella P, Belpomme D, *et al.* 102 cas de cancers primitifs de l'ovaire traités depuis 1974. II Place et rôle de la chirurgie de réduction et intérêts des interventions de contrôle. *Rev Franç Gynéc* 1979; 74 : 577-585.
4. Belpomme D, Pappo F, Hacène K, *et al.* Advanced ovarian carcinoma : new therapeutic approaches based on tumoral residuum analysis at staging and second look Laparotomy. *Proc ESMO, 12th annual meeting,* Nice 1986 (Abst. 19).
5. Belinson J, McClure M, Ashikaga T, Krakoff I. Treatment of advanced and recurrent ovarian carcinoma with Cyclophosphamide, Doxorubicin and Cisplatin, *Cancer* 1984; 54 : 19-23.
6. Conte P, Bruzzone M, Chiara S, *et al.* A randomized trial comparing Cisplatin plus Cyclophosphamide Versus Cisplatin, Doxorubicin and Cyclophosphamide in advanced ovarian cancer. *J Clin Oncol* 1986; 4 : 965-971.
7. Belpomme D, Pappo F, Le Rol A, *et al.* Chimiothérapie des adénocarcinomes de l'ovaire : bilan de ces dix dernières années, nouveaux concepts et place dans la stratégie thérapeutique d'ensemble. *Contraception-Fertilité-Sexualité,* 1984; Supp. 12 : 303-313.
8. Belpomme D, Hacène K, Pappo F, *et al.* Pronostic evaluation in advanced ovarian carcinoma : individualization of a group of patients with potentially curable disease. *Cancer* 1991; à paraître.
9. Bugat R, Pinel MC, Martin Ph, *et al.* Apport du Carboplatine dans le traitement des adénocarcinomes ovariens de stade FIGO III-IV. Etude de faisabilité de la combinaison CACb-300. *Gynécologie* 1988; 39 : 191-196.
10. Martin Ph, Bugat R, Pinon G, *et al.* 300 mg/m^2 Carboplatin (Cb), Adriamycin (A), Cyclophosphamide (C) (CACb-300) Combination in advanced ovarian carcinoma : a feasability study. *Cancer Chemother-Pharmacol* 1989; 23 : 331-332.
11. Pinel MC, Bugat R, Belpomme D, *et al.* Carboplatin replacing Cis-Platinum for the treatment of advanced ovarian carcinoma : first interim analysis of a randomized phase III trial companing CAP and CACb-300 : an ARTAC study. *Proc. NCI-EORTC Symposium,* Amsterdam 1989; Abst 316.
12. Belpomme D. L'obstacle de la résistance en chimiothérapie anticancéreuse. Une théorie de l'induction-sélection. *Cancer Communication* 1991 à paraître.

13. Potier P, Guénard D, Zaval F. Résultats récents dans le domaine des alcaloïdes anti-tumoraux du groupe de la Vinblastine. Etudes biochimiques. *CR Soc Biol* 1979; 173 : 414-424.
14. Mangeney P, Andriamialisoa RZ, Lallemand JY, et al. 5'-Noranhydrovinblastine. Prototype of a new class of Vinblastine derivatives. *Tetrahedron* 1979; 35 : 2175-2179.
15. Mangeney P, Andriamialisoa RZ, Langlois N, et al. A new class of antitumor compounds : 5' Nor and 5'-6'- Seco derivatives of Vinblastine-type alkaloids. *J Org Chem* 1979; 44 : 3765-3768.
16. Meininger V. 1987, *communication personnelle*.
17. Maral P, Bourut C, Chenu E, Mathe G. Experimental antitumor activity of 5'-Nor-Anhydro-vinblastine, Navelbine. *Cancer lett,* 1984; 22 : 49-54.
18. Takoudju M, Gros S, Schaepelynck-Lataste H, et al. Comparative in vitro and in vivo study of Navelbine ditartrate (Nor-5'-Anhydrovinblastine) with the two antitumor compounds Vinblastine and Vincristine. *14th Intl Cong Chemother* (June 23-28, Kyoto) 1985; Abst S-2-10.
19. Mathe G, Reizenstein P. Phase I pharmacologic study of a new Vincaalkaloid : Navelbine. *Cancer Lett* 1985; 27 : 285-293.
20. George M, Heron JG, Kerbrat P, et al. Phase II study of Navelbine (NVB) in advanced ovarian carcinomas (ADOVCA). A cooperative study of French Oncology Centers. *Proc Am Soc Clin Oncol* 1988; 7 : Abst 553.
21. Foster BJ, Clagett-Carr K, Marsoni S, et al. Role of Hexamethylmelamine in the treatment of ovarian cancer : where is the needle in the Haystack ? *Cancer Treat Rep* 1986; 70 : 1003-1014.
22. Bruckner HW. Role of Hexamethylmelamine in the treatment of ovarian cancer : where is the needle in the Haystack ? (commentary) *Cancer Treat Rep* 1987; 71 : 666-667.
23. Bruidley C, Gescher A, Langdou SP, et al. Studies of the mode of action of antitumor triazines and triazines-III. Metabolism studies on Hexamethylmelamine. *Biochem Pharmacol,* 1982; 31 : 625-631.
24. Worzalla JF, Kaiman BD, Johnson BM, et al. Metabolism of Hexamethylmelamine-ring 14C in rats and man *Cancer Res* 1974; 34 : 2669-2674.
25. Wharton JT, Rutledge F, Smith JP, et al. Hexamethylmelamine : an evaluation of its role in the treatment of ovarian cancer. *Am J. Obstet Gynecol* 1979; 133 : 833-841.
26. Smith JP, Rutledge FN. Random study of Hexamethylmelamine, 5 Fluorouracil and Melphalan in treatment of advanced carcinoma of the ovary. *Natl Cancer Inst Monogr* 1975; 42 : 169-172.
27. Wilson WL, Schroeder JM, Bisel HF, et al. Phase II study of Hexamethylmelamine (NSC 13875) *Cancer* 1969; 23 : 132-136.
28. Wilson WL, Bisel HF, Cole D, et al. Prolonged low dosage administration of Hexamethylmelamine (NSC 13875). *Cancer* 1970; 25 : 568-570.
29. Bonomi PD, Mladineo J, Morin B, et al. Phase II trial of Hexamethylmelamine in ovarian carcinoma resistant to alkylating agents. *Cancer Treat Rep* 1979; 63 : 137-138.
30. Johnson BL, Fisher RI, Bender RA, et al. Hexamethylmelamine in alkylating agent-resistant ovarian carcinoma. *Cancer* 1978; 42 : 2157-2161.
31. Omura GA, Greco FA, Birch R. Hexamethylmelamine in mustard-resistant ovarian adenocarcinoma. *Cancer Treat Rep,* 1981; 65 : 530-531.
32. Stanhope CR, Smith JP, Rutledge F. Second trial drugs in ovarian cancer. *Gynecol Oncol* 1977; 5 : 52-58.
33. Bolis G, D'Incalci M, Belloni C, et al. Hexamethylmelamine in ovarian cancer resistant to Cyclophosphamide and Adriamycin. *Cancer Treat. Rep* 1979; 63 : 1375-1377.
34. Pinon G, Goudier MJ, Coiffier B, et al. Navelbine and chemotherapy regimen in advanced ovarian carcinoma : an ARTAC phase II study. *Proc. ECCO 5,* Londres, 1989; Abst 1107.

35. WHO Handbook for reporting results of cancer treatment. *WHO offset publication N° 48*, World Health Organization, Geneva 1979.
36. Gehan EA. The determination of the number of patients required in a preliminary and a follow-up trial of a new chemotherapeutic agent. *J. Chronic Diseases* 1961; 13 : 346-353.
37. Lee YJ, Staquet M, Simon R, *et al.* Two-stage plans for patient accrual in phase II cancer clinial trials. *Cancer Treat Rep,* 1979; 63 : 1721-1726.
38. Belpomme D, Heritier F, Gisselbrecht C, *et al.* Long duration of response with Vindesine, Mitoxantrone, Mitomycine C (VMMc) combination chemotherapy in metastatic breast cancer : a pilot phase II study. *Cancer Treat Rep* 1987; 71 : 845-847.
39. Belpomme D, Gisselbrecht C, Marty M, *et al.* Traitement des cancers du sein métastasés par la combinaison VMMc (Vindésine, Mitoxantrone, Mitomycine C) : incidence sur la survie et étude des résistances croisées par rapport aux traitements antérieurs. *CR Therap Pharm Cl* 1987; 55 : 1-25.
40. Belpomme D, Gisselbrecht C, Marty M, *et al.* Les cancers du sein métastasés sont-ils potentiellement curables par chimiothérapie ? *Gynecologie* 1988; 39 : 197-204.
41. Goldie JH, Coldman J. Application of theoritical models to chemotherapy protocol design. *Cancer Treat Rep* 1986; 70 : 127-131.
42. Belpomme D, Heritier F, Ressayre C. Goldie Coldman hypothesis revisited : an induction-selection theory of chemoresistance. *Proc Am Soc Clin Onc,* San Francisco 1989; Abst 316.
43. Belpomme D, Schwartzenberg L, Bohu A, *et al.* Administration de Vincaleucoblastine à fortes doses dans les cancers de l'ovaire évolués : résultats préliminaires d'un essai thérapeutique phase II. *Rev Franç Gynéc* 1979; 74 : 597-601.
44. Bohu A, Belpomme D. Association de Cis-diammine dichloroplatinum et d'Hexaméthylmélamine pour le traitement des cancers de l'ovaire évolués devenus chimiorésistants. *Rev Franç Gynec* 1979; 74 : 603-607.
45. Stehman F, Ehslich C, Williams S, Einhorm L. Cisplatin, Vinblastine and Bleomycin as second-trail therapy in ovarian carcinoma. A pilot study of the gynecologic Oncology Group. *Am J Clin Oncol* 1985; 8 : 27-31.

C. Lymphomas

29

Phase II study of vinorelbine (Navelbine®) in previously treated Hodgkin's disease and non-Hodgkin's lymphomas

H. EGHBALI

Fondation Bergonié, 180, rue de Saint-Genès, 33076 Bordeaux, France

Vinca alkaloids are widely used in the first line treatment of non-Hodgkin's lymphomas and Hodgkin's disease. A phase II study was conducted using vinorelbine (Navelbine®) in patients previously treated with vinca alkaloids (vinblastine, vincristine and vindesine) and exhibiting resistance not only to these agents but also to most of the cytostatics currently used against lymphomas.

Patients and methods

Objective of the study

This open multicentre phase II study was designed to assess the anti-tumor activity of Navelbine® by evaluating the quality and duration of the responses observed in patients with malignant non-Hodgkin's lymphomas or Hodgkin's disease. The study was also intended to evaluate cross-reactivity with other vinca alkaloids and any side effects noted in a pretreated patient population included in no other therapeutic protocol.

Indications, inclusion and exclusion criteria

Indications

The study included patients with relapsed or refractory Hodgkin's disease, low grade or aggressive non-Hodgkin's lymphomas.

Inclusion criteria

Tumors must be histologically proven and beyond conventional salvage treatment or for which no treatment has been established. Tumors must be measurable or evaluable, and in clinically confirmed progression. Patients were required to have a performance status ≤ 2 (WHO scale) with an expected survival of at least 3 months without treatment and no clinical or electromyographical signs of peripheral neuropathy (apart from disorders attributable to the tumor). Normal blood chemistry tests were required (polymorphonuclear neutrophils $\geq 2.10^9/l$, platelets $\geq 100.10^9/l$, hemoglobin ≥ 6.8 mmol/l) in addition to normal hepatic and renal function (apart from bone marrow or hepatic involvement).

Exclusion criteria

Patients aged over 75 years, patients with only one previously irradiated tumor site and patients receiving chemo- or radiotherapy during the month immediately before the study were excluded.

Patients were also excluded if they presented with peripheral neuropathy (clinically or electromyographically confirmed), central nervous system or meningeal involvement, an intercurrent infection, a second cancer, if they had received treatment likely to produce an anti-neoplastic effect, or if follow-up could not be guaranteed throughout the study.

Treatment

Vinorelbine was given alone in all cases by a direct i.v. injection followed by flushing of the vein. After the first patients treated complained of venous toxicity, the i.v. mode of administration was modified to a 15-20 minute infusion in 250 ml isotonic glucose solution, giving a planned dose of 30 mg/m^2. Treatment was given weekly, with a minimum of 4 injections in high-grade lymphomas, and 8 in low-grade lymphomas and Hodgkin's disease. In the event of grade 3-4 leukopenia, the injection was postponed until the leukocyte count recovered. With repeated toxicity, the dose was cut to 25 mg/m^2.

Diagnostic methods and evaluation of response

WHO/EORTC/NCI criteria were used to establish the therapeutic response from one or two-dimensional measurements taken before and after treatment. The complete disappearance of the lesion and its signs was taken as complete response or complete remission (CR), more than 50 % reduction in lesion size as a partial response (PR), less than 50 % reduction as stabilization (STAB) and lesion growth as progression (P).

Toxicity

Clinical and biological toxicity were evaluated according to standard WHO criteria.

Results

Fifty-three patients were included in this study in accordance with the established criteria. Two patients were excluded due to major violations of the protocol (1 treated at the end of a post-chemotherapy aplasia and in the other case, treatment was reduced to a twice-monthly half-dose injection and was therefore incompatible with requirement). Four patients could not be evaluated owing to insufficient information on dosage and the biological effects of treatment.

Of the 47 patients actually included in the study, neither response nor toxicity were evaluated in 12 cases : 8 premature deaths occurred between days 5 and 20 of treatment (2 cases of mediastinal compression linked to tumor progression in an irradiated region, 1 case of pulmonary embolism preceded by phlebitis and confirmed by ECG, 1 case of hypercalcemia linked to lymphoma progression, 1 case of meningeal involvement linked to high-grade lymphoma, 2 cases of tumor-related respiratory distress, and 1 case of massive hemoptysis from a mediastinal tumor). Two patients discontinued treatment prematurely and were therefore not evaluated : 1 after the third injection owing to acute angina pain during infusion and 1 (a splenectomized patient) following the development of a serious lung infection after the second injection. The other 2 patients were not evaluated due to exclusive bone marrow

Table I. Non-evaluable patients : 12.

Premature death :	
Mediastinal compression	2
Pulmonary embolism	1
Hypercalcemia	1
Blastic meningitis	1
Acute respiratory failure	2
Massive hemoptysis	1
Discontinuation of treatment due to complications :	
Angina pectoris	1
Severe pneumopathy	1
Non-evaluable lesion (bone marrow)	2

involvement (*Table I*) and the absence of other measurable or evaluable lesions. Thirty-five patients were included in the analysis of efficacy and toxicity (17 cases of Hodgkin's disease and 18 cases of non-Hodgkin's lymphoma).

Hodgkin's disease

The 15 males and 2 females included in this group were aged between 22 and 74 years (mean : 36 years) and all had received prior polychemotherapy and extended irradiation. They had taken a mean of eight different drugs (rang : 6-11) before receiving vinorelbine; all had been treated with vinblastine and 15 with both vinblastine and vincristine under such standard regimens as MOPP, ABVD, CEP and CVPP. Most had undergone extended radiotherapy for the first tumor episode (2 cases of locoregional irradiation, 5 cases of mantle field irradiation, 9 cases of subtotal lymph node irradiation and 1 case of total body irradiation prior to an autologous bone marrow transplantation. All these patients exhibited relapsed or progressive disease including visceral tumor sites (4 - liver, 4 - lungs, 1 - bone marrow, 5 - isolated lymph nodes in previously irradiated areas) and 6 patients were suffering from systemic disorders (5 cases of biliary retention and 1 case of thrombocytopenia featuring bone marrow involvement) (*Table II*).

Table II. Patients with Hodgkin's disease : 17.

Mean age :	36 years (22-74)
Sex :	15 males
	2 females
Initial stage :	
I et II	7
III et IV	10
Initial chemotherapy :	17/17
MOPP, ABVD, CEP, CVPPP, etc.	
Initial radiotherapy :	17/17
Locoregional	2
Mantle field	5
Mantle + para-aortic field	2
Mantle + inverted Y field	7
Total body irradiation	1
Predominant tumor site :	
Lymph nodes only	5
Lymph node + spleen	2
Visceral : Lung	4
Liver	4
Bone	1
Bone marrow	1
Blood chemistry anomalies :	
Serum alkaline phosphatase > 3N	5
Pancytopenia	1

Non-Hodgkin's lymphomas

This group included 7 males and 11 females aged between 35 and 75 years (mean: 61 years) with the following histopathological types: 9 high-grade (3 transformations of low-grade lymphoma) and 9 low-grade lymphomas according to the Kiel classification or the Working Formulation.

All had previously undergone combination chemotherapy including a mean of 8 different drugs (range: 3-16) but had received less radiotherapy than the Hodgkin's group (no previous radiotherapy in 7 cases, isolated cervical irradiation in 5 cases, para-aortic in 4 cases and abdominal in 2 cases). All patients were in progression or relapse (*Table III*).

Table III. Patients with non-Hodgkin's lymphomas: 18.

Mean age:	61 years (range 36-75)
Sex:	7 males
	11 females
Low grade non-Hodgkin's lymphoma:	9
High grade non-Hodgkin's lymphoma:	9 (3 from low grade)
Initial stage:	
I	4
III	6
IV	8
Initial chemotherapy:	18/18
CVP	
CHOP	
M-BACOD	
Promace-MOPP, etc.	
Initial radiotherapy:	11/18
Locoregional	9
Abdominal	2
Predominant tumor site:	
Lymph nodes only	8
Spleen	3
Lymph nodes + spleen	1
Visceral (lung, liver, bone marrow)	5
Breast	1
Blood chemistry anomalies:	0

Therapeutic response

Fourteen patients in the Hodgkin's group received the full course of vinorelbine treatment established under the protocol. Three did not complete the course (1 patient refused to continue after the third injection and 2 patients exhibited progression after 5 and 7 injections respectively). Although 2 patients completed the course (8 injections) within 8 weeks (56 days), this period was protracted in the other cases due to poor hematologic tolerance (mean duration of treatment : 77 days = 11 weeks; range : 56-180 days. Fourteen responses were obtained, 8 stabilizations or minimal responses lasting 13-22 weeks (mean : 16.5 weeks) and 6 partial responses lasting 8-30 weeks (mean : 17.3).

Six patients in the non-Hodgkin's group (1 low - and 5 high-grade lymphomas) did not complete the course owing to progression. Twelve patients completed the course (mean duration : 78 days = 11.2 weeks; range : 60-112 days). Fourteen responses were obtained : 8 stabilizations or minor responses lasting 8-16 weeks, 5 partial responses lasting 8-16 weeks and 2 complete remissions lasting 9 and 11 weeks (*Table IV*).

Response rates were therefore 34 % in the Hodgkin's group and 38 % in the non-Hodgkin's group. The overall mean response rate for all patients entered was therefore 36 %, with a mean duration of 12 weeks.

Table IV. Therapeutic response.

	Number of patients	Mean duration (weeks)
Hodgkin's disease	17	
Failure of treatment	3	
Stabilization or minor response (13, 13, 15, 16, 16, 18, 21, 22 wks)	8	16.6
Partial response (8, 8, 8, 20, 30, 30 wks)	6	17.3
Non-Hodgkin's lymphomas		
Of low grade malignancy	9	
Failure of treatment	1	
Stabilization	4	12
Partial response	4	12
Of high-grade malignancy	9	
Failure of treatment	5	
Stabilization	1	14
Partial response (90 %)	1	8
Complete response	2	10

Toxicity

Toxicity was evaluated in 35 patients, irrespective of the nature of the response, according to WHO criteria (*Table V*).

Table V. Toxicity.

Gastrointestinal	Nausea-vomiting	0
	Constipation	3
	Biological	0
Alopecia	Grade 3	1
	Grade 1	7
Cardiovascular		(1?)
Hematologic	Grade 1 thrombocytopenia	4
	Grade 3 leukopenia	19* ⎫
	Grade 4 leukopenia	12* ⎭

* Grade 3 or 4 episodes in the same patients.

Gastrointestinal toxicity

Although no cases of treatment-related nausea were reported, 2 patients complained of nausea before treatment and between cycles (related to liver disease and ascites). Grade 1 and 2 constipation was seen in 2 and 3 patients respectively; all 5 were bedridden, with poor performance status (2 or 3) and this constipation was temporary.

Alopecia

Five patients presented with grade 3 alopecia before treatment, eight other cases were reported : 1 grade 3 and 7 grade 1 alopecia.

Venous toxicity

Since venous toxicity was seen at the very start of the study with the i.v. injections, the mode of administration was modified to a 15-minute infusion in 250 ml isotonic glucose solution. Two cases of venous thrombosis were detected in recipient veins (iliac and subclavian).

Cardiovascular toxicity

One patient (who was not evaluable and was excluded from analysis) complained of anginal pains upon administration and treatment was therefore discontinued. No EGG anomalies were observed.

Neurologic toxicity

Tendon reflexes were abolished in all patients previously treated with vincristine and/or vinblastine. Electromyogram examinations were performed on 12 patients at the start of anti-tumor treatment but were not repeated.

Hematologic toxicity

WBC was subnormal in all patients at the time of inclusion in the study (leukocytes $\geq 2.10^9/1$, platelets $\geq 100.10^9/1$). There were no reported cases of severe thrombocytopenia. In 4 patients with low platelet counts ($100.10^9/1$), a slight decrease in platelets was noted. At least 1 leukopenic episode was seen in 23 of the 35 patients (12 patients experienced 17 grade 4 episodes and 19 patients experienced 30 grade 3 episodes). These episodes were probably attributable to the injections, although no infection was reported.

Of those patients presenting repeated grade 3 and 4 leukopenias (> 2 episodes), 3 had hepatic involvement and a significant elevation in serum alkaline phosphatase, 2 had previously undergone supra and infra diaphragmatic extended field irradiation, 10 had bone marrow involvement and 2 were aged over 65 years.

Discussion

This study was conducted in a group of patients pretreated with vinca alkaloid-based polychemotherapy. Some had also undergone radiotherapy and were in relapse in the irradiated areas, particularly those with Hodgkin's disease. Among the 8 patients who died prematurely and could not therefore be evaluated, 5 Hodgkin's patients in relapse suffered acute respiratory failure and mediastinal compression. Although these patients were not evaluated, we believe that tumor relapses in irradiated areas may be relatively unresponsive to this drug, irrespective of the nature of the response seen at other sites in the same patient.

Patients with Hodgkin's disease, especially those with non-irradiated visceral impairment, achieved stabilization, or at best partial responses, the quality of the result varying according to the site. A wider range of responses was seen in the patients with non-Hodgkin's lymphomas. Those with low-grade lymphomas and slow progression responded in a similar fashion to the Hodgkin's patients, achieving stabilization or partial responses. Failures were more often seen in high-grade lymphomas, complete and almost complete responses were also obtained in this group.

The safety of this drug therefore proved highly satisfactory. While leukopenia represented the main limiting factor, it did not produce too many complications and no infections were detected. Leukopenia can often be "predicted" in irradiated patients, especially patients with Hodgkin's disease who have undergone extended field irradiation, patients with biliary retention (which thus influences the fate of vinorelbine) and, of course, patients with depressed bone marrow function (which often occurs in non-Hodgkin's malignant lymphomas and where bone marrow involvement is the major limiting factor). Therapeutic reductions and prolonged intervals between injections are not indicated in such cases.

In summary, vinorelbine seems to be effective against Hodgkin's and non-Hodgkin's lymphomas. Its hematologic toxicity is limited even in highly pretread patients. Though it appears to be more active against aggressive lymphomas.

30

Clinical study of Navelbine® activity in Hodgkin's disease. Phase II study

S. BENCHEKROUN [1], Z. CHOUFFAI [1], M. HARIF [1], A. QUESSAR [1],
M. LAABID [1], A. TRACHLI [1], N. BENCHEMSI [1], M. BESENVAL [2],
A. HERRERA [2]

[1] Service d'Hématologie et d'Oncologie pédiatrique, CHU Ibn Rochd, Casablanca, Maroc
[2] Laboratoire Pierre-Fabre Oncologie, 192, rue Lecourbe, 75015 Paris, France

Navelbine® (NVB) (vinorelbine 5, nor-anhydrovinblastine) is a new semi-synthetic vinca alkaloid. A phase I study (Pr Mathé *et al.*) demonstrated that the maximum tolerated dose varies between 27.5 and 35.4 mg/m^2 in heavily pretreated patients. NVB has been screened in a phase II study in Hodgkin's disease (HD) since 1986 in the hematology and oncology department at the CHU Ibn Rochd in Casablanca, Morocco. The purpose of the study is to demonstrate the efficacy of this new antitumor agent in non-pretreated HD. At the beginning of the study only disease stages III and IV that had progressed during at least 6 months have been included. Withdrawal from the study has been decided when no signs of disease regression was observed during at most 15 days.

Patients and methods

Thirthy-two patients with previously untreated HD have been included in the study. Median age was 25 (5-60) years. Diagnosis of HD was made by nodal biopsy in all cases. Type 2 and 3 are predominant (69 %) (*Table I*).

Table I. Sex, stages and histological types in 32 cases of HD (ND : Non determined).

Sex :	
M	20
F	12
Stages :	
I, II	10*
III	6
IV	16
Histological types :	
Type 1	8
2	12
3	10
4	1
ND	1

* These patients were included after encouraging results were obtained for advanced stages.

Pre-treatment evaluation included :
— complete history and physical examination;
— assessment of the extent of disease by chest X ray, CT scan when possible, lymphangiogram, bone marrow biopsy in two sites and trephine needle biopsy of the liver;
— complete peripheral blood count (CBC) with differential, coagulation workup, erythrocyte sedimentation rate, and protein electrophoresis;
— other investigations are performed according to tumor sites such as pleura or skin biopsy etc.

According to the Ann Arbor classification, stage IV disease was observed in 50 % and B and b symptoms in 88 % (*Table II*).

Table II. Site of extra-nodal disease.

Bone marrow	6
Liver	8
Lung	2
Pleura	2
Skin	2

Navelbine® protocol

Pre-chemotherapy laboratory tests included CBC with platelet SGOT, SGPT, alkaline phosphatase, uric acid, creatinine and BUN. These tests are repeated prior to each NVB treatment. The treatment consisted of NVB 30 mg/m^2 weekly. Four injections were given when CBC, liver and renal functions were normal prior to each injection. On day 15 a clinical examination determined whether or not treatment should be continued. NVB was discontinued when no signs of response were observed. A week after the fourth injection (Day 28) a new disease assessment was made, and MOPP/ABVD protocol was started.

Therapeutic results

One hundred and twenty-eight doses were given to 32 patients. Encouraging results observed in the first patients led us to include earlier stages (I and II) and patients with B symptoms or ichthyosis.

The average dose of NVB was 30.1 + 1.7 mg/m^2. The interval between injections was seven days in 89.2 % of cases, between 8 and 14 days in 8.6 % and over 15 days in 2.2 % of cases. A 90 % response rate to treatment was noted. Remission was complete (CR) in 1 case, and incomplete (MR) in 27 cases. There was a minor response (MR) in 3 cases. Results were unevaluable (measurements were not made at the end of treatment or loss to follow up) in 2 patients, and they were excluded from the study (*Table III*).

Therapeutic efficacy was usually seen after the first injection. An objective response was noted between 6 and 21 days with an average of 10 days. Response has been observed within eight days in 19 patients.

Neutropenia was observed in 17 cases and was the single complication of therapy. Vomiting was mild and alopecia was observed in only one case. There has been no neurotoxicity.

Table III. Therapeutic results according to stage.

Results	Stages			
	IA-IB-II n = 7	IIB-IIIA n = 8	IIIB n = 1	IV n = 14
CR	1	—	—	—
PR	3	8	1	14
MR	3	—	—	—

Conclusion

Navelbine® used as a single therapeutic agent provided high clinical response (90 %). This has been achieved with 4 doses administered weekly. Progressive disease was not observed. Therapeutic efficacy was usually noticed following the first injection and few side effects, mainly hematologic, occurred. Thus, NVB appears to be a major drug in the treatment of HD. It could replace other vinca alkaloids used in standard protocols for HD in order to increase their efficacy in advanced stages. It could be used as well in rescue protocols for relapsing or progressive disease.

31

Navelbine® : Conclusions and new trends

M. MARTY

Medical Oncology Department, Hôpital Saint-Louis, 1, avenue Claude-Vellefaux, 75010 Paris, France.

We can draw three sets of conclusions at the end of this seminar on Navelbine®, which both partially conclude the pre-clinical and pharmacological development of the molecule and open the therapeutic phase as it becomes available to the physicians and patients for the treatment of non small cell lung cancers.

Navelbine®

Some characteristics of the molecule are unique not only within the vinca-alkaloid family but also within the whole group of cytotoxic anticancer drugs in general.

It is a semi-synthetic molecule generated by the application of a novel chemical reaction (modified Polonovski reaction). Thus the catharanthine variety has been modified leading to this original molecule, while in the past chemists considered the modification of the vindoline variety to be the only significant ones.

Its experimental anti-tumour spectrum of activity is broad : all human cancer cell lines studied *in vitro*, with the exception of those carrying a pleiotropic resistance phenotype (NCI Dr Cros) are sensitive to Navelbine® concentrations obtained *in vivo*. Similarly, its activity is generally at least equal to that exhibited by the most active vinca-alkaloids on grafted murine tumours and human tumour nude mice xenografts. Nevertheless, at present one cannot but note the parallel between this broad experimental spectrum of activity in the new NCI screening pannel of human cell line and the current clinical anti-tumour spectrum of activity. The predictive value of this model has yet to be established.

General and specific toxicological studies are more predictive and predict almost exclusively for hematological toxicity that is dominated by dose-dependent, non-cumulative and reversible neutropenia. Neurotoxicity appears to be less marked in all animal species, and especially in primates. Investigation of other systems does not suggest any other types of toxicity.

The modalities of Navelbine® binding with tubulin and tubulin-associated proteins defining the specificity of the mitotic spindle and axonal tubulin are highly characteristic : binding is virtually specific to mitotic tubulin and excludes the axonal component. Not only does this represent the basis for its specific toxicological profile in animals and man, but it also offers a potential method for rapidly sifting other tubulo-affine agents : the inhibition of tubulin polymerization correlates with the probability of cytotoxic activity while the formation of paracrystalline structures may predict neurotoxicity. And last but not least these studies emphasize the physiological role of tubulin-bound proteins and stress the need to study them more systematically in both normal and cancer cells; they potentially represent differential targets for anti-tumour drugs.

Pharmacokinetic studies conducted by Professor Cano's team have shown :

— That plasma pharmacokinetics are relatively unaffected by its specific structural modification; and the terminal half-life of Navelbine® is between those of vincristine and vindesine. This confirms the absence of any clear correlation between the plasma pharmacokinetics and neurotoxicities of vinca-alkaloids.

— That extensive hepatic up-take and metabolism is involved. These facts have been well clarified following isolated liver perfusion studies and incubation of viable hepatocytes in the presence of the compound. Similar results have also been obtained with other vinca-alkaloids and these elegant models have therefore enabled us to improve our understanding of the metabolism of members of this class.

— Unlike other vinca-alkaloids, Navelbine® is absorbed from the GI tract in both animals and man with slight variations within and between subjects. This route may prove of value in cases where infusions are difficult or contra-indicated.

— Finally, tissue distribution studies have demonstrated a high concentration of the molecule in target tissues. An investigation of the differential concentrations in tumour cells and their healthy counterparts would probably clarify its anti-tumour spectrum of activity.

Phases I and II studies have unquestionably established that this molecule exhibits good safety, not only in terms of less severe but poorly tolerated adverse reactions (nausea, vomiting, hair loss) but also in the sense that visceral toxicity is virtually restricted to reversible neutropenia. It is true that in these studies we only used a weekly dose regimen. No clear determination of the maximum tolerated single dose was defined and the relationship between this dose and adverse effects, pharmacokinetic parameters and activity is not yet established. This would be important, according to the specific relationship noted between the surviving fraction of murine lymphoma cells and vinca-alkaloid concentration, which exhibits a plateau corresponding to a saturation of the cytotoxic effect. The same study with Navelbine® would be particularly valuable. Additionally, it should be possible to abrogate this toxic neutropenia by using hematopoiesis stimulating factors (CSF) and administer high doses using a different regimen (single dose or repeat dose after 3-5 days). Moreover, a precise definition of this dose would enable us to investigate the myelosuppressant combinations which appear too difficult to manage in initial lung

Navelbine® : Conclusions and new trends

cancer studies. The investigation of anti-tumour activity in man is at an early stage. Navelbine® shows a spectrum of activity that is unusual for vinca-alkaloids and has previously only been observed with anthracyclines and alkylating agents. Indeed, while such apparently remarkable activity in Hodgkin's disease and possibly in non-Hodgkin's lymphomas is not unexpected for this class of compound its high activity in non small cell lung cancers is not frequent for this class (only vindesine has shown activity to date). Such marked activity (comparable with that observed with the most active agents in advanced breast cancer) is quite unusual. If subsequent studies confirm its significant activity in ovarian adenocarcinomas, Navelbine® will indeed boast a highly specific and extensive spectrum of activity. It is therefore essential to define its activity in the other major indications of vinca-alkaloids but it is difficult to carry out studies in this area (acute lymphoid leukemia, embryonic carcinomas) as well as in indications generally unusual for this class of drugs (advanced adenocarcinomas, sarcomas and epidermoid cancers).

We have also to reconsider the most extensively studied tumour types. In non-small cell lung cancers, a response rate of about 30 % is well supported by the significant duration of the response. The fact that the combinations in question barely exceeded these rates (or not at all) is only apparently paradoxical : these combinations have only been given to subjects in stages III and IV of the disease. In terms of activity, they are very comparable with the most efficacious combinations reported which improve both survival and quality of life. Since these results have been obtained in less than 2 years, they cannot be regarded as optimal and definitive. Activity appears to be inversely related to the number of previous treatments for breast cancer : it also relates to visceral, skeletal and soft tissue metastases and was increased in a preliminary study with the fluorouracil/Navelbine® combination. This all confirms that this molecule is an important and novel agent in this type of tumour and that research should be extended to other possible combinations. Finally, the studies which should enable us to confirm or reject its activity in lymphomas (Hodgkin's disease in particular) and ovarian adenocarcinomas are more difficult to design. In these two cases, they should perhaps be aimed at initially resistant forms so that confirmation of even a slight activity would constitute significant clinical progress.

We can already state that, in view of its particularly favourable therapeutic index, Navelbine® represents a valuable addition to the therapeutic arsenal available for certain types of tumour. Laboratoires Pierre Fabre Oncologie are already collaborating closely with clinical research groups concerned with each tumour type in an attempt to establish an exact definition of the optimum application for each indication.

Current development plan

The development of Navelbine® does in fact exhibit most of the characteristics specifically stated by the European Commission for Proprietary Medicinal Products.
 1) The use of different pharmacological models characterizing cytotoxic activity in tumour cells, established human lines and murine and human grafted tumours : comparison of these three systems has yet not enabled their respective advantages to be evaluated in a clear fashion.

Although the investigation of established human cell lines does provide an impression of a broad spectrum of activity, the established lines used by the NCI are still far from providing information on human pathology. Breast and ovarian adenocarcinomas in particular are highly under-represented.

2) A general toxicological study supplemented by a specific toxicology (neurotoxicity) study relating to vinca-alkaloids, incorporating possibilities for studying a specific toxicological feature if suggested as a result of clinical trials.

3) The use of isolated differential organ and cell models : pharmacokinetic investigation of the molecule has revealed the value of these models which have made it possible to characterize the metabolism of all vinca-alkaloids, an aspect which has been inadequately understood for the past twenty years.

4) Definition of pharmacological models : in particular, does the differential study of the capacity to modify tubulin polymerization and induce para-crystalline structures constitute a useful tool for the characterization of other tubulo-affine and slightly neurotoxic or non-neurotoxic agents ? We are far from being able to predict cytotoxic activity using these models, although they have made it possible to define the adverse reactions and therapeutic index of this molecule.

5) Clinical trials have necessarily been conducted in a more classical manner : phase I trials have only employed one regimen. However, the application of methods suited to establishing the lower limit of expected activity (two stage design and grouped sequential designs, here applied to the field of oncology for the first time) in a small sample of patients during certain phase II trials will enable the spectrum of activity of this molecule to be characterized.

Classification of anti-cancer agents

Navelbine® constitutes an interesting example of the problems raised in the study of molecules that are « analogues » of known molecules. The difficulties encountered in actually defining an analogue are summarized below :

What degree of stuctural similarity is required for the definition of an analogue ? In the case of Navelbine®, it is evident that the modification of the catharantine nucleus gives the molecule binding properties for different substrates which are unusual for all other vinca-alkaloids and would allow the molecule to be regarded as « original » from the start of these studies.

— The adverse reactions associated with Navelbine® differ considerably from those typical of vincristine or vindesine but cannot be used to support the « analogue » claim.

— Its pharmacokinetics (which are not particularly predictive), activity and adverse reactions do not therefore help to characterize an « analogue » nature.

— And finally, the spectrum of activity, still only partially defined, is already highly specific to this molecule.

We should once again stress the originality of this molecule with respect not only to other vinca-alkaloids but also to other cytotoxic agents, and repeat that, notwithstanding significant structural and pharmacological similarities, it is better to regard all novel anti-tumour substances as original molecules.

IMPRIMERIE LOUIS-JEAN
BP 87 — 05003 GAP Cedex
Tél. : 92.51.35.23
Dépôt légal : 405 — Mai 1991
Imprimé en France